Copyright © 2013 by Culinary Nutrition Publishing, LLC, Chicago, IL 60613

Library of Congress Cataloging-in-Publication Data

Powers, Catharine. Hess, Mary Abbott
    Essentials of Nutrition for Chefs / Catharine Powers, Mary Abbott Hess
      p.cm
    ISBN 978-0-9816769-4-4
    1. Nutrition

                  201 129 2515

Limit of Liability/Disclaimer of Warranty: While the publisher and authors have used their best efforts in preparing this book, they make no representations or warranties with respect to the accuracy or completeness of the content of this book and specifically disclaim any implied warranties of merchantability or fitness for a particular purpose. The advice and strategies contained herein may not be suitable for your situation. You should consult with a professional where appropriate. Neither the publisher nor authors shall be liable for any loss of profit or any other commercial damages, including but not limited in special, incidental, consequential or other damages.

Cover photos: Front cover by Tami Petitto. Back cover purchased through istockphoto.com, contributed by PeaFactory.

For more information or permission to reprint contact
Culinary Nutrition Publishing, LLC

www.nutritionforchefs.com

www.culinarynutritionpublishing.com

$65.00

ISBN 978-0-9816769-4-4

Table of Contents

Foreword

Everyone, from energetic young children to adults in their sunset years, should have healthful food choices wherever they eat. Schools, colleges and universities, employee dining rooms, entertainment venues, restaurants of all sorts, healthcare facilities, and congregate or group feeding sites share a responsibility to provide appetizing, healthful foods. As a culinary professional, you have an opportunity to show that planning, preparing and serving nourishing and appealing foods to guests is not only the right thing to do but also makes good business sense.

Adventuresome diners, innovative technology and an abundance of healthful ingredients – fruits, vegetables, whole grains, beans, lean meats, low-fat dairy products, nuts, seeds, herbs and spices – make this an exciting time to be a culinary professional. Basic nutrition knowledge mixed with creativity will position you to meet the needs of a challenging marketplace. We designed *Essentials of Nutrition for Chefs* as a roadmap for your journey with fundamental nutrition information plus charts, diagrams, sidebars and practical applications.

Today, I work with foodservice operators across the country, from school foodservice operators to restaurants, training others how to put healthful cooking into practice. The 14 years I spent at The Culinary Institute of America, Hyde Park developing and teaching the CIA's cutting-edge nutrition program gave me insight into what today's culinary students and professionals need to know about nutrition. We put this knowledge into practice at the institute's St. Andrew's Cafe, a living laboratory that tested and validated healthy cooking concepts.

So many individuals have inspired and motivated me and shaped my food and nutrition knowledge as well as my culinary skills. Special thanks and admiration go to my coauthor, Mary Abbott Hess, whose life motto, "Just do it!" inspires me to take risks and do more. Many culinary and nutrition colleagues, especially those at The Culinary Institute of America, have generously shared their expertise and passion for food with me throughout the years. All of you truly have enriched my life.

A very personal thanks goes to my mom, Charlene Powers Huber, a retired registered dietitian, for her constant support while I have pursued non-traditional dietetic roles and for her encouragement and role modeling each step of the way. Finally, I would like to acknowledge my sons, Andrew and William, who have taught me the practical side of preparing healthful foods for kids and who have always been eager taste-testers.

Catharine Powers
Medina, Ohio

As a result of my leadership in both the American Dietetic Association (now the Academy of Nutrition and Dietetics) and The American Institute of Wine & Food, one of my professional and personal goals coalesced around the intersection of nutrition science and the culinary arts. Chefs can give us wonderful food that nourishes both body and soul, but to do so, they often need more thorough nutrition education. Thus, my focus became supporting the culinary expertise of fellow dietitians while also increasing nutrition knowledge among chefs.

Within the Academy of Nutrition and Dietetics, the Food & Culinary Professionals Dietary Practice Group has had a transformative influence on many registered dietitians. More and more dietitians are now working in the food industry, and a number of them have told me that we need better ways to share nutrition knowledge with chefs. As an author, educator and nutrition communications consultant, I saw this need as an opportunity to create a resource to help chefs, food writers, cooking teachers and other culinary professionals combine today's nutrition knowledge with their culinary skills to create healthful foods that meet high standards for taste and quality.

My coauthor, Cathy Powers, is the most accomplished culinary nutritionist I know. In *Essentials of Nutrition for Chefs* we address contemporary nutrition issues and offer solutions to some of the daily "cooking healthy" challenges facing chefs. Within these pages are answers to hundreds of questions chefs have asked us over the years, the most current nutrition thinking and facts, and virtually everything chefs should know to create healthful foods. To go beyond the science and look at nutrition through the lens of food and food choices, we invited experts – chefs, fellow dietitians and food professionals – to share their advice, recipes and best practices. These experts add a unique dimension to the book.

We have been delighted by response to the first edition of *Essentials of Nutrition for Chefs*. The book has been adopted by many culinary programs and received top honors in the Health and Special Diets category at the 2011 International Association of Culinary Professionals (IACP) book awards and was a finalist in the Professional Kitchens category. In 2011, I was part of a team that used the first edition of *Essentials of Nutrition for Chefs* to teach a course on nutrition for chefs at the Washburne Culinary Institute in Chicago. With this experience, input from chef instructors and responses from students, we have made the second edition of the book even better.

My thanks go to the amazing team listed in the acknowledgments. Special personal thanks go to Chef William Reynolds for enriching both my culinary education and my life as well as critically reviewing this book from the perspective of a chef; to The American Institute of Wine & Food and the memory of Julia Child who remains an inspiration and guardian angel; and to the Food & Culinary Professionals Dietetic Practice Group, the International Association of Culinary Professionals and Les Dames D' Escoffier International – three strong networks of generous colleagues who have supported my culinary education and this venture.

Mary Abbott Hess
Chicago, Illinois

Preface

Essentials of Nutrition for Chefs is unique because it offers a look at nutrition through the lens of food. This textbook provides essential nutrition information for culinary professionals as well as guidance on practical application. A longstanding criticism of healthful cooking is that removing fat, salt and sugar results in foods that are bland, boring and lacking in flavor and texture. Omitting these classic flavor-enhancing ingredients makes creating wonderful tastes and textures more challenging. *Essentials of Nutrition for Chefs* is designed to help chefs meet this challenge by preparing food that nourishes both body and soul.

Building on the positive response and acknowledged excellence of the first edition, which received the 2011 International Association of Culinary Professionals Cookbook Award in the Health and Special Diets category, this second edition is even better.

Chef William Reynolds, an experienced chef educator and winner of the Foodservice Educator Network International's *2011 Award for Excellence in Culinary Education*, reviewed the entire text with a critical eye to what chefs need to know and understand about nutrition. He used the first edition in classes and provided valuable suggestions from the perspective of a chef and educator.

New information on *Dietary Guidelines for Americans*, *MyPlate*, the National Restaurant Association *Chef Survey: What's Hot in 2012*, the International Food Information Council (IFIC) *2012 Food & Health Survey: Consumer Attitudes Toward Food Safety, Nutrition & Health* and the Academy of Nutrition and Dietetics *Nutrition and You:Trends 2011* report and other sources are included. New charts, website resources, chef interviews and case studies are also included.

What Lies in Store

Chapter 1, *The Power of Food*, focuses on marrying the science of nutrition with the art of preparing food and discusses the foodservice industry's responsibility to offer plenty of healthful food choices for today's consumers. The heart of the second chapter, *Nutrition Guidelines and Tools*, is the *Dietary Guidelines for Americans, 2010* Report and the applications of that document are reflected throughout the book. Additional tools include the Nutrition Facts panel on food labels and the *MyPlate* guide to a healthful diet which replaces *MyPyramid*. Chapters 3 through 7 review the six classes of nutrients – carbohydrates, fats, protein, water, vitamins and minerals. Chapters 8 through 10 are all about putting nutrition into practice by planning healthful menus, recognizing the importance of flavor and using healthful cooking techniques. Chapter 11 focuses on communicating nutrition to guests and looks at the impact of healthcare reform on nutrition in restaurants. Finally, Chapters 12 and 13 deal with nutrition for various age groups and for those with special dietary and health needs.

Each chapter begins with learning objectives – the knowledge readers can expect to glean from the pages that follow. Throughout each chapter, charts, tables and sidebars present information in a concise, learner-friendly format. Chefs working in a variety of operations around the country talk about how nutrition fits into their life and work in features titled *A Word from the Chef*, which are sprinkled throughout the book. Another recurring feature, *Case by Case*, highlights practical applications from a variety of operational viewpoints, including schools, healthcare, restaurants, and business and industry. Each chapter concludes with *Opportunities for Chefs*, hands-on *Learning Activities* and a list of additional resources for more in-depth information. Key words are in bold italics for easy identification and definitions are found in the glossary.

Principles in Practice

Essentials of Nutrition for Chefs also contains 38 recipes illustrating concepts discussed in each chapter. All the recipes, which the various chefs and dietitians featured in the book have been kind enough to share, have been standardized and tested. From starters to desserts, from summer to winter, from simple to complex, from fruits to nuts, the recipes reflect a range of cooking techniques and showcase nutrient-rich ingredients.

Select nutrient data (calories, fat, saturated fat, trans fat, cholesterol, sodium, carbohydrates, dietary fiber and protein) are listed with each recipe. These data are rounded using Food and Drug Administration rounding rules for labeling. Most nutrient data presented in charts are also rounded. Recipes for this book were analyzed using ESHA Genesis R & D software. Optional recipe ingredients are not included in the analyses. The analyses do not include suggested accompaniments. Recipes were taste-tested and many include salt; if lower sodium levels are desired, salt can be omitted.

Acknowledgments

It is hard to believe how many hearts, hands and minds have touched this text from inception to printing. Thank you to everyone who encouraged and supported us in writing and revising *Essentials of Nutrition for Chefs*, especially:

Jane Grant Tougas, who assisted at every step of the process from brainstorming and shaping the book's vision to editing, writing and endless re-writing. Her skill and attention to detail gave this book one voice.

Tami Petitto, a superbly creative designer who gave color to ordinary words and brought energy to every page. Her aesthetic and functional sensibilities are outshone only by her patience. The cover photo is an example of her ability to see beauty in simple things and her eye for just the right angle.

William N. Reynolds, who shared his passion, his expertise and his critical eye. He offered a thorough and careful review of each page of the text from the viewpoint of the chef. One of three chefs who is an honorary member of the Academy of Nutrition and Dietetics, he has always given freely of his time in training dietitians and others on the importance of healthful cooking that is also delicious.

Mary Kimbrough, RD, LD, our Culinary Nutrition Associates, LLC business partner who showed support while we worked on our book project and who offered a very practical view of nutrition.

Deborah McBride whose copyediting skills made sure we crossed every "t" and dotted every "i" and offered guidance in publishing.

All the outstanding contributors who offered their expertise and experience to make this book more practical for chefs, foodservice operators, recipe developers, cooking teachers and other culinary professionals.

Chefs and Culinary Professionals

Jeremy Bearman, Executive Chef, Rouge Tomate, New York, New York

Timothy Cipriano, Executive Director of Food Services, New Haven Public Schools, New Haven, Connecticut

Ann Cooper, "The Renegade Lunch Lady," Director of Nutrition Services, Boulder Valley School District, Boulder, Colorado

Ron DeSantis, CMC, AAC, CHE, Director of Culinary Excellence, Yale University, New Haven, Connecticut

Jean Duane, Alternative Cook, LLC, Centennial, Colorado

Brad Farmerie, Executive Chef, AvroKO Hospitality Group, New York, New York

Brian Garam, Le Cordon Bleu College of Culinary Arts, Chicago, Illinois

En Ming Hsu, Pastry Chef Consultant, Las Vegas, Nevada

Wook Kang, Le Cordon Bleu College of Culinary Arts, Chicago, Illinois

Graham Kerr, Culinary and Television Personality, Camano Island, Washington

Kristy Lambrou, MS, RD, Culinary Nutritionist, Rouge Tomate, New York, New York

Deborah Madison, Chef, Author and Educator, Santa Fe, New Mexico

Philip Papineau, The Culinary Institute of America, Hyde Park, New York

Denise Pierchalski, Chef, Pittsburgh Premier Catering, Pittsburgh, Pennsylvania

Ina Pinkney, Ina's, Chicago, Illinois

Nora Pouillon, Restaurant Nora, Washington, DC

William N. Reynolds, Chef and Culinary Educator, Chicago, Illinois

Brent Ruggles, CEC, Regional Executive Chef, Las Colinas Country Club, Irving, Texas

Joel Schaefer, President and Chef, Allergy Chefs, Inc., Jacksonville, Florida

Sarah Stegner, Chef/Owner, Prairie Grass Café, Northbrook, Illinois

Scott Uehlein, Corporate Chef, Canyon Ranch, Tucson, Arizona

Kevin Watson, CEC, PCC, CDM, CFPP, Lead Instructor, Pennsylvania Culinary Institute; Owner, Pittsburgh Premier Catering; Personal Chef, Pittsburgh Steelers, Pittsburgh, Pennsylvania

Marvin Woods, Culinary and Television Personality, Atlanta, Georgia

Registered Dietitians and Food and Nutrition Experts

Jacqueline R. Berning, PhD, RD, CSSD, Associate Professor and Chair, Biology Department, University of Colorado, Colorado Springs, Colorado

Leslie Bonci, MPH, RD, LDN, CSSD, Director of Sports Nutrition, University of Pittsburgh Medical Center, Pittsburgh, Pennsylvania

Joseph M. Carlin, MS, MA, RD, LND, FADA, Public Health Nutritionist, Administration for Community Living, Boston, Massachusetts

Nancy Clark, MS, RD, CSSD, Sports Nutritionist, Brookline, Massachusetts

Margaret Condrasky, EdD, RD, CCE, Associate Professor of Food Science and Human Nutrition, Clemson University, Clemson, South Carolina

Becky Dorner, RD, LD, Becky Dorner & Associates, Akron, Ohio

Cheryl Forberg, RD, Nutritionist for NBC's "The Biggest Loser," Napa, California

Penny M. Kris-Etherton, PhD, RD, FADA, Distinguished Professor of Nutrition, Pennsylvania State University, State College, Pennsylvania

Georgia Kostas, MPH, RD, LD, President, Georgia Kostas & Associates, Inc., Dallas, Texas

Carolyn Leontos, MS, RD, CDE, Professor Emeritus Retired, University of Nevada Cooperative Extension, Las Vegas, Nevada

Marilyn Majchrzak, MS, RD, Corporate Menu Development Manager, Canyon Ranch, Tucson, Arizona.

Mariam Majeed, formerly with Islamic Food and Nutrition Council of America, Park Ridge, Illinois

Jill Nussinow, MS, RD, The Veggie Queen™, Santa Rosa, California

Maggie Powers, PhD, RD, CDE, Research Scientist, International Diabetes Center at Park Nicollet, St. Louis Park, Minnesota

Tina Wasserman, BS, MA, Cooking and More, Dallas, Texas

Donna L. Weihofen, MS, RD, Senior Clinical Nutritionist, University of Wisconsin Comprehensive Cancer Center, Madison, Wisconsin

Renee Zonka, CEC, RD, CHE, MBA, Dean, Kendall College, Chicago, Illinois

Foodservice Operations/Experts

Canyon Ranch, Tucson, Arizona

Fletcher Allen Health Care, Burlington, Vermont

Hallmark Cards, Kansas City, Missouri

Ina's, Chicago, Illinois

IPic Entertainment, Chicago, Illinois

Janet Helm, Chief Food and Nutrition Strategist, North America, Weber Shandwick Public Relations, Chicago, Illinois

New Haven Public Schools, New Haven, Connecticut

Oberlin College, Oberlin, Ohio

Panera Bread Company, Richmond Heights, Missouri

Parkland Memorial Hospital, Dallas, Texas

Rouge Tomate, New York City, New York

Seasons 52, Orlando, Florida

The Spice House, Chicago, Illinois

Reviewers

Garrett Berdan, RD, LD, Consultant, Bend, Oregon

Susan Braverman, MS, RD, CDN, FADA, Director of Dietetic Internship, Department of Family, Nutrition, & Exercise Sciences, Queens College, Flushing, New York

Patty Erd, The Spice House, Chicago, Illinois

Mary Kimbrough, RD, LD, Partner, Culinary Nutrition Associates, LLC, Dallas, Texas

Kathy King, RD, LD, Helm Publishing, Lake Dallas, Texas

Carolyn Leontos, MS, RD, CDE, Consultant, Las Vegas, Nevada

William N. Reynolds, Chef and Culinary Educator, Chicago, Illinois

Janet Sass, MS, RD, Assistant Dean and Associate Professor, Hospitality & Nutrition, Northern Virginia Community College, Annandale, Virginia

Debbie F. Swanson, RD, CHE, Culinary Instructor, The Art Institute of Colorado, Denver, Colorado

Carole Zucco, PhD, Hess & Hunt, Inc., Nutrition Communications, Chicago, Illinois

The Power of Food

LEARNING OBJECTIVES

After completing this chapter, you should be able to:

- Summarize the factors that influence food selection
- Discuss the importance of providing healthier food options to your guests
- List general food recommendations for providing nutritious meals
- Discuss how American's eating habits have changed in the last 30 years
- List the operational implications of cooking healthfully
- Define essential nutrients
- List the six classes of nutrients
- Identify the nutrients that provide energy (calories)
- Describe the factors that influence daily calorie needs
- Explain nutrient density and list examples of foods that are nutrient dense and foods that have a low nutrient density

Food, glorious food: Cooking it and eating it are as much a part of our culture as art, music, dance, theater, poetry, prose and other creative pursuits. We cook and eat to celebrate, to mourn, to court, to impress, to console and to calm. Look closely and you will see that just about every human emotion has an associated food ritual or behavior. Granted, some may be more constructive than others; regardless, the depth of emotion tied to food speaks to feeding the soul as well as the body.

Long before the emergence of nutrition science as we know it today, people learned through experience that food and wellness share a close bond. Based on the four classical elements – fire, air, water and earth – early Greek physicians prescribed "hot, cold, wet and dry foods" to treat illness. Different foods or food combinations were thought to create disease-fighting substances in the body. It was the Greek physician Hippocrates who famously said: "Let food be your medicine and medicine be your food."

With the 20th century emergence of nutrition as a science, food garnered new respect as an evidence-based health promoter and disease preventer. But as history has shown many times, people don't always do what they know to be best for their health and well being. So it has been with food. Although science has repeatedly demonstrated the health benefits of nutritious food eaten in moderation, modern lifestyles and calorie-laden food options don't often support healthful choices.

Fortunately, however, we are living in a time of profound transition in the public's attitude toward food and health. For example, foodservice trend watcher the Mintel Group observes that while it's unlikely consumers will start demanding absolutely healthy menus, they do want choices. Menus will continue to feature indulgent options, but will be balanced with healthier, better-for-you options. [1] As a chef who understands the role of nutrition and possesses the expertise to deliver food that is both healthy and delicious, you can help lead this march into the future of food and health. As Nora Poullion, chef/owner of the acclaimed Washington, DC, restaurant Nora – the nation's first certified-organic restaurant – notes, "Chefs from every kind of foodservice operation have the power to change the health of the country."

Essentials of Nutrition for Chefs is a tool to help you do just that. With knowledge and skills in place, you will be ready to meet the growing need for healthier food options while becoming a stronger, more versatile and better prepared foodservice professional. Keep in mind that this book is not a comprehensive nutrition text; rather, it presents nutrition basics for culinarians and foodservice operators: what you need to know to cook and serve healthful, delicious food that guests want to purchase over and over again. That is the bottom line – for you, for your patrons and for the success of your operation.

A Word from the Chef
Still Galloping After All These Years

Chef Graham Kerr – aka the "Galloping Gourmet" – has educated and entertained several generations of cooks and "foodies" with his television shows, books and personal appearances. And he is still going strong. A keen observer of American culture and the national food scene, Graham sees some serious change on the horizon.

"Over the next decade, we must gain control over healthcare costs and to do so, we're going to have to make some serious adjustments in our lifestyle choices," he predicts. "We are facing a tsunami of sickness and we must get to higher ground. Right now, our medical model is based on intervention; we need to turn that around and focus on prevention." Graham himself is currently working on the ways in which we as a nation can increase fruit and vegetable consumption by at least 100% before the year 2020.

It's not surprising that Graham believes talking down to people with rules, regulations and restrictions isn't the way to go. "We do much better talking person to person, neighbor to neighbor," he says. "Social networking tools like Facebook, Twitter, Pinterest and Tumblr are driving the paradigm shift toward prevention. Where does the chef come in? People are going to make wiser menu choices, and we'll see some radical change over the next 10 years. Every restaurant will have a registered dietitian on call."

The menu itself, Graham explains, is a "sales piece for the senses." It's where the chef meets the customer. "Holding the menu, seeing your choices and making one is part and parcel of dining away from home," he says. "It's all about the right brain and tantalizing the senses."

Although Graham is not a big fan of including nutrition information on the menu, he does believe every restaurant should voluntarily work for the common good by making nutrition numbers available for diners who are trying choose foods that meet their individual needs. "This is an opportunity for chefs to demonstrate that they want to delight and 'do less harm,' " he explains.

Butternut Squash Ginger Cheesecake

Graham Kerr
Media Personality, Educator and Celebrity Chef

Serves: 10

Greek yogurt is firmer than regular yogurt and a compact source of protein, calcium and other nutrients. In addition to its pleasing flavor, it is thicker in consistency and makes an excellent base for creamy dips, dressings and toppings. The figs in this crust add flavor, texture and fiber and replace the need for added fat. This versatile unbaked pastry crust can be used in many desserts. The butternut squash filling is a creative way to use this nutrient-rich vegetable.

Fig Crust

Dried figs, stalk ends removed	7	ounces
Gingersnap cookies, broken	1	cup

Filling

Butternut squash, cut in half and seeded	1	medium
Gelatin, unflavored	2	packets
Water	½	cup
Brown sugar	¾	cup
Cottage cheese, 2% fat	1 ½	cup
Cinnamon, ground	½	teaspoon
Ginger, ground	½	teaspoon
Cloves, ground	¼	teaspoon
Yogurt, Greek or strained	¾	cup

Garnish

Crystallized ginger, chopped finely	1	tablespoon

Per Serving

Calories	240		Cholesterol	5	mg
Fat	4	g	Sodium	200	mg
Saturated Fat	2	g	Carbohydrates	45	mg
Trans Fat	0	g	Dietary Fiber	4	mg
Sugar	31	g	Protein	8	g

Start the filling:

1. Preheat the oven to 350° F (180° C). Place the squash halves face down on a baking sheet and bake in the preheated oven for 40 minutes. Remove and let cool.

2. Scoop out 2 cups of the flesh for this recipe and pat dry.

For the crust:

1. Process the figs in a food processor for a few seconds, add the broken gingersnaps and continue processing until they clump together in a sticky ball. Don't process too long or the cookies will lose their texture.

2. Press the crust mixture into the bottom and up the sides of a lightly greased, high-sided, 7-inch (18 cm) springform pan. Dip your fingers into a bowl of cold water to alleviate any stickiness.

For the filling:

1. Sprinkle the gelatin over the water in a small saucepan and allow to soften for 1 minute. Warm over low heat, stirring, until the gelatin is completely dissolved, about 3 minutes.

2. Place the squash, softened gelatin and the remaining filling ingredients in the processor and whiz until smooth, about 2 minutes.

3. Pour the filling into the prepared crust, pop into the refrigerator and chill until set, about 3 hours.

To serve:

1. Unmold, slice into 8 to 10 servings with a warm knife and garnish each piece with the crystallized ginger.

It's All About the Food

In 2010, the *Journal of the American Medical Association* published article titled "Dietary Guidelines in the 21st Century – a Time for Food." [2] As the authors note, "The relatively recent focus on nutrients parallels an increasing discrepancy between theory and practice: the greater the focus on nutrients, the less healthful foods have become." Furthermore, "In contrast with discrete nutrients, specific foods and dietary patterns substantially affect chronic disease risk. . . . Fruits, vegetables, whole grains and nuts are consistently associated with lower risk of disease. Fish consumption reduces risk of cardiac mortality."

In other words, the public relates to food, not to nutrients. Although nutrition is a complex and evolving science, choosing and preparing healthier foods is, by contrast, rather straightforward. As a foodservice professional, you will be well on your way to providing nutritious meals to your guests if you remain focused on preparing meals with foods that are inherently healthier and served in appropriate portions. Core food recommendations throughout this text include:

- Increase fruit
- Increase vegetables, including legumes
- Increase whole grains
- Substitute healthier fats for less-healthful fats and reduce total fats used
- Increase fish and seafood
- Decrease foods with added sugars
- Limit sources of sodium, especially salt
- Decrease processed and packaged foods

The message is clear: Reducing fats and sugars helps diners lower the many health risks caused by overweight and obesity, while increasing vegetables, legumes, fruits, fish and whole grains leads to better health. Your charge is to select, prepare and serve these important foods in ways that delight and satisfy your guests.

An Alliance of Taste and Health

Taste and health have been jockeying for position for years. Many believed you had to choose one over the other. Was "good" food tasty or healthful? Why not both? While many chefs ate and served healthful foods, and many in the nutrition community valued artfully prepared, flavorful dishes, advice on healthful eating tended to be very restrictive for many years. Eventually, Julia Child, one of the founders of The American Institute of Wine & Food (AIWF), became concerned about a growing "fear of food" in America. In October 1990, AIWF held a groundbreaking conference, *Resetting the American Table: Creating a New Alliance of Taste and Health*, to address this issue.

At this conference, 50 culinary and nutrition leaders – including co-author of this book Mary Abbott Hess, LHD, MS, RD, LDN, FADA, who was president of The American Dietetic Association (now The Academy of Nutrition and Dietetics) at the time – sought to build an alliance or at least achieve peaceful coexistence. A consensus document, *Standards for Food and Diet Quality*, was created under the umbrella tenet, "In matters of taste, consider nutrition. In matters of nutrition, consider taste. And in all cases, consider individual needs and preferences." The intent was to move Americans toward a more healthful diet without giving up the pleasures of the table. The document, with statements on nutrition, physical activity, food availability, quality and preparation, food safety, and education, was compiled and released by AIWF in 1993 (Appendix A). Twenty years later, many of its components have been incorporated into public policy and many of its core concepts have become the foundation of healthful cooking.

It just makes good sense for dietitians and chefs to work together. We are all concerned about proper eating habits. If we join and work together, we can help each other in reaching our common goal – healthful, good-tasting food.

Julia Child
The American Dietetic Association 1991
Annual Meeting

Attitudes Toward Healthful Eating

Until recently, lowering dietary fat (especially trans fat and saturated fat) was the primary focus of much health advice. While moderating fat remains important, today's healthful diet also includes getting plenty of the vitamins, minerals, antioxidants, phytochemicals and fiber from a variety of fruits, vegetables and whole grains. With 65% of American adults and as many as a third of American children either overweight or obese, calories are also a major issue. [3, 4] Reflecting these concerns, the healthy diet paradigm has shifted from restriction to balance – seeking positive nutrients and balancing the number of calories consumed with the number burned. Contemporary menus reflecting this shift feature less processed and more whole foods, healthful cooking techniques, and portion control. And with so many restaurants serving very large portions, downsizing has the dual benefit of reducing food costs while promoting healthful eating.

Research from The Academy of Nutrition and Dietetics shows that consumers are changing the way they eat – or recognizing the need to make improvements. AND has conducted a nationwide consumer nutrition trends survey eight times since 1991 to measure attitudes, knowledge, beliefs and behaviors regarding food and nutrition, to identify trends and to understand how consumers' attitudes and behavior have evolved over time. [5]

Respondents are categorized into one of three segments reflecting overall attitudes toward maintaining a healthy diet and getting regular exercise:

- **I'm Already Doing It:** Consumers who feel that maintaining a healthy diet and regular exercise are very important; are concerned about diet, nutrition and overall fitness; and feel they are doing all they can to eat a healthy diet.

- **I Know I Should:** Consumers who feel that maintaining a healthy diet and regular exercise are very important, but may not have taken significant actions to do all they can to eat a healthy diet.

- **Don't Bother Me:** People who do not feel diet and exercise are very important to them and are the least concerned with their overall nutrition and fitness.

Over the past 20 years, the number of people in the "I Know I Should" category has remained relatively consistent, while the number of respondents in the "I'm Already Doing It" category has grown steadily. The number of "Don't Bother Me" respondents has steadily decreased.

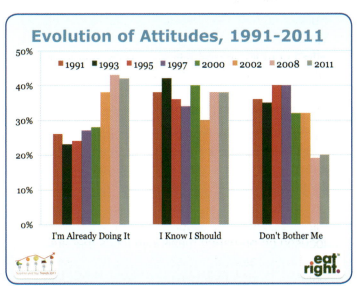

Source: Academy of Nutrition and Dietetics, Nutrition and You: Trends 2011, www.eatright.org/

Research from Mintel Menu Insights corroborates the AND's findings. More than eight in 10 adults told Mintel that it's very or somewhat important to them to eat healthfully; but when dining out, most people are really looking for taste, texture and experience. Although about 75% of people surveyed by Mintel said they would like to see more healthy options on menus, only 51% actually ordered from those selections. Clearly people don't always do what they say, but it is evident that there is a growing trend toward choosing healthier options. The introduction of mandatory calorie labeling on menus will no doubt help to make the choices clearer for consumers. [6]

Always in Season

Darden Restaurants, Inc., headquartered in Orlando, Florida, is the world's largest company-owned and operated full-service restaurant enterprise. The Darden family of restaurants features some of the most recognizable and successful brands in full-service dining – Red Lobster, Olive Garden, LongHorn Steakhouse, The Capital Grille and Bahama Breeze.

Darden's Seasons 52, opened in Orlando in early 2003. Seasons 52 now has 27 locations around the country and is continuing to grow. The fresh grill and wine bar concept is known for its lighter approach to dining. The menu changes four times a year with the seasons. Everything on the menu is less than 475 calories.

There's not a fryer to be found in the kitchen, and no butter or heavy cream in any dish. Fresh products are featured 52 weeks a year at their optimal flavor and freshness. "There is always a reason to come back," says Clifford Pleau, executive chef and director of culinary development. "We use authentic cooking techniques such as grilling over open mesquite or oak fires and caramelizing vegetables to enhance natural flavors without adding calories."

Clifford is passionate about "letting the product do the work" by using only high-quality, in-season ingredients. "After all," he says, "nothing ripens like the sun." Whether in the restaurant or at home, Clifford believes in celebrating and living well. He uses the freshest ingredients and cooking techniques, allowing the vibrant colors and natural flavors of the food to shine through.

"I see myself as an educator," Clifford says, which explains why in addition to his corporate training responsibilities, he, along with Seasons 52's master sommelier, George Miliotes, publishes the monthly Seasons 52 Fresh Intelligence newsletter online. Here they share their knowledge about the season's best food and wines, bringing culinary inspiration right into their patrons' kitchens.

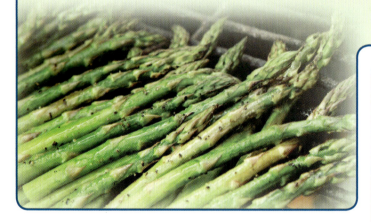

The Road to Wellness

Over the past 20 years, the Seattle-based Hartman Group, a health and wellness research firm, has published dozens of groundbreaking studies on consumer food and health trends. The group's "Road to Wellness" is an infographic tracing health and wellness milestones over the last 200 years. This journey through time demonstrates that today's health and wellness trend is not a fad; rather, it is another step in an evolving process of growth and awareness.

Reprinted with permission by The Hartman Group, www.hartman-group.com/hartbeat/infographic-the-road-to-wellness

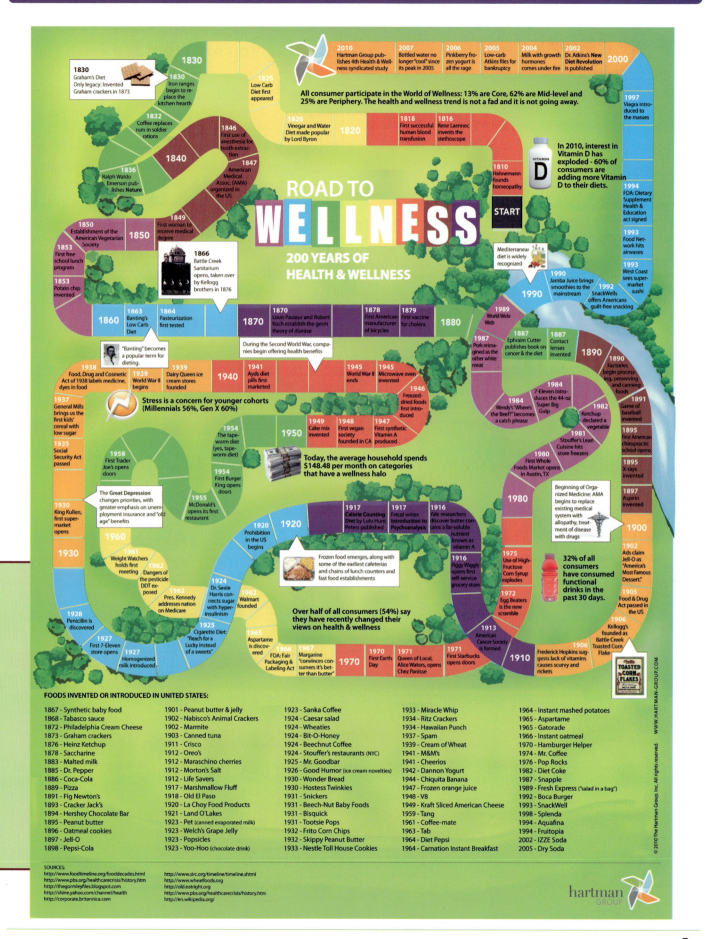

ROAD TO WELLNESS
200 YEARS OF HEALTH & WELLNESS

1830 Graham's Diet Only legacy: Invented Graham crackers in 1873

1830 Iron ranges begin to replace the kitchen hearth

1825 Low Carb Diet first appeared

1832 Coffee replaces rum in soldier rations

1846 First use of anesthesia for tooth extraction

1847 American Medical Assoc. (AMA) organized in the US

1836 Ralph Waldo Emerson publishes Nature

1849 First woman to receive medical degree

1850 Establishment of the American Vegetarian Society

1853 First free school lunch program

1853 Potato chip invented

1866 Battle Creek Sanitarium opens, taken over by Kellogg brothers in 1876

1863 Banting's Low Carb Diet

1864 Pasteurization first tested

1870 Louis Pasteur and Robert Koch establish the germ theory of disease

1878 First American manufacturer of bicycles

1879 First vaccine for cholera

"Banting" becomes a popular term for dieting.

During the Second World War, companies begin offering health benefits

1938 Food, Drug and Cosmetic Act of 1938 labels medicine, dyes in food

1939 World War II begins

1939 Dairy Queen ice cream stores founded

1941 Ayds diet pills first marketed

1945 World War II ends

1945 Microwave oven invented

1946 Freeze-dried foods first introduced

Stress is a concern for younger cohorts (Millennials 56%, Gen X 60%)

1937 General Mills brings us the first kids' cereal with low sugar

1954 The tapeworm diet (yes, tapeworm diet)

1949 Cake mix invented

1948 First vegan society founded in CA

1947 First synthetic Vitamin A produced

1935 Social Security Act passed

1958 First Trader Joe's opens doors

1954 First Burger King opens doors

Today, the average household spends $148.48 per month on categories that have a wellness halo

The Great Depression changes priorities, with greater emphasis on unemployment insurance and "old age" benefits

1930 King Kullen, first supermarket opens

1955 McDonald's opens its first restaurant

1917 Calorie Counting Diet by Lulu Hunt Peters published

1917 Freud writes Introduction to Psychoanalysis

1916 Yale researchers discover butter contains a fat-soluble nutrient known as vitamin A

Beginning of Organized Medicine: AMA begins to replace existing medical system with allopathy, treatment of disease with drugs

1961 Weight Watchers holds first meeting

1920 Prohibition in the US begins

Frozen food emerges, along with some of the earliest cafeterias and chains of lunch counters and fast food establishments

1916 Piggly Wiggly opens first self-service grocery store

1975 Use of High-Fructose Corn Syrup explodes

1972 Egg Beaters is the new scramble

32% of all consumers have consumed functional drinks in the past 30 days.

1962 Dangers of the pesticide DDT exposed

1924 Dr. Seale Harris connects sugar with hyperinsulinism

1962 Walmart founded

Over half of all consumers (54%) say they have recently changed their views on health & wellness

1928 Penicillin is discovered

1925 Cigarette Diet: "Reach for a Lucky instead of a sweets"

1965 Aspartame is discovered

1966 FDA: Fair Packaging & Labeling Act

1967 Margarine "convinces consumers it's better than butter"

1970 First Earth Day

1971 Queen of Local, Alice Waters, opens Chez Panisse

1971 First Starbucks opens doors

1913 American Cancer Society is formed

1906 Frederick Hopkins suggests lack of vitamins causes scurvy and rickets

1927 First 7-Eleven store opens

1927 Homogenized milk introduced

1810 Hahnemann founds homeopathy

1818 First successful human blood transfusion

1816 Rene Laennec invents the stethoscope

1820 Vinegar and Water Diet made popular by Lord Byron

In 2010, interest in Vitamin D has exploded - 60% of consumers are adding more Vitamin D to their diets.

2010 Hartman Group publishes 4th Health & Wellness syndicated study

2007 Bottled water no longer "cool" since its peak in 2005

2006 Pinkberry frozen yogurt is all the rage

2005 Low-carb Atkins files for bankruptcy

2004 Milk with growth hormones comes under fire

2002 Dr. Atkins's New Diet Revolution is published

All consumer participate in the World of Wellness: 13% are Core, 62% are Mid-level and 25% are Periphery. The health and wellness trend is not a fad and it is not going away.

1997 Viagra introduced to the masses

1994 FDA: Dietary Supplement Health & Education act signed

1993 Food Network hits airwaves

1993 West Coast sees supermarket sushi

Mediterranean diet is widely recognized

1990 Jamba Juice brings smoothies to the mainstream

1992 SnackWells offers Americans guilt-free snacking

1989 World Wide Web

1987 Pork reimagined as the other white meat

1887 Ephraim Cutter publishes book on cancer & the diet

1887 Contact lenses invented

1890 Factories begin processing, preserving and canning foods

1984 7-Eleven introduces the 44-oz Super Big Gulp

1984 Wendy's "Where's the Beef?" becomes a catch phrase

1982 Ketchup declared a vegetable

1891 Game of baseball invented

1981 Stouffer's Lean Cuisine hits store freezers

1895 First American chiropractic school opens

1980 First Whole Foods Market opens in Austin, TX

1895 X-rays invented

1897 Aspirin invented

1900

1902 Ads claim Jell-O as "America's Most Famous Dessert."

1905 Food & Drug Act passed in the US

1906 Kellogg's founded as Battle Creek Toasted Corn Flake

TOASTED CORN FLAKES

START

VITAMIN D

FOODS INVENTED OR INTRODUCED IN UNITED STATES:

1867 - Synthetic baby food	1901 - Peanut butter & jelly	1923 - Sanka Coffee	1933 - Miracle Whip	1964 - Instant mashed potatoes
1868 - Tabasco sauce	1902 - Nabisco's Animal Crackers	1924 - Caesar salad	1934 - Ritz Crackers	1965 - Aspartame
1872 - Philadelphia Cream Cheese	1902 - Marmite	1924 - Wheaties	1934 - Hawaiian Punch	1965 - Gatorade
1873 - Graham crackers	1903 - Canned tuna	1924 - Bit-O-Honey	1937 - Spam	1966 - Instant oatmeal
1876 - Heinz Ketchup	1911 - Crisco	1924 - Beechnut Coffee	1939 - Cream of Wheat	1970 - Hamburger Helper
1878 - Saccharine	1912 - Oreo's	1924 - Stouffer's restaurants (NYC)	1941 - M&M's	1974 - Mr. Coffee
1883 - Malted milk	1912 - Maraschino cherries	1925 - Mr. Goodbar	1941 - Cheerios	1976 - Pop Rocks
1885 - Dr. Pepper	1912 - Morton's Salt	1926 - Good Humor (ice cream novelties)	1942 - Dannon Yogurt	1982 - Diet Coke
1886 - Coca-Cola	1912 - Life Savers	1930 - Wonder Bread	1944 - Chiquita Banana	1987 - Snapple
1889 - Pizza	1917 - Marshmallow Fluff	1930 - Hostess Twinkies	1947 - Frozen orange juice	1989 - Fresh Express ("salad in a bag")
1891 - Fig Newton's	1918 - Old El Paso	1931 - Snickers	1948 - V8	1992 - Boca Burger
1893 - Cracker Jack's	1920 - La Choy Food Products	1931 - Beech-Nut Baby Foods	1949 - Kraft Sliced American Cheese	1993 - SnackWell
1894 - Hershey Chocolate Bar	1921 - Land O'Lakes	1931 - Bisquick	1959 - Tang	1998 - Splenda
1895 - Peanut butter	1923 - Pet (canned evaporated milk)	1931 - Tootsie Pops	1961 - Coffee-mate	1994 - Aquafina
1896 - Oatmeal cookies	1923 - Welch's Grape Jelly	1932 - Frito Corn Chips	1963 - Tab	1994 - Fruitopia
1897 - Jell-O	1923 - Popsicles	1932 - Skippy Peanut Butter	1964 - Diet Pepsi	2002 - IZZE Soda
1898 - Pepsi-Cola	1923 - Yoo-Hoo (chocolate drink)	1933 - Nestle Toll House Cookies	1964 - Carnation Instant Breakfast	2005 - Dry Soda

SOURCES:
http://www.foodtimeline.org/fooddecades.html
http://www.pbs.org/healthcarecrisis/history.htm
http://thegormleyfiles.blogspot.com
http://shine.yahoo.com/channel/health
http://corporate.britannica.com
http://www.sirc.org/timeline/timeline.shtml
http://www.wheatfoods.org
http://old.eatright.org
http://www.pbs.org/healthcarecrisis/history.htm
http://en.wikipedia.org/

hartman GROUP

Health Risks

In 1902, human nutrition pioneer W. O. Atwater predicted: "The evils of overeating may not be felt at once, but sooner or later they are sure to appear – perhaps in an excessive amount of fatty tissue, perhaps in general debility, perhaps in actual disease." [7] In fact, within the last century, changes in diet and level of physical activity have been profound and have led to an increase in lifestyle diseases like heart disease, obesity and diabetes – to name a few.

Today, chronic diseases are the leading causes of death and disability in the United States. Five out of 10 deaths among Americans each year are from chronic diseases. Heart disease, cancer and stroke account for more than 50% of all deaths each year. About one-fourth of people with chronic conditions have one or more daily activity limitations. Four modifiable health risk behaviors – lack of physical activity, poor nutrition, tobacco use and excessive alcohol consumption – are responsible for much of the illness, suffering and early death related to chronic diseases and accidents. [8]

Obesity, which is an epidemic in America, contributes to many chronic diseases. In its report to the nation, the 2010 Dietary Guidelines Committee called obesity the greatest threat to public health in this century. [9] Six different types of cancer are associated with being overweight or obese. [10] Although a single dietary element is often tagged as the cause of a chronic disease – for example, saturated fat and heart disease or salt and high blood pressure – research over the past three decades shows that a cluster of dietary elements is usually at the root of the problem. [11]

Historically, people from nations that consume plant-based diets have lower incidences of diet-related diseases and disorders than Americans. Many of these diets are based on rice, grains, beans, legumes, nuts, fruits and vegetables. Foods are minimally processed with greater emphasis on seasonal and local produce. Immigrants living in the United States, however, typically adopt Western food practices – such as eating more processed foods – that lead to increased disease risk.

It's True: You Are What You Eat

What people consume as infants, toddlers, young children and teens builds the body they take into adulthood. In fact, five of the 10 leading causes of death are related to lifelong dietary choices (bolded in the list below). And although not in the top 10, cirrhosis of the liver and osteoporosis are also triggered by food choices made over time. The good news is that it's never too late to improve nutrition.

Leading Causes of Death in the U.S.

1. **Heart disease**
2. **Cancer**
3. Chronic lower respiratory disease
4. **Stroke**
5. Accidents
6. Alzheimer's disease
7. **Diabetes**
8. Influenza and pneumonia
9. **Kidney disease**
10. Suicide

Source: National Center for Health Statistics, Centers for Disease Control and Prevention, U.S. Department of Health and Human Services. National Vital Statistics Report. December 2011. Deaths: Final Data for 2009. http://www.cdc.gov/nchs/data/nvsr/nvsr60/nvsr60_03.pdf.

Why We Eat What We Eat

At the most basic level, the purpose of food is to provide the nutrients and energy the body needs to grow and function. But many variables influence food choice.

Taste, Cost and Convenience

According to The International Food Information Council (IFIC) *2012 Food & Health Survey: Consumer Attitudes Toward Food Safety, Nutrition & Health*, taste remains the main driver behind purchasing foods and beverages. Eighty-seven percent of consumers surveyed listed taste as their priority in choosing foods. Consumers are not willing, nor should they have to, sacrifice taste for nutrition. Healthful foods can taste good too. [12]

Price and convenience continue as significant factors, also. Food selection is driven in large part by economics – the cost of food. Contrary to the beliefs of some, however, preparing healthier food does not have to cost more. For example, whole grains and legumes are relatively inexpensive. Fruits and vegetables served in season are often less expensive than imported, out-of-season produce. The most expensive part of the meal, the animal protein source, can be served in a smaller portion. Shifting the balance of the plate to include more grains, fruits and vegetables, and less animal protein, helps control food costs while providing healthful options.

That convenience plays a significant role in food selections is evidenced by the prevalence of quick-service restaurants as well as carryout and delivered meals. For many consumers, the time available for home meal preparation and consumption is limited – and so are cooking skills. This combination of circumstances creates many opportunities for the foodservice industry to provide convenient and healthful meals.

Healthfulness

According to the IFIC survey, healthfulness is a major influencer for 61% of consumers in their decision to buy foods and beverages. Concern about nutrition is influenced by age, gender and education. AND's *Nutrition and You: Trends 2011* survey showed that

as people age, diet and nutrition become increasingly important. [5] The most health conscious consumers belong to the 65+-year-old age group. Foodservice operators whose primary audience is the elderly must develop menus with the older person's needs in mind. At the other end of the spectrum, operators feeding school children must respond to an entirely different set of preferences and health considerations.

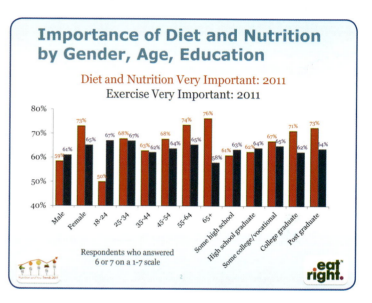

The IFIC 2012 survey indicates that regional and ethnic preferences play an important role in food selection. For example, rice and beans are served across the United States but in many different ways with different seasonings. In Louisiana, red beans and rice is a staple. In the South, Hoppin' John (black-eyed peas and rice) rules. In the Southwest, pinto beans and rice are a favorite. The popularity of ethnic cuisines has emboldened consumers to try new seasonings and flavors. This curiosity has brought greater diversity to the American diet and introduced many new options to replace fats and salt for flavor. Ethnicity and religion can dictate food selections on a daily basis, on specific holidays or during certain seasons. Chefs should understand the food practices, customs and holiday food traditions of the populations they serve and try to use the most healthful ingredients and cooking techniques available to their foodservice organization.

Sustainability

According to the 2012 IFIC survey, 35% of Americans say that sustainability is important to them. Americans see "ensuring a sufficient food supply" as the most important aspect of sustainability. Reducing the amount of pesticides used to produce food, maximum food output with minimal use of natural resources, optimal land and water use and efficiency, and less food and energy waste as important concerns as well.

Marketing

Marketing also influences food selections. Food choices are influenced by the description of menu items on signage or printed menus. Even the location of an item on the menu can affect selection. Comments made by servers also can influence guests' choices. An enthusiastic description of a dish, knowledge of ingredients and preparation methods, and helping the customer make a food selection (especially when the guest has food restrictions) makes the server a partner in the customer's successful dining experience and influences the patron to form a positive impression and become a repeat customer.

Social Interaction

Remember that people also use mealtime for social interaction. Dining with others offers many benefits beyond meeting nutrient needs. Eating together enhances quality of life and creates a time for sharing cultural values. In an issue of the *AIWF Journal of Gastronomy* titled "Taste, Health and the Social Meal," Margaret Mackenzie, PhD, RN, writes, "Virtually every anthropologic study that focuses on food emphasizes that meals are vitally important symbols – and ways of strengthening – social connections. . . .Yet regular shared meals are under great pressure and, according to various reports, may be declining in our culture." She continues, "Families may need to find different ways to establish family meal rituals. One solution to the challenges of today's society is eating out." [13]

Marketing Food to Children

Marketing high-calorie, low-nutrient foods to children has garnered much attention and criticism over the last decade. In 2005, the Institute of Medicine (IOM) released *Food Marketing to Children and Youth: Threat or Opportunity?* The study, which was requested by Congress and sponsored by the U.S. Centers for Disease Control and Prevention, provided a comprehensive review of the scientific evidence on the influence of food marketing on diets and the diet-related health of children and youth. The report found that current food and beverage marketing practices place children's long-term health at risk. If America's children and youth are to develop eating habits that help them avoid early onset of diet-related chronic diseases, they have to reduce their intake of high-calorie, low-nutrient snacks, fast foods and sweetened drinks.

The IOM report found that more than $10 billion is spent each year for marketing food and beverages to children and youth in America, and that the majority of products marketed are processed foods – high in calories, sugars, salt and fat, and low in nutrients. The report's recommendations for the foodservice industry include:

- Use creativity, resources, and the full range of marketing practices to promote healthful meals for children and youth.

- Expand and actively promote healthier food, beverage, and meal options for children and youth.

- Provide calorie content and other key nutrition information, as possible, on menus and packaging that is prominently visible at the point of choice and use.

Source: Food Marketing to Children and Youth: Threat or Opportunity? www.iom.edu/Reports/2005/Food-Marketing-to-Children-and-Youth-Threat-or-Opportunity.aspx

Restaurants today are popular because they are intense food-sharing enterprises necessary now that the home is losing its traditional importance as a place where food is prepared and served to a group.

Lionel Tiger
The Pursuit of Pleasure

Choosing Healthful Foods

The 2012 IFIC *Food & Health Survey: Consumer Attitudes Toward Food Safety, Nutrition & Health* survey also showed a shift toward healthier eating. [12] Seventy-five percent of respondents said they have made an effort to increase their consumption of whole-grain foods; 87% said they were eating more fruits and vegetables. Asked if they had decreased their consumption of foods with solid fats, sugar and salt, 76% said they had done so; 75% said they were choosing foods with more whole grains. Gender and education level influence food choices and what people think about food and health. In the AND survey, 73% of women said that diet and nutrition are very important compared to only 59% of men. People with a college education and beyond were more likely to say diet and nutrition are very important than were people with a high school degree or less formal education. It's important to point out, however, that this survey shows what people say and not necessarily what they do.

Consumption of Specific Foods in Past Five Years

Foods	% Increase	% Decrease	% Stayed the Same
Vegetables	49	6	45
Whole-grain foods	48	7	45
Fish	46	11	42
Chicken	44	8	49
Fruits	41	12	48
Dairy products	17	22	61
Beef	12	39	49
Pork	11	35	52

Source: Academy of Nutrition and Dietetics, *Nutrition and You: Trends 2011,* www.eatright.org/Media/content.aspx?id=7639.

People usually think they eat less that than really do. In fact, it is very difficult to determine what is actually eaten. Even when food records are kept, perception seldom precisely matches consumption, especially when snacks and alcohol are involved. What people say they want is often not what they choose. Many customers say they want healthful choices but don't select these items when they are offered, often because they believe the healthful or low-calorie options will not taste as good. Some restaurants are integrating healthful choices throughout the menu, rather than calling them out as healthy options. Food manufacturers use this "stealth health" approach, too, quietly reducing (but not eliminating) fat, salt and sugar in processed foods. Restaurants like Subway, however, have increased sales by highlighting and heavily advertising specific healthful or low-calorie choices.

As restaurant food labeling is implemented, perceptions may change. Faced with the facts on calories, will customers make different choices? Some observers say that consumers do not want to be "confronted" with nutrition information when they eat out because it detracts from full enjoyment and celebration; others opine that consumers appreciate and use the information to make more healthful, lower-calorie choices.

The Academy of Nutrition and Dietetics and others in the world of food and nutrition have long supported the idea that "all foods fit." While all foods can fit, moderation and balance present a challenge. For even a few foods high in fat, salt, sugar and calories to "fit" in the daily diet, plenty of healthful nutrient-dense, fairly low-calorie foods are needed to offset them. While the concept that there are no good or bad foods and that what really counts is the total diet sounds good, it is not that useful – unless, of course, you are making a case for "bad foods." One has to make many excellent choices in order to fit in a daily soft drink or French fries. The reality of weight control and disease prevention is simple: It all boils down to calories. That makes balance and moderation among the chef's greatest challenges.

Nutrients in Foods

It is becoming increasingly important that chefs know what is in the food they make and serve. That does not mean that everything must fit a healthful profile, but knowing calorie count and some information about nutritional benefits and risks enables the chef to create balance and moderation across the total menu. Knowledge provides power – the power to make informed choices and to create positive change.

Foods provide a vast array of substances that are necessary to sustain life and health. There are six classes of essential nutrients:

- Carbohydrates
- Fats
- Proteins
- Vitamins
- Minerals
- Water

To be an essential nutrient, a substance must meet three criteria:

1. It must be needed by the human body.
2. It cannot be made by the body (or made in sufficient quantity) to meet bodily needs; thus, it must be provide by food sources.
3. If absent, it will create a deficiency disease or medical problem.

Essential nutrients are discussed in greater detail in later chapters.

All calories – the body's fuel – come from carbohydrates, proteins, fats and alcohol. Water and the many vitamins and minerals, each with specific functions, are vital to life and health but do not provide calories. Alcohol does provide calories but is not a nutrient.

Essential Nutrients

Carbohydrates	Fats	Protein	Vitamins	Minerals	Water
Fiber	Linoleic acid	Essential amino acids:	B_6	Calcium	Water
Glucose	Linolenic acid	Histidine	B_{12}	Chloride	
		Isoleucine	Biotin	Chromium	
		Leucine	Folate	Copper	
		Lysine	Niacin	Fluoride	
		Methionine	Pantothenic acid	Iodine	
		Phenylalanine	Riboflavin	Iron	
		Threonine	Thiamin	Magnesium	
		Tryptophan	Vitamin A	Manganese	
		Valine	Vitamin D	Molybdenum	
			Vitamin E	Phosphorus	
			Vitamin K	Potassium	
			Vitamin C	Selenium	
				Sodium	
				Sulfur	
				Zinc	

Energy Balance

Energy is measured in calories. Teens and adults need about 2,000 to 3,000 calories from food each day. Calorie needs are dependent on activity level, age, height, physical health and body composition. Calories are used to fuel physical activity, basic body functions and digestion.

Energy is needed to make and fuel cells of the body that are necessary for all life-sustaining activities – blood circulation, breathing, temperature maintenance, nerve activity and hormone secretion. These activities, taken together at the cellular level, are called **basal metabolism**. Age, gender, genetics, body composition and size affect basal metabolic energy needs, which account for 50% to 65% of total calorie needs.

In addition, energy also supports activities such as walking, working the line, serving guests, running,

Calculating Calories from Foods

Calories are the unit used to measure the energy in food. The energy-yielding nutrients in food (protein, fats and carbohydrates) are measured in grams. Foods are usually a mixture of protein, fat, carbohydrates and water. Few foods contain just one nutrient.

Nutrient	Calories per Gram
Carbohydrate	4
Fat	9
Protein	4
Alcohol	7

A teaspoon of oil weighs about 5 grams and contains approximately 5 grams of fat and 45 calories:

5 grams fat x 9 calories per gram = 45 calories

A cup of low-fat milk weighs about 245 grams and contains approximately 8 grams of protein, 12 grams of carbohydrates and 2.5 grams of fat. The balance of milk's weight comes from water (220 grams). One cup of low-fat milk will have:

8 grams protein x 4 calories/gram = 32 calories from protein

12 grams carbohydrate x 4 calories/gram = 48 calories from carbohydrate

2.5 grams fat x 9 calories/gram = 22.5 calories from fat

Total calories = 102.5

Factors Affecting the Basal Metabolic Rate

Your BMR is influenced by a number of factors working in combination, including:

Body size - larger adult bodies have more metabolizing tissue and a higher BMR.

Age - metabolism slows with age due to a loss in muscle tissue and hormonal and neurological changes. BMR declines about 2% per decade after 30.

Gender - generally, men have faster metabolisms than women because they tend to have more muscle tissue and muscle tissue burns more calories.

Amount of body fat - fat cells are sluggish and burn far fewer calories than most other tissues.

Infection or illness - BMR increases because the body has to work harder to build new tissues and to create an immune response.

Crash dieting, starving or fasting - eating too few calories encourages the body to slow down the metabolism to conserve energy; BMR can drop by up to 15%. Lean muscle tissue is also lost, which further reduces the BMR.

cycling, rock climbing, skating, etc. Depending on the individual, this activity may account for 25% to 50% of total energy needs. Sedentary people need fewer calories because they burn fewer supporting daily activities.

Energy is also needed to break food down into the small components that go into the bloodstream and later to cells. This process is called the **thermic effect** of food and accounts for 5% to 10% of total energy needs.

If you consume more calories than you need, you gain weight. If you consume fewer than you need, you lose weight. Because total calorie needs decline after early adulthood, even maintaining the same eating habits and levels of calories consumed will cause weight gain. Many people need fewer calories than they think they do, and most underestimate the number of calories that they eat. This combination results in weight gain over time.

Estimated Calorie Needs per Day by Age, Gender and Physical Activity Level

Estimated amounts of calories[a] needed to maintain calorie balance for various gender and age groups at three different levels of physical activity. The estimates are rounded to the nearest 200 calories. An individual's calorie needs may be higher or lower than these average estimates.

Age (years)	Male			Female[c]		
	Activity Level[b]					
	Sedentary	Moderately Active	Active	Sedentary	Moderately Active	Active
2	1,000	1,000	1,000	1,000	1,000	1,000
3	1,200	1,400	1,400	1,000	1,200	1,400
4	1,200	1,400	1,600	1,200	1,400	1,400
5	1,200	1,400	1,600	1,200	1,400	1,600
6	1,400	1,600	1,800	1,200	1,400	1,600
7	1,400	1,600	1,800	1,200	1,600	1,800
8	1,400	1,600	2,000	1,400	1,600	1,800
9	1,600	1,800	2,000	1,400	1,600	1,800
10	1,600	1,800	2,200	1,400	1,800	2,000
11	1,800	2,000	2,200	1,600	1,800	2,000
12	1,800	2,200	2,400	1,600	2,000	2,200
13	2,000	2,200	2,600	1,600	2,000	2,200
14	2,000	2,400	2,800	1,800	2,000	2,400
15	2,200	2,600	3,000	1,800	2,000	2,400
16-18	2,400	2,800	3,200	1,800	2,000	2,400
19–20	2,600	2,800	3,000	2,000	2,200	2,400
21–25	2,400	2,800	3,000	2,000	2,200	2,400
26–30	2,400	2,600	3,000	1,800	2,000	2,400
31–35	2,400	2,600	3,000	1,800	2,000	2,200
36–40	2,400	2,600	2,800	1,800	2,000	2,200
41–45	2,200	2,600	2,800	1,800	2,000	2,200
46–50	2,200	2,400	2,800	1,800	2,000	2,200
51–55	2,200	2,400	2,800	1,600	1,800	2,200
56–60	2,200	2,400	2,600	1,600	1,800	2,200
61–65	2,000	2,400	2,600	1,600	1,800	2,000
66–75	2,000	2,200	2,600	1,600	1,800	2,000
76+	2,000	2,200	2,400	1,600	1,800	2,000

a. Based on Estimated Energy Requirements (EER) equations, using reference heights (average) and reference weights (healthy) for each age-gender group. For children and adolescents, reference height and weight vary. For adults, the reference man is 5 feet 10 inches tall and weighs 154 pounds. The reference woman is 5 feet 4 inches tall and weighs 126 pounds. EER equations are from the Institute of Medicine. Dietary Reference Intakes for Energy, Carbohydrate, Fiber, Fat, Fatty Acids, Cholesterol, Protein, and Amino Acids. Washington, DC: The National Academies Press; 2002.

b. Sedentary means a lifestyle that includes only the light physical activity associated with typical day-to-day life. Moderately active means a lifestyle that includes physical activity equivalent to walking about 1.5 to 3 miles per day at 3 to 4 miles per hour, in addition to the light physical activity associated with typical day-to-day life. Active means a lifestyle that includes physical activity equivalent to walking more than 3 miles per day at 3 to 4 miles per hour, in addition to the light physical activity associated with typical day-to-day life.

c. Estimates for females do not include women who are pregnant or breastfeeding.

Source: Britten P, Marcoe K, Yamini S, Davis C. Development of food intake patterns for the MyPyramid Food Guidance System. J Nutr Educ Behav 2006;38(6 Suppl):S78-S92.

Nutrient Density

Nutrient density is a measure of positive nutrients to calories. Nutrient-dense foods pack a lot of essential nutrients into relatively few calories. In other words, they are particularly healthful food choices and ingredients. Vegetables, fruits, whole grains, fish, eggs, low-fat milk, lean meat, beans and poultry prepared without added solid fats or sugars are nutrient dense. Nutrient-dense foods are often described as **nutrient rich**. The *Dietary Guidelines for Americans* suggest getting the most nutrition from calories consumed and eating a variety of nutrient-dense foods and beverages within and among the basic food groups. Foods that have low nutrient density supply calories but relatively small amounts of vitamins and minerals. For example, whole-wheat bread is nutrient dense, but a croissant has a low nutrient density.

Numerous researchers and organizations have developed approaches based on nutrient density that can be used as tools to help consumers improve their dietary patterns by selecting more nutritious food items. This approach, called **nutrient profiling**, is the process of ranking foods based on their nutrient content. Some of the models developed focus on nutrients to limit (giving higher scores to foods low in fat, sugar and salt); others have factored in nutrients known to be beneficial to health (giving higher scores to foods rich in vitamins, minerals and fiber). Some models are a combination of both (with a calculation that adds points for essential nutrients and removes points for those substances that should be limited). Several nutrient profiling approaches are described in the next chapter.

What We Eat vs. What We Should Eat

On average, about 35% of calories consumed are from solid fats and added sugars (SoFAS). It is recommended, however, that no more than 5% to 15% of total calories come from SoFAS for most individuals.

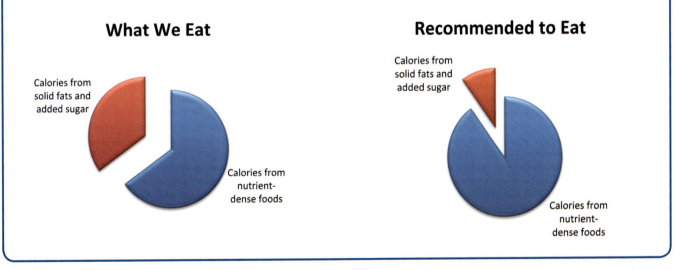

What We Eat

Calories from solid fats and added sugar

Calories from nutrient-dense foods

Recommended to Eat

Calories from solid fats and added sugar

Calories from nutrient-dense foods

Source: Report of the Dietary Guidelines Advisory Committee on the Dietary Guidelines, 2010. Available at www.cnpp.usda.gov/DGAs2010-DGACReport.htm

What's 'Good' and What's 'Bad'?

Nutritional composition tables that compare similar foods are a traditional tool for determining "good" and "bad" choices. Most of the available databases are derived from information compiled by the U.S. Department of Agriculture. Over the past few years, calculating nutrient density has emerged as a new way to compare foods. Nutrient density "scores" are popping up on food labels throughout the supermarket.

A best-selling book by David Zinczenko with Matt Goulding called *Eat This Not That!* (Rodale Books, 2012) compares similar brand-name foods and gives caloric values plus nuggets of nutrition information. Many of these comparisons are startling even to experienced dietitians and nutritionists. For example:

- At Dunkin Donuts, the ham/egg/cheese breakfast sandwich has 190 fewer calories than the multigrain bagel with "lite" cream cheese.

- The Super Roast Beef at Arby's has 370 fewer calories than the healthier-sounding Roast Beef and Swiss Market Fresh Sandwich.

- At Ruby Tuesday, a full steak dinner (7-oz sirloin, green beans and sauteed mushrooms) has less than half the calories of a turkey burger with fries.

- Even similar-sounding menu items (such as the Quiznos Honey Bourbon Chicken on Wheat Bread Sub at 310 calories and its Honey Mustard Chicken Sub at 550 calories) can have dramatically different calorie counts.

Chefs perusing this and similar books will find ideas on healthful ingredients and advice on how to modify recipes and accompaniments to reduce calories, fat and sodium.

Portion Distortion

Many chefs are very interested in nutrition and believe they are serving (mostly) healthful food. Recent surveys conducted by Clemson University have reported that although chefs recognize the importance of nutrition in menu planning, they are serving meals that are inconsistent with the current *Dietary Guidelines for Americans*. A key area of concern is portion size. A survey of 300 chefs attending culinary and research chef meetings revealed that 76% thought they served "regular" portions, but they actually served portions two to four times larger than recommended serving sizes. Although chefs say they know that large portions pose problems for weight management, many believe that customers expect large portions and that it is each customer's responsibility to eat an appropriate amount. Many customers, however, have a "clean plate" mindset that drives them to eat everything on the plate. [14]

Over the past two decades, portion sizes of individually packaged foods have grown, too. Consequently, customers now think large portions are normal. This "portion distortion" can hinder efforts to control weight and improve health. [15] One of the goals of this book is to help chefs understand *appropriate* portions and provide food that is satisfying, healthful and delicious. Later chapters will explore portions and strategies for focusing on food quality rather than excessive quantity. Every chef wants to make customers happy and improve the dining experience. Helping customers (and themselves) stay healthy is a bonus.

Portion sizes and corresponding calories have increased over the last 20 years. Here are some examples.

Portions and Calories - 20 Years Later

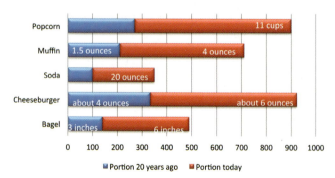

Source: Portion Distortion Quiz, Dept. of Health & Human Services, National Institutes of Health, and National Heart, Lung, and Blood Institute. Available at http://hp2010.nhlbihin.net/portion.

A Place for Healthful Food in Foodservice

After years of courtship, culinary professionals and nutritionists have come together in a way that will benefit both – as well as the people they serve. There is agreement: Healthy foods can taste good, and tasty foods can be healthful. In fact, all types of foodservice operations are incorporating healthful items across their menus. Onsite dining facilities, fast casual and quick-service restaurants, chains, and full-service and fine dining restaurants are offering healthier foods. Some establishments that were once concerned only with taste are now mindful of nutrition and health as well and are preparing foods that nourish the body as much as they feed the senses.

Traditional providers of healthful meals – schools, colleges and universities, hospitals, and long-term care (or senior care) facilities – are very aware that healthful meals also must taste good and look good. When a person eats all or most meals in one foodservice venue, consistently healthful food is particularly important. Fine dining establishments often have health-conscious diners, but nutrition is of less concern for the occasional celebratory meal.

Operational Implications

Preparing and serving healthier foods requires some changes in labor and training, equipment, and purchasing. Changing menus seasonally and using local products may demand more menu-planning time. In some situations – for example, in a hospital – developing specific seasonal menus may be challenging. Featuring "seasonal green vegetables" provides some wiggle room. Healthier menu items may require nutrient data calculation and seeking new ingredients with lower levels of sodium, sugar or fat. Buying local, seasonal products may necessitate a larger vendor list. Creating standardized recipes, and following them exactly, will ensure that customers are served the calories listed on the menu. But flexibility is important, too. If a school lists fresh peaches on the menu for August, but the local crop is late, a menu substitution will be needed.

Preparing healthier foods may also entail equipment changes. For example, baking or roasting rather than deep-frying (think oven-baked sweet potato strips or roasted vegetables) can take more time and certainly requires more oven space. Fresh or frozen vegetables require more refrigeration or freezer space than canned varieties as well as different equipment for pre-prep. Steamers or grills may be needed, and healthier food preparation may mean more *a la minute* cooking.

Staffing changes also may be necessary. More labor may be needed to pre-prep fruits and vegetables. On he other hand, using items such as pre-shredded carrots and cabbage or diced red peppers or onions that already have the labor cost built in makes it easier to define costs. Kitchen staff may need additional training in using standardized recipes and in measuring procedures, especially if calories and grams of fat are posted for customers.

Even though adding healthier items to the menu may require some operational realignment in the kitchen, the change can be good for business. According to research from the Mintel Group, consumers are demanding greater transparency from restaurants in terms of ingredients, processes and preparation. These expectations have been driven in part by a greater awareness and understanding of healthy eating. Operators have responded with a slew of healthy offerings in terms of ingredients, preparations, portion sizing and menuing to meet varying definitions of "healthy." [16] This change demonstrates an important attitude adjustment among consumers. The notion of food deprivation is giving way to a feeling of healthful enjoyment.

The Alliance of Taste and Health Moves Forward

Taste and health, together, can lead to better, healthier foods for all. We continue to move forward, incorporating healthful food choices in all aspects of our lives and culture. The foodservice industry is an important participant in the effort to help America become a healthier nation. Here are some recent changes that have moved us in a positive direction.

- Nutrition education and healthful cooking techniques are included in culinary school curricula.

- Chef certification now requires knowledge of nutrition.

- Chefs, restaurateurs and dietitians collaborate in many work settings.

- Healthful cooking and baking classes are growing in popularity for professional chefs as well as home cooks.

- Food and culinary expertise has grown within the profession of dietetics.

- Food and culinary topics are increasingly popular continuing education topics for maintaining the registered dietitian credential.

- Nutrition advice has become more taste-conscious, moving away from prohibitive, restrictive diets and toward more emphasis on positive food components.

- Improved technology allows more exact nutrient calculation and evaluation of recipes.

- Readership of magazines such as *Cooking Light* and *Eating Well* and of books on flavorful, healthful cooking has increased.

- Many excellent cookbooks feature plant-based diets

- Customers in schools, colleges and universities, and other foodservice settings are demanding healthful foods.

- Farmers markets, organic farming, seasonal foods and "eating local" continue to grow in popularity.

Nutrition Isn't an Afterthought

"Nutrition is an important part of what we teach students," notes William Reynolds, retired provost, Chicago's Washburne Culinary Institute. Established in 1937, Washburne is the nations' oldest culinary program. "Nutrition is not what most students are thinking about when registering," Bill continues, "but by graduation, nutrition should be as much a consideration as ingredient quality, preparation method and flavor."

Bill, who is an honorary member of the Academy of Nutrition and Dietetics and an active member of the Academy's Food & Culinary Professionals Dietetic Practice Group, believes that most chefs don't give nutrition the priority it deserves: "We need to get away from 'taking stuff out' after the fact to make a recipe more healthful. Nutrition should be a consideration from the beginning of the process. You don't make the food and then remake it to be more nutritious," he explains. "From the outset, use the cooking method and ingredients that give the best taste and the most nutrition."

- Jamie Oliver, Rachael Ray, Alice Waters, Mario Batali, Art Smith and other celebrity chefs have become advocates for healthful foods in schools and communities.

- Media interest in healthy foods and cooking has grown as evidenced by documentaries and books that expose unhealthy food choices and/or food production practices.

- More companies are introducing single-portion, 100-calorie snacks.

- Beverages are available in smaller single-serve containers.

- Many major food companies are voluntarily reducing sodium across their product lines and offering more reduced-sodium ingredients.

- The *Dietary Guidelines for Americans* encourage restaurants and the food industry to offer health-promoting foods that are low in sodium; limited in added sugar, refined grains and solid fat; and served in small portions.

What Is a Registered Dietitian?

A *registered dietitian (RD)* is a food and nutrition expert who has met established minimum academic and professional requirements and has passed a comprehensive national examination to qualify for the credential "RD." Continuing education hours are necessary to maintain the RD credential. To help protect the public from charlatans, some states also license or certify dietitians and other nutrition experts. The majority of RDs work in the treatment and prevention of disease (administering medical nutrition therapy, often as part of medical teams) in hospitals, HMOs, private practice or other health care facilities. In addition, a large number of RDs work in community and public health settings, academia and research. A growing number of RDs work in the food and nutrition industry, business, journalism, sports nutrition and corporate wellness programs.

Partnering with a Registered Dietitian

The culinary professional or chef and the registered dietitian (RD) or nutritionist have an opportunity to work as partners in planning, preparing and serving healthier foods to consumers across the country in a variety of foodservice venues. A culinary registered dietitian can be a valuable resource when a chef has questions about nutrition or needs nutrient calculation for a recipe. A culinary RD also can review menus and help fine-tune menu offerings with an eye toward nutritional health. Some dietitians are trained as chefs and some own restaurants or food businesses with a health focus. Chefs can request assistance finding a local RD with the needed expertise from The Academy of Nutrition and Dietetics Food & Culinary Professionals Dietetic Practice Group (FCP) by simply contacting the group's administrator (www.foodculinaryprofs.org/) and asking to post a query on the FCP website.

Three chefs have been granted honorary membership by the Academy of Nutrition and Dietetics, thereby recognizing their commitment to healthful cooking. They include celebrity chef Graham Kerr; president-emeritus of the Culinary Institute of America, Ferdinand Metz; and retired provost from Chicago's Washburne Culinary Institute, William Reynolds.

Typical American Diet Compared to Recommended Intake Levels or Limits

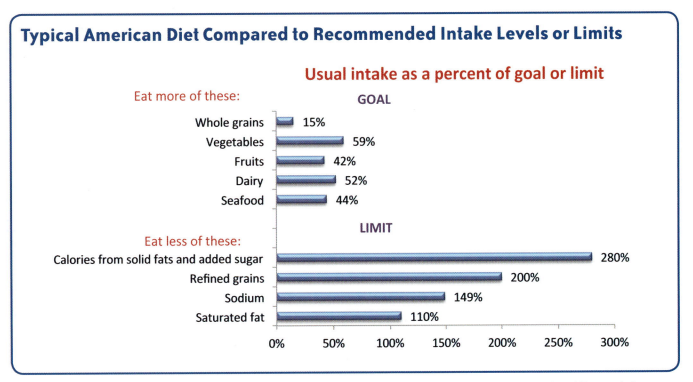

Source: *Dietary Guidelines for Americans, 2010.* Based on data from: U.S. Department of Agriculture, Agricultural Research Service and U.S. Department of Health and Human Services, Centers for Disease Control and Prevention. *What We Eat in America,* NHAMES 2001-2004 and 2005-2006.

Opportunities for Chefs

Nutrition should never be an afterthought for the chef. Rather, it should be an integral part of the menu development process. Food professionals have an opportunity to help change the way consumers eat and to have a positive impact on the overall health of people.

The focus on nutritional health has shifted from restriction to balance – that is, seeking positive nutrients and balancing the number of calories consumed with the number burned. Food can taste good and be healthful – especially when the focus is on what you *can* eat, not on what you should avoid. Contemporary menus reflecting this shift feature less processed and more whole grains, vegetables, fruits, legumes, low-fat dairy products and lean protein foods, healthful cooking techniques, and portion control. The chef who can make healthful food with great taste and texture, as well as provide a good dining experience, is positioned well for the changing times.

Learning Activities

1. Select a menu from a foodservice operation that you work in or visit frequently. Identify the nutrient-dense menu items.

2. Using the categories of consumers identified by the Academy of Nutrition and Dietetics trend survey – "I'm Already Doing It," "I Know I Should," and "Don't Bother Me" - determine the label that best fits you and explain why.

3. Based on your age, gender and activity level, identify the calorie level that will maintain your healthy weight.

For More Information

- Academy of Nutrition and Dietetics, www.eatright.org

- Food & Culinary Professionals, a dietetic practice group of the Academy of Nutrition and Dietetics, www.foodculinaryprofs.org

- *Gastronomica: The Journal of Food and Culture*, www.gastronomica.org

- Hess MA. *Resetting the American Table*. J Am Diet Assoc. 1991;91(2):228-30.

- International Food Information Council, www.ific.org

- Montanari M. *Food Is Culture*. New York: Columbia University Press; 2006.

- National Restaurant Association, www.restaurant.org

- Nestle M. *What to Eat*. New York: North Point Press; 2006.

- U.S. Department of Agriculture Food Composition Tables, www.nal.usda.gov/fnic/foodcomp/search

- Wansink B. *Mindless Eating: Why We Eat More Than We Think*. New York: Bantam Dell; 2007.

CHAPTER 2

Nutrition Standards and Tools

LEARNING OBJECTIVES

After completing this chapter, you should be able to:

- Explain the function of the recommended Dietary Reference Intakes
- Describe and discuss the *Dietary Guidelines for Americans* and identify challenges for chefs
- List the food groups found in *MyPlate* and recommended servings from each group
- Explain how *MyPlate* encourages variety, proportionality and moderation
- Read and analyze food labels, nutrient claims and health claims
- Discuss the attributes and limitations of various food rating systems

This chapter explores the various U.S. government standards and tools developed for the greater good – that is, to promote the health of Americans as a population. Keep in mind that each person has unique nutrition needs based on his/her history, environment, personal taste, ethnicity, and cultural values and beliefs. This chapter also looks at various tools and food label terminology that help chefs and consumers make informed food choices.

Some nutrition standards refer to adequacy and recommend levels of intake based on research; some identify actions that promote moderation; others describe components of a healthful diet. All of the commonly used standards and tools are based on four cornerstones:

- **Adequacy** means providing or eating foods that supply all of the essential nutrients needed for life and health. For those with severe dietary restrictions or intolerances, dietary supplements can fill nutrient gaps.

- **Balance** means that the whole diet should provide enough, but not too much, of each of the essential nutrients. Balance also means including foods from all of the food groups, which requires considerable planning.

- **Moderation** means serving and eating adequate, appropriate portions. In light of today's tendency toward over-consumption, moderation is critical to a healthy diet and menu planning. It often requires recalibrating the menu to reduce portions of meat and high-fat, high-sugar, highly salted foods while still meeting the consumer's desire for value.

- **Variety** means serving different foods within each food group to increase the likelihood of a nutritionally adequate diet. Different food groups provide different essential nutrients as do a variety of foods within each group. Variety also refers to incorporating different cooking methods, flavors and temperatures to create healthful and enjoyable meals.

Dietary Reference Intakes

The **Dietary Reference Intakes** (DRIs), developed by the Food and Nutrition Board of the Institute of Medicine, National Academy of Sciences, are based on medical research and food intake surveys. DRIs refer to minimum recommended and maximum safe levels of many nutrients by age and gender. DRIs aim to prevent chronic diseases and promote optimal health. They are used primarily by dietitians and other health professionals to assess and plan diets for healthy individuals and groups. Each DRI category (minimum, recommended and maximum) refers to average daily intake over time – at least one week for most nutrients. The concept of "nutrient intake adequacy over time" means that a specific level does not have to be met each and every day.

Programs such as school nutrition must meet a certain percentage of the DRIs. Correctional and long-term care facilities, however, must develop menus that meet the total nutrient needs of residents. Most chefs do not need to be particularly concerned about DRI levels other than to know their intended use. Generally, planning menus using the *Dietary Guidelines for Americans* and *MyPlate* will meet DRI requirements. (See Appendix B for a DRI chart.)

Daily Values

Daily Values (DVs), which are used on all food and supplement labels, are derived from recommended levels of nutrients in the DRIs based on a 2,000-calorie diet. The DV amounts for total fat, saturated fat, cholesterol and sodium are maximum amounts per day. The DVs for total carbohydrate and dietary fiber are minimum amounts per day. (See Appendix C.) A food that has 20% of a DV is an excellent source of that nutrient; a food that has 10% to 19% of a DV is a good source of that nutrient; while a food that has 0% to 5% DV of a nutrient is a poor source of that nutrient.

Dietary Guidelines for Americans 2010

The **Dietary Guidelines for Americans** (www. dietaryguidelines.gov), which are targeted to those over 2 years of age living in the United States, identify actions that will help the public meet the Dietary Reference Intakes. They provide science-based advice to promote health and reduce risk for chronic disease through diet and physical activity. The Department of Health and Human Services (HHS) and the U.S. Department of Agriculture (USDA) have published the guidelines every five years since 1980. Because of their focus on health promotion and risk reduction, the *Dietary Guidelines* form the basis of federal food, nutrition education and information programs. They also set some nutrition standards used by the food industry such as specifications for foods served in federally funded feeding programs.

The current edition of the guidelines includes recommendations for the general population as well as specific recommendations for certain populations such as racial/ethnic groups, vegetarians and others with special dietary needs. The *Dietary Guidelines for Americans 2010* also recognize that in recent years nearly 15% of American households have been unable to acquire adequate food to meet their needs. The guidelines can help these people maximize the nutritional content of their meals.

The *Dietary Guidelines for Americans 2010* are developed from the *Report of the Dietary Guidelines Advisory Committee* (www.cnpp.usda.gov/DGAs2010-DGACReport.htm), a document based on review of the scientific literature and evidence-based research. This publication also acknowledges that the majority of Americans, although overweight or obese, are also undernourished in several key nutrients.

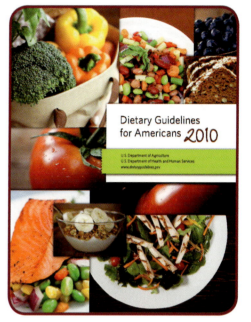

The *Dietary Guidelines for Americans 2010* recommendations are based on two overarching concepts:

- **Maintain calorie balance over time to achieve and sustain a healthy weight.** People who are most successful at achieving and maintaining a healthy weight do so through continued attention to consuming only enough calories from foods and beverages to meet their needs and by being physically active. To curb obesity and improve health, many Americans must decrease the calories they consume and increase the calories they expend through physical activity.

- **Focus on consuming nutrient-dense foods and beverages**. A healthy eating pattern emphasizes nutrient-dense foods and beverages such as vegetables, fruits, whole grains, fat-free or low-fat milk and milk products, seafood, lean meats and poultry, eggs, beans and peas, and nuts and seeds. Today, however, Americans consume too much sodium and too many calories from solid fats, added sugars and refined grains, thereby displacing nutrient-dense foods and beverages and making it difficult to achieve recommended nutrient intake while controlling calories and sodium intake.

The *Dietary Guidelines* recommendations that follow are the most important in terms of their implications for improving public health. To benefit fully, individuals should follow all of the *Dietary Guidelines* recommendations as part of an overall healthy eating pattern (www.cnpp.usda.gov/dietaryguidelines.htm).

- **Balancing calories to manage weight**. Prevent and/or reduce overweight and obesity through improved eating habits and physical activity.

  - Control total calorie intake to manage body weight. For people who are overweight or obese, this means consuming fewer calories from foods and beverages.

  - Increase physical activity and reduce time spent in sedentary behaviors.

  - Maintain appropriate calorie balance during each stage of life – childhood, adolescence, adulthood, pregnancy and breastfeeding, and older age.

- **Foods and nutrients to increase**. Individuals should meet the following recommendations as part of a healthy eating pattern while staying within their calorie needs.

  - Increase vegetable and fruit intake.

  - Eat a variety of vegetables, especially dark green, red and orange vegetables, and beans and peas.

  - Consume at least half of all grains as whole grains. Increase whole-grain intake by replacing refined grains with whole grains.

  - Increase intake of fat-free or low-fat milk and milk products, such as milk, yogurt, cheese or fortified soy beverages.

  - Choose a variety of protein foods, which include seafood, lean meat and poultry, eggs, beans and peas, soy products, and unsalted nuts and seeds.

  - Increase the amount and variety of seafood consumed by choosing seafood in place of some meat and poultry.

  - Replace protein foods that are higher in solid fats with choices that are lower in solid fats and calories and/or are sources of oils.

  - Use oils to replace solid fats where possible.

  - Choose foods that provide more potassium, dietary fiber, calcium and vitamin D – all of which are nutrients of concern in American diets. These foods include vegetables, fruits, whole grains, and milk and milk products.

- **Foods and food components to reduce.**

  - Reduce daily sodium intake to less than 2,300 milligrams. People who are 51 and older and those of any age who are African American or have hypertension, diabetes or chronic kidney disease should further reduce intake to 1,500 milligrams per day. This recommendation applies to about half of the U.S. population, including children and the majority of adults.

  - Consume less than 10% of calories from saturated fat. Replace saturated fat with monounsaturated and polyunsaturated fats.

  - Consume less than 300 milligrams per day of dietary cholesterol.

  - Keep trans fatty acid consumption as low as possible by limiting foods that contain synthetic sources of trans fats (such as partially hydrogenated oils) and by limiting other solid fats.

  - Reduce the intake of calories from solid fats and added sugars.

  - Limit consumption of foods that contain refined grains, especially those that also contain solid fats, added sugars and sodium.

  - If alcohol is consumed, it should be consumed in moderation – up to 1 drink per day for women and 2 drinks per day for men – and only by adults of legal drinking age.

- **Building healthy eating patterns.** Select an eating pattern that meets nutrient needs over time at an appropriate calorie level.

  - Account for all foods and beverages consumed and assess how they fit within a total healthy eating pattern.

  - Follow food safety recommendations when preparing and eating foods to reduce the risk of foodborne illnesses.

Nutrition Guidelines in Real Life

It only makes sense that a hospital would serve healthful food – but that is not always the case. Hospital cafeteria food does not necessarily have a healthy reputation. At Parkland Memorial Hospital (www.parklandhospital.com) in Dallas, one of the country's largest and busiest public hospitals, it's a different story.

In 2009, Parkland's 20-year contract with a major fast food chain expired and in the bid for vendor foodservices, the final selection was made in favor of UFood Grill (www.ufoodgrill.com), a popular eatery franchised/licensed by Fort Worth-based Puente Enterprises, Inc. The final decision was made by a selection committee including, among others, registered dietitians, registered nurses and a cardiologist.

UFood Grill had to meet a rigorous set of nutrition, variety and return-on-investment standards. "Although it is a quick-service restaurant, UFood Grill is inherently great-tasting 'fresh-for-you,' 'better-for-you' concepts," explains Gina Puente-Brancato, owner of Puente Enterprises. "Nevertheless, we had to make some changes to meet Parkland's strict nutrition standards. Sodium and saturated fat were the biggest challenges." Although prices are slightly higher than in the past, UFood Grill has been a hit with customers.

Parkland Hospital Baseline Nutrition Requirements

A minimum of 30% of the posted menu items for each menu line should meet all of the following criteria:

- less than 30% of calories from fat
- less than 7% of calories from saturated fat
- less than 1% of calories from trans fat
- less than 100 milligrams of cholesterol per serving
- less than 800 milligrams of sodium per serving
- No single menu item sold and served to the customer could provide greater than 50% of the calories from fat or contain more than 33 grams of fat.
- No single menu item sold and served to the customer should provide greater than 1,600 milligrams of sodium.

As healthcare reform measures strengthen the national focus on disease prevention, hospitals will be under increasing pressure to set an example for healthful eating in their communities. In Dallas, Parkland Health & Hospital Systems and Puente Enterprises have demonstrated the impact of commitment and collaboration.

MyPlate

Over the years there have been many guides to healthful eating. Since 1943, government guidance for healthful eating has evolved from the Basic 7, to the Basic 4, to the Food Guide Pyramid, to *MyPyramid* and now to *MyPlate*, which uses a familiar image – a place setting for a meal – to illustrate the five food groups that are the building blocks for a healthy diet.

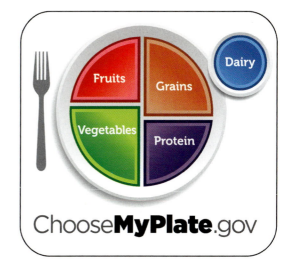

The new *MyPlate* icon emphasizes the proportions of fruit, vegetable, grains, protein and dairy food groups to be consumed daily. *MyPlate* supports the *Dietary Guidelines for Americans* with consumer-relevant themes and easy-to-understand, action-oriented messages, which focus on key behaviors including:

- Balancing Calories
  - Enjoy your food, but eat less.
  - Avoid oversized portions.
- Foods to Increase
  - Make half your plate fruits and vegetables.
  - Make at least half your grains whole grains.
  - Switch to fat-free or low-fat (1%) milk.
- Foods to Reduce
  - Compare sodium in foods like soup, bread and frozen meals and choose foods with lower numbers.
  - Drink water instead of sugary drinks.

MyPlate Portions

Fruit

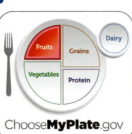

ChooseMyPlate.gov

What Is in the Fruit Group?

Any fruit or 100% fruit juice counts as part of the Fruit Group. Fruits may be fresh, canned, frozen or dried and may be whole, cut-up or pureed.

How Much Is Needed?

The amount of fruit needed depends on age, sex and level of physical activity. Amounts range from 1 to 2 cups.

What Counts as a Cup?

In general, 1 cup of fruit or 100% fruit juice, or ½ cup of dried fruit can be considered 1 cup from the Fruit Group. One small apple, orange, pear or banana also equals 1 cup.

Health Benefits of Fruit

- Eating a diet rich in fruit as part of an overall healthy diet may reduce risk for heart disease, including heart attack and stroke.

- Eating a diet rich in fruits as part of an overall healthy diet may protect against certain types of cancers.

- Diets rich in foods containing fiber, such as fruits, may reduce the risk of heart disease, obesity and type 2 diabetes.

- Eating fruits rich in potassium as part of an overall healthy diet may lower blood pressure, reduce the risk of developing kidney stones and help decrease bone loss.

- Eating foods such as fruits that are lower in calories per cup instead of higher-calorie foods may be useful in helping lower calorie intake.

Nutrients in Fruit

- Most fruits are naturally low in fat, sodium and calories. None contain cholesterol.

- Fruits contain essential nutrients that are lacking in the diets of many Americans, including potassium, dietary fiber, vitamin C and folate (folic acid).

- Diets rich in potassium may help maintain healthy blood pressure. Fruit sources of potassium include bananas, prunes and prune juice, dried peaches and apricots, cantaloupe, honeydew melon, and orange juice.

- Dietary fiber from fruits, as part of an overall healthy diet, helps reduce blood cholesterol levels and may lower risk of heart disease. Fiber is important for proper bowel function. It helps reduce constipation and diverticulosis. Fiber-containing foods such as fruits help provide a feeling of fullness with fewer calories. Whole or cut-up fruits are sources of dietary fiber; fruit juices contain little or no fiber.

- Vitamin C is important for growth and repair of all body tissues, helps heal cuts and wounds and keeps teeth and gums healthy.

- Folate (folic acid) helps the body form red blood cells. Women of childbearing age who may become pregnant should consume adequate folate from foods and in addition take folate supplements (often in the form of a prenatal vitamin) to reduce the risk of neural tube defects, spina bifida and anencephaly during fetal development.

Grains

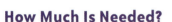

ChooseMyPlate.gov

What Is in the Grains Group?

Any food made from wheat, rice, oats, cornmeal, barley or other cereal grain is a grain product. Bread, pasta, oatmeal, breakfast cereals, tortillas and grits are examples of grain products.

Grains are divided into two subgroups: whole grains and refined grains. Whole grains contain the entire grain kernel — the bran, germ and endosperm. Examples include:

Brown rice	Whole cornmeal
Bulgur (cracked wheat)	Whole-grain breakfast cereal
Oatmeal	Whole-wheat flour

Refined grains have been milled, a process that removes the bran and germ to give grains a finer texture and improve shelf life. Refining also removes dietary fiber, iron and many B vitamins. Most refined grains are enriched, meaning certain B vitamins (thiamin, riboflavin and niacin) and iron are added back after processing. Fiber is not added back to enriched grains. Check the ingredient list on refined-grain products to make sure that the word "enriched" is included in the grain name. Some food products are made from mixtures of whole grains and refined grains. Examples of refined-grain products include:

Cornflakes (and other breakfast cereals)
De-germed cornmeal
White bread
White flour
White rice

How Much Is Needed?

The amount of grain needed depends on age, sex and level of physical activity. Amounts range from 3 to 8 ounce equivalents. Most Americans consume enough grains, but not enough whole grains. At least half of all the grains eaten should be whole grains.

What Counts as a 1 Ounce Equivalent?

In general, 1 slice of bread, ½ of a small sandwich bun or English muffin, 1 cup of ready-to-eat cereal, or ½ cup of cooked rice, cooked pasta, or cooked cereal or grain, or 1 small slice of pizza (crust is bread equivalent) can be considered a 1 ounce equivalent from the Grains Group. Many sandwich buns, rolls and pizza slices are quite large and can be 3 or 4 ounce equivalents.

Health Benefits of Whole Grains

- Consuming whole grains as part of a healthy diet may reduce the risk of heart disease.

- Consuming foods containing fiber, such as whole grains, as part of a healthy diet, may reduce constipation.

- Eating whole grains may help with weight management.

- Eating grain products fortified with folate before and during pregnancy helps prevent neural tube defects during fetal development.

Nutrients in Whole Grains

- Grains are important sources of many nutrients, including dietary fiber, several B vitamins (thiamin, riboflavin, niacin and folate) and minerals (iron, magnesium and selenium).

- Dietary fiber from whole grains or other foods may help reduce blood cholesterol levels and may lower risk of heart disease, obesity and type 2 diabetes. Fiber is important for proper bowel function; it helps reduce constipation and diverticulosis. Fiber-containing foods such as whole grains help provide a feeling of fullness with fewer calories.

- The B vitamins thiamin, riboflavin and niacin play a key role in metabolism, helping the body release energy from protein, fat and carbohydrates. B vitamins are also essential for a healthy nervous system. Many refined grains are enriched with B vitamins.

- Folate (folic acid) helps the body form red blood cells. Women of childbearing age who may become pregnant should consume adequate folate from foods and in addition take folate supplements (often in the form of a prenatal vitamin) to reduce the risk of neural tube defects, spina bifida and anencephaly during fetal development.

- Iron is used to carry oxygen in the blood. Many teenage girls and women in their childbearing years have iron-deficiency anemia and should eat foods high in heme-iron (meats) or other iron- containing foods along with foods rich in vitamin C, which can improve absorption of non-heme iron. Whole and enriched refined-grain products are major sources of non-heme iron in American diets.

- Whole grains contain magnesium and selenium. Magnesium is a mineral used in building bones and releasing energy from muscles. Selenium protects cells from oxidation and is important for a healthy immune system.

Vegetables

What Is in the Vegetable Group?

Any vegetable or 100% vegetable juice counts as a member of the Vegetable Group. Vegetables may be raw or cooked; fresh, frozen, canned or dried/dehydrated; and whole, cut-up or mashed.

Vegetables fall into five subgroups based on their nutrient content: dark green vegetables, orange vegetables, beans and peas, starchy vegetables, and other vegetables.

Dark Green Vegetables

Bok choy (and other Asian deep green leafy vegetables)

Broccoli

Collard greens

Dark green leafy lettuces

Kale

Mesclun

Mustard greens

Romaine lettuce

Spinach

Turnip greens

Watercress

Orange Vegetables

Acorn squash

Butternut squash

Carrots

Hubbard squash

Pumpkin

Red and orange peppers

Sweet potatoes

Tomatoes

Tomato juice

Beans and Peas

Black beans

Black-eyed peas

Garbanzo beans (chickpeas)

Kidney beans

Lentils

Lima beans (dried, white)

Navy beans

Pinto beans

Soybeans

Split peas

White beans

Starchy Vegetables

Cassava

Corn

Green bananas

Green peas

Lima beans (green)

Potatoes

Taro

Water chestnuts

Other Vegetables

Artichokes

Asparagus

Avocado

Bean sprouts

Beets

Brussels sprouts

Cabbage

Cauliflower

Celery

Cucumbers

Eggplant

Green beans

Green peppers

Iceberg (head) lettuce

Leeks

Mushrooms

Okra

Onions

Parsnips

Peapods

Rutabagas

Sugar snap peas

Summer squash

Turnips

Wax beans

Zucchini

ChooseMyPlate.gov

How Much Is Needed?

The amount of vegetables needed depends on age, sex and level of physical activity. Amounts range from 1 to 3 cups daily. Most adults should have 3 cups of vegetables every day. While potatoes count as a starchy vegetable and have some nutrients, deep green and orange vegetables have far more nutrients and fewer calories, especially when compared to fried potatoes.

What Counts as a Cup?

In general, 1 cup of raw or cooked vegetables or vegetable juice, or 2 cups of raw leafy greens can be considered 1 cup from the Vegetable Group.

Health Benefits of Vegetables

- Eating a diet rich in vegetables as part of an overall healthy diet may reduce risk for heart disease, including heart attack and stroke.

- Eating a diet rich in certain vegetables as part of an overall healthy diet may protect against colon and other types of cancers.

- Diets rich in foods containing fiber, such as some vegetables, may reduce the risk of heart disease, obesity and type 2 diabetes.

- Eating vegetables rich in potassium as part of an overall healthy diet may lower blood pressure, reduce the risk of developing kidney stones and help to decrease bone loss.

- Eating foods such as vegetables that are lower in calories per cup instead of some other higher-calorie food may be useful in helping lower calorie intake.

Nutrients in Vegetables

- Most vegetables are naturally low in fat and calories. None contain cholesterol. (Sauces, butter or oils used in cooking, however, add fat, calories and/or cholesterol.)

- Vegetables are important sources of many nutrients, including potassium, dietary fiber, folate (folic acid), vitamin A and vitamin C.

- Diets rich in potassium may help to maintain healthy blood pressure. Vegetable sources of potassium include sweet potatoes, white potatoes, white beans, tomato products (paste, sauce and juice), beet greens, soybeans, lima beans, spinach, lentils and kidney beans.

- Dietary fiber from vegetables, as part of an overall healthy diet, helps reduce blood cholesterol levels and may lower risk of heart disease. Fiber is important for proper bowel function. It helps reduce constipation and diverticulosis. Fiber-containing foods such as vegetables help provide a feeling of fullness with fewer calories.

- Folate (folic acid) helps the body form red blood cells. Women of childbearing age who may become pregnant should consume adequate folate from foods and in addition take folate supplements (often in the form of a prenatal vitamin) to reduce the risk of neural tube defects, spina bifida and anencephaly during fetal development.

- Vitamin A keeps eyes and skin healthy and helps to protect against infections.

- Vitamin C is important for growth and repair of all body tissues, helps heal cuts and wounds, and keeps teeth and gums healthy.

More about Beans and Peas

Beans and peas are the mature forms of legumes. They include kidney beans, pinto beans, black beans, lima beans, black-eyed peas, garbanzo beans (chickpeas), split peas and lentils. Available in dry, canned, refrigerated and frozen forms, beans and peas are excellent sources of plant protein and provide other nutrients such as iron and zinc. Because they are similar to meats, poultry and fish in their nutrient composition, they are considered part of the Protein Foods Group. Many people use beans and peas as vegetarian alternatives for meat. They are also considered part of the Vegetable Group because they are excellent sources of dietary fiber and nutrients such as folate and potassium, which are often low in the diet of many Americans.

Green peas, green lima beans, wax beans, peapods and green (string) beans are not considered part of the beans and peas subgroup. Green peas and green lima beans are grouped with other starchy vegetables. Green beans, wax beans and peapods are grouped with other vegetables such as onions, lettuce, celery and cabbage.

Protein Foods

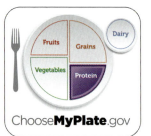

ChooseMyPlate.gov

What Is in the Protein Foods Group?

All foods that come from meat, poultry, seafood, beans and peas, eggs, processed soy products, and nuts and seeds are considered part of the Protein Foods Group. Beans and peas are also part of the Vegetable Group. Select a variety of protein foods to improve nutrient intake and health benefits, including at least 8 ounces of cooked seafood per week. Young children need less, depending on their age and calorie needs. The advice to consume seafood does not apply to vegetarians. Vegetarian options in the Protein Foods Group include beans and peas, processed soy products, and nuts and seeds. Meat and poultry choices should be lean or low-fat. Some commonly eaten choices in the meat and beans group are:

Lean cuts of
Beef
Ham
Lamb
Pork
Veal

Game meats
Bison
Buffalo
Rabbit
Venison

Lean ground meats
Beef
Pork
Lamb

Organ meats
Liver
Giblets

Poultry
Chicken
Duck
Goose
Turkey
Ground chicken and turkey

Eggs (chicken and duck)

Beans and peas
Black beans
Black-eyed peas
Chickpeas (garbanzo beans)
Falafel
Kidney beans
Lentils
Lima beans (mature)
Navy beans
Pinto beans
Soybeans
Split peas
Tofu (and other soy products)
White beans

Bean burgers (garden or veggie burgers)

Tempeh

Texturized vegetable protein (TVP)

Nuts and seeds
Almonds
Cashews
Hazelnuts (filberts)
Mixed nuts
Peanuts
Peanut butter
Pecans
Pistachios
Pumpkin seeds
Sesame seeds
Sunflower seeds
Walnuts

Fish
Finfish
Catfish
Cod
Flounder
Haddock
Halibut
Herring
Mackerel
Orange roughy
Pollock
Porgy
Salmon
Sea bass
Snapper
Swordfish
Tilapia
Trout
Tuna

Shellfish
Clams
Crab
Crayfish
Lobster
Mussels
Octopus
Oysters
Scallops
Squid (calamari)
Shrimp

Canned fish
Anchovies
Clams
Mackerel
Sardines
Salmon
Tuna

How Much Is Needed?

The amount of food from the Protein Foods Group needed depends on age, sex and level of physical activity. Most Americans eat more than enough food from this group but need to make leaner and more varied selections. Needs range from 2 to 6½ ounce equivalents per day depending on age.

What Counts as a 1 Ounce Equivalent?

In general, 1 ounce of cooked meat, poultry or fish, ¼ cup cooked beans, 1 egg, 1 tablespoon of peanut butter, or ½ ounce of nuts or seeds can be considered a 1 ounce equivalent from the Protein Foods Group.

Health Benefits of Protein Foods

- Meat, poultry, fish, beans and peas, eggs, and nuts and seeds supply protein, B vitamins (niacin, thiamin, riboflavin, and B_6), vitamin E, iron, zinc and magnesium.

- Proteins function as building blocks for bones, muscles, cartilage, skin, blood, enzymes, hormones and vitamins. Proteins are one of three nutrients that provide calories (the others are fat and carbohydrates).

- B vitamins help the body release energy, play a vital role in the function of the nervous system, aid in the formation of red blood cells and help build tissues.

- Iron is used to carry oxygen in the blood. Teenage girls and women in their childbearing years who have iron-deficiency anemia should eat foods high in heme-iron (meats) or eat other iron-containing foods along with a food rich in vitamin C, which can improve absorption of non-heme iron.

- Magnesium helps build bones and release energy from muscles.

- Zinc is necessary for biochemical reactions and helps the immune system function properly.

- Docosahexaenoic acid (DHA) and eicosapentaenoic acid (EPA) are omega-3 fatty acids found in seafood. Eating 8 ounces per week of seafood may help reduce the risk for heart disease.

Nutrients in Protein Foods

- Diets that are high in saturated fats raise "bad" cholesterol – LDL (low-density lipoprotein) – levels in the blood, which increases the risk for coronary heart disease. Some food choices in this group are high in saturated fat, including fatty cuts of beef, pork and lamb; regular (75% to 85% lean) ground beef; regular sausages, hot dogs and bacon; some luncheon meats, such as regular bologna and salami; and some poultry, such as duck.

- Diets that are high in cholesterol can raise LDL cholesterol levels in the blood. Cholesterol is found only in foods from animal sources. Foods especially high in cholesterol include egg yolks (egg whites are cholesterol-free) and organ meats such as liver and giblets. To help keep blood cholesterol levels healthy, limit the amount of these foods. Generally, one whole egg or egg yolk per day does not raise cholesterol, but eating a three-egg omelet every day may.

- Including a large amount of dietary fat from meats and other sources in the diet makes it difficult to avoid consuming more calories than are needed.

Benefits of Eating 8 Ounces of Seafood per Week

- Seafood contains a range of nutrients, including the omega-3 fatty acids EPA and DHA. Eating about 8 ounces per week of a variety of seafood contributes to the prevention of heart disease. Smaller amounts of seafood are recommended for young children.

- The health benefits of seafood outweigh the health risk associated with consuming small amounts of mercury, a heavy metal found in seafood in varying levels.

- The seafood varieties commonly consumed in the United States that are higher in EPA and DHA and lower in mercury include salmon, anchovies, herring, sardines, Pacific oysters, trout, and Atlantic and Pacific mackerel (but not king mackerel, which is high in mercury).

Benefits of Eating Nuts and Seeds

- Eating peanuts and certain tree nuts (such as walnuts, almonds and pistachios) may reduce the risk of heart disease when consumed as part of a diet that is nutritionally adequate and within calorie needs. Nuts and seeds are high in calories and should be consumed in small portions. They can replace other protein foods in the diet, such as meat or poultry. Unsalted nuts and seeds help reduce sodium intake.

Dairy

What Is in the Dairy Group?

All fluid milk products and many foods made from milk are considered part of this food group. Most Dairy Group choices should be fat-free or low-fat. Foods made from milk that retain their calcium content are part of this group; foods made from milk that have little to no calcium, such as cream cheese, cream and butter, are not. Calcium-fortified soymilk (soy beverage) is part of the Dairy Group, which also includes:

All fluid milk

Fat-free (skim)

Low-fat (1%)

Reduced-fat (2%)

Whole milk

Buttermilk

Flavored milks

Chocolate

Strawberry

Kefir

Lactose-reduced or lactose-free milks

Milk-based desserts

Puddings made with milk

Ice milk

Frozen yogurt

Ice cream

Hard natural cheese, such as:

Cheddar

Mozzarella

Swiss

Parmesan

Soft cheeses, such as:

Ricotta

Cottage cheese

All yogurts

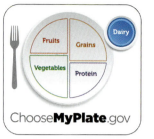

ChooseMyPlate.gov

How Much Is Needed?

The amount of food needed from the Dairy Group depends on age. Amounts range from 2 to 3 cups of liquid milk per day.

What Counts as a Cup?

In general, 1 cup of milk, yogurt or soymilk (soy beverage), 1 ½ ounces of natural cheese, 2 ounces of processed cheese, ½ cup ricotta cheese, 2 cups cottage cheese, 1 cup pudding made from milk or 1 cup frozen yogurt can be considered 1 cup from the Dairy Group.

Health Benefits of Dairy Foods

- Dairy products are linked to improved bone health and may reduce the risk of osteoporosis.

- Dairy products are especially important to bone health during childhood and adolescence, when bone mass is being built.

- Dairy products are associated with a reduced risk of cardiovascular disease and type 2 diabetes and with lower blood pressure in adults.

Nutrients in Dairy Products

- Calcium is used for building bones and teeth and maintaining bone mass. Dairy products are the primary source of calcium in American diets. Diets that provide 3 cups or the equivalent of dairy products per day may improve bone mass.

- Diets rich in potassium help to maintain healthy blood pressure. Dairy products, especially yogurt, fluid milk and soymilk (soy beverage), provide potassium.

- Vitamin D helps the body maintain proper levels of calcium and phosphorous needed to build and maintain bones. Milk and soymilk (soy beverage) that are fortified with vitamin D are good sources of this nutrient. Other sources include vitamin D-fortified yogurt and vitamin D-fortified ready-to-eat breakfast cereals.

- Many cheeses, whole milk and products made from them are high in saturated fat. Diets high in saturated fat raise LDL (low-density lipoprotein) or "bad" cholesterol levels in the blood. High LDL cholesterol increases the risk for coronary heart disease. Read labels and choose lower-fat cheeses and other dairy products most of the time.

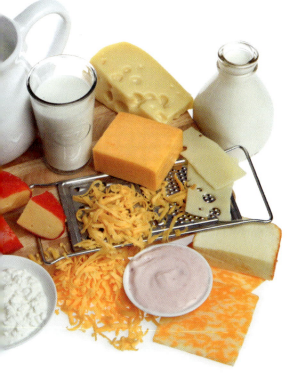

Oils

Although oils are not a food group, they do provide essential nutrients and thus are included in USDA's food patterns. *Oils* are fats that are liquid at room temperature – for example, the vegetable oils used in cooking. Oils come from many different plants and also from fish. Some commonly eaten oils include:

Canola oil

Corn oil

Cottonseed oil

Olive oil

Safflower oil

Soybean oil

Sunflower oil

Some oils are used mainly as flavorings, such as walnut oil and sesame oil. Foods naturally high in oils include:

Nuts

Olives

Some fish

Avocados

A person's allowance for oils depends on age, sex and level of physical activity. Amounts range from 3 to 7 teaspoons per day; most Americans eat more than that. This total includes all oils used in cooking, in salad dressings and in prepared foods.

Chefs will surely notice that certain foods such as cream, butter, bacon, processed meats, charcuterie, sugar, sweetened beverages, most baked desserts, jams, and other foods and ingredients are not found on *MyPlate*. The *Dietary Guidelines for Americans 2010* recommend limiting these foods and substituting more healthful options. The authors of this book take a more liberal approach and recommend using high-fat, high-saturated fat and high-sugar foods ingredients sparingly and only as necessary to make delicious food and serving small to moderate portions of foods containing such ingredients.

Daily Amounts of Food from Each Group in *MyPlate*

These amounts are appropriate for individuals who get less than 30 minutes per day of moderate physical activity, beyond normal daily activities. Those who are more physically active may be able to consume more while staying within calorie needs.

	Age	Fruit	Vegetable	Grains	Protein Food	Dairy	Oils Allowance
Children	2-3 years	1 cup	1 cup	3 ounce equivalents	2 ounce equivalents	2 cups	3 teaspoons
	4-8 years	1-1 ½ cups	1½ cups	5 ounce equivalents	4 ounce equivalents	2 ½ cups	4 teaspoons
Girls	9-13 years	1 ½ cups	2 cups	5 ounce equivalents	5 ounce equivalents	3 cups	5 teaspoons
	14-18 years	1 ½ cups	2½ cups	6 ounce equivalents	5 ounce equivalents	3 cups	5 teaspoons
Boys	9-13 years	1 ½ cups	2½ cups	6 ounce equivalents	5 ounce equivalents	3 cups	5 teaspoons
	14-18 years	2 cups	3 cups	8 ounce equivalents	6 ½ ounce equivalents	3 cups	6 teaspoons
Women	19-30 years	2 cups	2½ cups	6 ounce equivalents	5 ½ ounce equivalents	3 cups	6 teaspoons
	31-50 years	1 ½ cups	2½ cups	6 ounce equivalents	5 ounce equivalents	3 cups	5 teaspoons
	51+ years	1 ½ cups	2 cups	5 ounce equivalents	5 ounce equivalents	3 cups	5 teaspoons
Men	19-30 years	2 cups	3 cups	8 ounce equivalents	6 ½ ounce equivalents	3 cups	7 teaspoons
	31-50 years	2 cups	3 cups	7 ounce equivalents	6 ounce equivalents	3 cups	6 teaspoons
	51+ years	2 cups	2½ cups	6 ounce equivalents	5 ½ ounce equivalents	3 cups	6 teaspoons

Healthy Eating Plate (an alternative view)

Nutrition experts at the Harvard School of Public Health (HSPH) have developed the Healthy Eating Plate, a visual guide similar to *MyPlate*. At first glance, the HSPH plate looks like *MyPlate*. It recommends that half the plate contain vegetables and fruits and that whole grains be included in the diet. In addition, however, it stresses heart-healthy oils and specific protein sources and significantly limits potatoes, fruit juices, red meat, refined grains, butter, milk and dairy products and advises avoidance of processed meats, trans fats and sugary drinks. The intent of both plates is similar, but the HSPH plate is a more aggressive plan for disease prevention and recommends more dietary restrictions.

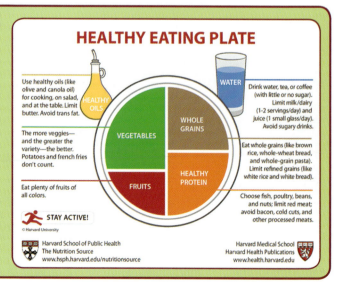

Food Pyramids

As mentioned previously, *MyPlate* was preceded by *MyPyramid*. Various groups developed alternative pyramids to reflect special needs. The Mediterranean Diet Pyramid illustrated the healthy traditional food and dietary patterns of the Mediterranean region. Other globally influenced dietary pyramids include the Latin American and the Asian Diet pyramids, which represent the traditional food models of populations with historically low incidences of chronic, diet-related diseases. Pyramids also have been developed for children and other age groups and for specific health concerns. Oldways Preservation Trust developed a series of Heritage Pyramids that can be viewed at oldwayspt.org/resources/ heritage-pyramids.

Food Labels

Although fresh ingredients used in preparing menu items in foodservice do not carry a package label, processed and packaged products are required to have a label with useful information. All food labels must include the common or usual name of the product; the name and address of the manufacturer, packer or distributor; net contents in weight, measure or count; the Nutrition Facts panel; and the ingredients listed in descending order of predominance by weight. The label also might feature health claims, allergy warnings, nutrient claims, organic designation and/or country of origin.

Nutrition Facts Panel

The **Nutrition Facts panel** is required on most packaged foods. A simplified format can be used when a food contains insignificant amounts of seven or more of the mandatory nutrients and total calories. Foods with a small label area may also use a simplified format. Baby foods have a simplified format because there are no Daily Values for infants.

The **Nutrition Labeling and Education Act of 1990** (NLEA: Public Law 101-535) created the nutrition label and initiated education to help consumers use the label to make better food choices. The list required on the Nutrition Facts panel focuses on the nutrients and food components of greatest public

health concern as determined by the *Dietary Guidelines for Americans*. There have been some changes in the food labeling law over time, such as the addition of information on trans fats, sugars and labeling for common allergens. USDA is currently revising regulations for nutrition information on food labels. Until then, we will see the following Nutrition Panel:

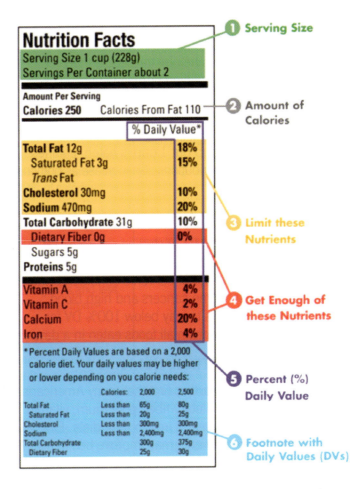

Source: http://www.fda.gov/Food/ResourcesForYou/Consumers/ucm079449.htm

1. Serving Size

Serving sizes are given in familiar units, such as cups or pieces, followed by weight in grams. The serving size listed on the label, however, is not necessarily the portion size consumed. A **portion** is how much food is actually eaten at one time, whether in a restaurant, on the go from a package, or at home. A serving size is the amount of food listed on a product's Nutrition Facts panel.

Sometimes the portion size and serving size match, but often they do not. The serving size is not a

Other Nutrient-Content Claims

Claims such as "lean ground beef," "excellent source of vitamin C," "extra fiber" or "contains antioxidants" relate to the nutrient content of foods.

Claim	Requirement
High, rich in or excellent source of	Contains 20% or more of the Daily Value
Good source, contains or provides	10% – 19% of the Daily Value
More, fortified, enriched, added, extra or plus	10% or more of the Daily Value; used for vitamins, minerals, protein, dietary fiber and potassium
Lean	On meat, poultry and fish products that contain less than 10 grams total fat, 4.5 grams or less saturated fat and less than 95 milligrams cholesterol per serving
Extra lean	On meat, poultry, and fish products that contain less than 5 grams total fat, less than 2 grams saturated fat and less than 95 milligrams cholesterol per serving
Contains antioxidant(s)	• A Recommended Dietary Intake (RDI) must be established for each of the nutrients that are the subject of the claim. • Each nutrient must have existing scientific evidence of antioxidant activity. • The level of each nutrient must be sufficient to meet the definition for "high," "good source" or "more." • Beta-carotene may be the subject of an antioxidant claim when the level of vitamin A present as beta-carotene in the food is sufficient to qualify for the claim.

Health Claims

Health claims describe a relationship between a food, food component or dietary supplement ingredient and reducing the risk of a disease or health-related condition. The Food and Drug Administration (FDA) approves health claims, which must be supported by significant scientific evidence and undergo a lengthy approval process. Claims change from time to time as scientific consensus validates the relationship of a substance in food to its effect on health. In addition, wording varies on different products.

FDA currently permits ***qualified health claims***, each of which is considered on an individual basis. These claims do not meet the "significant scientific" standard. Rather, they are based on emerging, but not conclusive, evidence for a relationship between a food, food component or dietary supplement and reduced risk of disease or health-related condition. These claims require a disclaimer, such as "scientific evidence suggests but does not prove that . . . ."

For example, a qualified health claim might say, "Green tea may reduce your risk of cancer*." The disclaimer might say, "*Very limited and preliminary scientific research suggests green tea reduces risk of cancer. The FDA concludes that there is little scientific evidence supporting this claim."

Health Claims Report Card

The following four-tiered ranking system is used to categorize the quality and strength of scientific evidence for qualified health claims.

Grade	Level of Confidence in Health Claim	Label Disclaimers Required by the FDA
A	High: significant scientific agreement	The health claims do not require disclaimers.
B	Moderate: evidence not entirely conclusive	"Although there is scientific evidence supporting this claim, the evidence is not conclusive."
C	Low: evidence limited and inconclusive	"Some scientific evidence suggests [health claim]. However, the FDA has determined that this evidence is limited and not conclusive."
D	Extremely low: little scientific evidence	"Very limited and preliminary scientific research suggests [health claim]. The FDA concludes that there is little scientific evidence supporting this claim."

Health claims based on authoritative statements allow certain health claims to be used on foods based on an authoritative statement from a scientific body of the government or the National Academy of Sciences. **Structure/function claims** may be used without FDA permission. Claims such as "fiber maintains bowel regularity" or "calcium builds strong bones" are examples of this type of claim.

FDA has approved 12 health claims and four health claims based on authoritative statements for use on food labels. Each claim must meet specific guidelines for amount of the specific nutrient mentioned. Additional claims are being evaluated. (www.fda. gov/Food/LabelingNutrition/LabelClaims/default.htm)

Health Claims Supported by Science and Generally Accepted by Health Experts

Approved Claims	Requirements for Food	Model Claim/Statement
Calcium and osteoporosis	High in calcium	Regular exercise and a healthy diet with enough calcium help teens and young adult white and Asian women maintain good bone health and may reduce their high risk of osteoporosis later in life.
Sodium and hypertension	Low sodium	Diets low in sodium may reduce the risk of high blood pressure, a disease associated with many factors.
Dietary fat and cancer	Low fat or extra lean	Development of cancer depends on many factors. A diet low in total fat may reduce the risk of some cancers.
Dietary saturated fat and cholesterol and risk of coronary heart disease	Low fat or extra lean, low saturated fat, and low cholesterol	While many factors affect heart disease, diets low in saturated fat and cholesterol may reduce the risk of this disease.
Fiber-containing grain products, fruits, and vegetables and cancer	Grain product, fruit or vegetable that contains dietary fiber; low fat and good source of dietary fiber (without fortification)	Low fat diets rich in fiber-containing grain products, fruits, and vegetables may reduce the risk of some types of cancer, a disease associated with many factors.

Approved Claims	Requirements for Food	Model Claim/Statement
Fruits, vegetables and grain products that contain fiber, particularly soluble fiber, and risk of coronary heart disease	Fruit, vegetable or grain product that contains fiber; low fat, low saturated fat, low cholesterol	Diets low in saturated fat and cholesterol and rich in fruits, vegetables, and grain products that contain some types of dietary fiber, particularly soluble fiber, may reduce the risk of heart disease, a disease associated with many factors.
Fruits and vegetables and cancer	Fruit or vegetable that is low fat and a good source (without fortification) of at least one of the following: vitamin A or C or dietary fiber	Low fat diets rich in fruits and vegetables (foods that are low in fat and may contain dietary fiber, vitamin A or vitamin C) may reduce the risk of some types of cancer, a disease associated with many factors. Broccoli is high in vitamin A and C, and it is a good source of dietary fiber.
Folate and neural tube defects	At least 40 micrograms of folate per serving	Healthful diets with adequate folate may reduce a woman's risk of having a child with a brain or spinal cord defect.
Dietary non-carcinogenic carbohydrate sweeteners and dental caries	Sugar free	Frequent between-meal consumption of foods high in sugars and starches promotes tooth decay. The sugar alcohols in [name food] do not promote tooth decay.
Soluble fiber from certain foods and risk of coronary heart disease	Low saturated fat and cholesterol; must contain one of more of following: oat bran, rolled oats, whole oat flour, whole-grain barley or dried millet barley	Soluble fiber from foods such as [name of soluble fiber source and, if desired, name of food product], as part of a diet low in saturated fat and cholesterol, may reduce the risk of heart disease. A serving of [name food] supplies __ grams of the [necessary daily dietary intake for the benefit] soluble flour from [name of soluble fiber source] necessary per day to have the effect.
Soy protein and risk of coronary heart disease	At least 6.25 grams of soy protein per serving; low fat, saturated fat and cholesterol	• 25 grams of soy protein a day, as part of a diet low in saturated fat and cholesterol, may reduce the risk of heart disease. A serving of [name food] supplies __ grams of soy protein. • Diets low in saturated fat and cholesterol that include 25 grams of soy protein a day may reduce the risk of heart disease. One serving of [name food] provides __ grams of soy protein.

Approved Claims	Requirements for Food	Model Claim/Statement
Plant sterol/stanol esters and risk of coronary heart disease	At least 0.65 gram of plant sterol esters per serving of spread and salad dressings; at least 1.7 grams of plant stanol esters per serving of salad dressings, snack bars and dietary supplements; low saturated fat and cholesterol	• Foods containing at least 0.65 gram of vegetable oil sterile esters, eaten twice a day with meals for a daily total intake of at least 1.3 grams, as part of a diet low in saturated fat and cholesterol, may reduce the risk of heart disease. A serving of [name food] supplies __ grams of vegetable oil sterol esters. • Diets low in saturated fat and cholesterol that include two servings of foods that provide a daily total of at least 3.4 grams of plant stanol esters in two meals may reduce the risk of heart disease. A serving of [name food] supplies __ grams of plant stanol esters.
Whole-grain foods and risk of heart disease and certain cancers (based on authoritative claims)	51% or more whole-grain ingredients by weight per serving; low fat; dietary fiber	Diets rich in whole grain foods and other plant foods and low in total fat, saturated fat, and cholesterol, may reduce the risk of heart disease and some cancers.
Potassium and the risk of high blood pressure and stroke (based on authoritative claims)	Good source of potassium; low sodium, total fat, saturated fat and cholesterol	Diets containing foods that are a good source of potassium and that are low in sodium may reduce the risk of high blood pressure and stroke
Fluoridated water and reduced risk of dental carries (based on authoritative claims)	Bottled water meeting all general requirements for health claims with the exception of minimum nutrient contribution; fluoride	Drinking fluoridated water may reduce the risk of dental caries or tooth decay.
Saturated fat, cholesterol and trans fat, and reduced risk of heart disease (based on authoritative claims)	Low saturated fat and cholesterol; quantitative trans fat labeling; limits on trans fat and total fat	Diets low in saturated fat and cholesterol, and as low as possible in trans fat, may reduce the risk of heart disease

Labeling Exemptions

The following foods are currently exempt from label requirements:

- Packages with less than 12 square inches for labeling (must have address or phone number, but not full labeling)

- Foods produced by small businesses – for example, businesses with food sales of less than $50,000/year and businesses with fewer than 100 full-time equivalent employees that have sales of fewer than 100,00 units annually

- Restaurant food, unless a health claim is made

- Food served for immediate consumption (vending machines, hospital cafeterias, airplanes, shopping malls and sidewalk vendors)

- Ready-to-eat food that is not for immediate consumption but is prepared primarily on site (bakery, deli and candy store items)

- Foods shipped in bulk but not for sale in that form to consumers

- Medical foods

- Plain tea, coffee, spices and foods with no significant amount of any nutrient

- Nutrient supplements, herbs and related products

What Puts the 'Whole' in Whole-Wheat Bread?

Bread with whole-wheat flour first on the ingredients list contains more whole-wheat flour than any other flour or ingredient. If flour or enriched flour is listed first, and whole-wheat flour is second or lower, the bread is not whole-wheat bread. Recently white whole-wheat flour has come to market. Although it grinds to a white-colored flour, it does contain the whole grain.

Ingredient List

A food label must include a list of ingredients in descending order by weight. The ingredient that weighs the most is listed first, and the ingredient that weighs the least is listed last. Ingredients are always listed by their common or usual name – for example, sugar versus sucrose. The ingredient list also includes, when appropriate, identification of Food and Drug Administration-certified food additives, sources of protein hydrolysates used as flavors or enhancers, a declaration that casein is a milk derivative and the total percentage of juice in juice beverages.

Allergen Labeling

The *Food Allergen Labeling and Consumer Protection Act (FALCPA) of 2004* is an amendment to the Federal Food, Drug, and Cosmetic Act. It requires that the label of a food that contains an ingredient that is or contains protein from a major food allergen declare the presence of that allergen. This act was passed to make it easier for people with food allergies to identify and avoid the eight major food allergens that account for 90% of food allergic reactions and are the sources from which many other ingredients are derived. The eight foods identified by the law are:

- Milk
- Eggs
- Fish (e.g., bass, flounder, cod)
- Crustacean shellfish (e.g., crab, lobster, shrimp)
- Tree nuts (e.g., almonds, walnuts, pecans)
- Peanuts
- Wheat
- Soybeans

Ingredients Most Likely to Be of Concern to Customers

Vegetable sources of saturated fat

Coconut oil, palm kernel oil, palm oil, coconut oil, some hydrogenated oils, vegetable shortenings, margarines and sources of trans fatty acids

Animal sources of saturated fat

Lard, beef fat, bacon fat, salt pork, butterfat, milk-fat, cheese, cream cheese, dried or frozen liquid whole eggs, and egg yolks (not egg whites)

Primary sources of sweeteners

Glucose (glucose, dextrose, corn syrup); fructose (fructose, fruit sugar, fructose corn syrup, levulose); honey (honey, raw honey, unpasteurized honey, invert sugar, invert sugar syrup, tupelo honey); maltose (maltose, malted syrup, maltodextrin, dextrins); sorghum (sorghum molasses, grain sorghum syrup); lactose (milk sugar, whey); sugar alcohols (sorbitol, manitol, xylitol).

Primary sources of sodium

Sodium chloride (salt), monosodium glutamate (MSG), calcium disodium phosphate, EDTA, whey, dried buttermilk powder, cheeses, Dutch-processed cocoa, soy sauce, baking powder, baking soda, Worcestershire sauce, barbecue sauce, pickles and pickled foods,

Potential allergens

Milk, eggs, fish, shellfish, peanuts, tree nuts, wheat and soy in all forms, tartrazine and other artificial colors, monosodium glutamate (MSG), sulfites, casein, and nitrites.

FALCPA has designated these eight foods and any ingredient that contains protein derived from one or more of them as major food allergens. Even small amounts of these foods – as whole foods, ingredients or contaminants – can be dangerous to a person with a food allergy. (For more on food allergies see Chapter 13.)

The law requires that food labels identify source names of all major food allergens used to make the product. This requirement is met if the common or usual name of an ingredient (e.g., buttermilk) already identifies the name of the allergen's food source – in this case, milk. Otherwise, the allergen's food source name must be declared at least once on the food label in one of two ways.

- In parentheses following the name of the ingredient.

  Examples: "lecithin (soy)," "flour (wheat)" and "whey (milk)"

- Immediately after or next to the list of ingredients in a "contains" statement. Example: "contains wheat, milk and soy"

Organic and Natural Labeling

USDA's **National Organic Program** (NOP) (www.ams.usda.gov/nop) regulates standards for any farm, wild crop harvesting or handling operation that wants to sell an agricultural product as organically produced. NOP also accredits certifying agents (foreign and domestic) who inspect organic production and handling operations to ensure that they meet USDA standards.

The **Organic Foods Production Act**, which was included in the 1990 Farm Bill, and the National Organic Program assure consumers that the organic agricultural products they purchase are produced, processed and certified to consistent national organic standards. Except for operations whose gross income from organic sales totals $5,000 or less, farm and processing operations that grow and process organic agricultural products must be certified by USDA-accredited certifying agents.

Organic is a labeling term that indicates that the food or other agricultural product has been produced through approved methods that integrate cultural, biological and mechanical practices that foster cycling of resources, promote ecological balance and conserve biodiversity. The USDA organic seal verifies:

- **In crops:** Irradiation, sewage sludge, synthetic fertilizers, prohibited pesticides and genetically modified organisms were not used.

- **In livestock:** Producers met animal health and welfare standards, did not use antibiotics or growth hormones, used 100% organic feed, and provided animals with access to the outdoors.

- **In multi-food ingredients:** The product has 95% or more certified organic content.

Organic labeling requirements apply to raw, fresh and processed products that contain organic agricultural ingredients. Labeling requirements are based on the percentage of organic ingredients in a product.

- Products labeled **100% organic** must contain only organically produced ingredients and processing aids (excluding water and salt). The USDA Organic Seal may be used on the product package.

- Products labeled **organic** must consist of at least 95% organically produced ingredients (excluding water and salt). Any remaining product ingredients must consist of nonagricultural substances approved on the national list including specific non-organically produced agricultural products that are not commercially available in organic form. The USDA Organic Seal may be used on the product package.

- Processed products that contain at least 70% organic ingredients can use the phrase **made with organic ingredients** and list up to three of the organic ingredients or food groups on the principal display panel. For example, soup made with at least 70% organic ingredients and only organic vegetables may be labeled either "soup made with organic peas, potatoes and carrots" or "soup made with organic vegetables." The USDA Organic Seal may not be used on the product package.

- Processed products that contain less than 70% organic ingredients cannot use the term organic anywhere on the principal display panel; however, they may identify the specific ingredients that are organically produced on the ingredients statement on the information panel.

USDA has defined *natural* for meat and poultry only. Meat and poultry products that contain no artificial ingredients or added color and that are minimally processed (the raw product not fundamentally altered) may be labeled natural. The label must explain the use of the term natural – for example, "no added colorings or artificial ingredients" or "minimally processed."

For all other food products and processed products, there is no legal definition of the term natural. It is left to the producer or manufacturer to create its own definition. The term often suggests that a food is healthful, but it may not be. Many fried, sweet and salty snacks are marketed as natural.

When purchasing food and ingredients, remember that the "organic" label is not an indicator of a food being more nutritious – it simply signifies a type of food production. The current body of research shows no significant difference in the nutritional content or safety between organic and conventionally produced foods.

Front-of-Package (FOP) Nutrition Labeling

In response to public interest in identifying healthier foods, some manufacturers have voluntarily added nutrition information and ratings to the front of food packages. The large number of different FOP approaches and messages, however, confuses consumers and is ultimately counterproductive. FOP labeling systems are linked to differing sets of nutritional criteria developed by a manufacturers, supermarket chain, trade organization or health organization. Many FOP programs are regional or specific to a particular chain of stores.

Some manufacturers that make high-fat products use labels to promote low sugar content, while some manufacturers of high-sugar products promote

them as being fat-free – but neither type of product is a truly healthful choice. In addition to confusing consumers, this selective FOP labeling may give an impression of healthfulness that can encourage overconsumption of products whose nutritional quality is mediocre at best.

In addition, FDA has found when a product has FOP or shelf labeling, consumers are less likely to check the more complete Nutrition Facts panel on the back or side of the package. FDA is on the lookout for FOP labels that appear to be misleading and for symbols that imply nutrient content claims.

The Institute of Medicine (IOM) along with the Centers for Disease Control and Prevention, the FDA, and USDA's Center for Nutrition Policy and Promotion formed a committee to study and report on FOP labeling. The committee concluded that it is time to move to one system "that encourages healthful food choice through simplicity, visual clarity and the ability to convey meaning without written information." [1]

The IOM committee recommended that FDA and USDA develop a standard FOP system for use on all food products. Suggested characteristics include:

- Calories in common household measure serving sizes
- A symbol system that shows saturated and trans fats, sodium and added sugars
- Information integrated with the Nutrition Facts panel so that they reinforce each other
- Similar labeling on all grocery products to allow consumers to compare food products across and within food categories

FDA is developing a proposed regulation to develop standardized, science-based nutrition criteria that must be met by manufacturers making broad FOP or shelf-label nutrition claims in text or via symbols. [2]

Various Front-of-Package Label Systems Currently Used

- **Symbols that broadly suggest that a food is "healthy," "good for you" or "a better choice."** The American Heart Association's Heart-Check Mark is an example.

- **Shelf-label symbols used by supermarkets that give foods a "grade."** Examples include Guiding Stars (the more stars, the "healthier" the food) and NuVal, which gives a numerical score based on several factors associated with the food.

- **Symbols that provide both specific nutrition information and gradations about positive or negative nutrient levels.** The British voluntary "traffic light" system is an example. Great Britain has neither mandatory nutrition labeling nor a mandatory format for nutrition labeling; however, if a claim is made, nutrition labeling is required.

- **Federal dietary guidance symbols that are intended to provide advice on how to construct a healthy diet.** The presence of logos such as *MyPlate* is not determined by the specific nutrient profile of a food. Questions have been raised about whether or not using such a logo implies that a food has healthy attributes, even if the total fat, saturated fat content, cholesterol and/or sodium content are high.

- **Symbols that list key nutrients found in the food on the front of the package.** *Facts Up Front* was developed by the Grocery Manufacturers Association and the Food Marketing Institute and is a nutrient-based labeling system that summarizes important information from the Nutrition Facts panel in a simple and easy-to-use format on the front of food and beverage packages.

The *Facts Up Front* icons (numbers on colored tabs) are designed to allow consumers to quickly see, understand and use key nutrient information as they peruse store shelves and navigate aisles. The basic *Facts Up Front* label lists calories and information about saturated fat, sodium and sugar – nutrients the *Dietary Guidelines for Americans* recommend limiting. The four nutrient facts are always presented together as a consistent set.

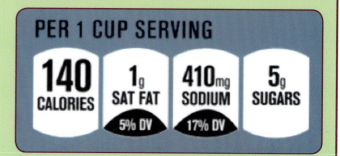

PER 1 CUP SERVING

140 CALORIES — 1g SAT FAT 5% DV — 410mg SODIUM 17% DV — 5g SUGARS

Manufacturers may also choose to include information on up to two "nutrients to encourage." These nutrients – potassium, fiber, protein, vitamin A, vitamin C, vitamin D, calcium and iron – are needed to build a nutrient-dense diet, according to the *Dietary Guidelines for Americans*. A "nutrients to encourage" designation can be placed on a package only when the product meets FDA requirements for a "good source" nutrient content claim.

A Word from the Chef
Building on a Classical Foundation

"Nutrition plays an important role in my personal cooking and my teaching," says Wook Kang, a graduate of and now chef instructor at the Le Cordon Bleu –Chicago, formerly the Cooking and Hospitality Institute of Chicago. "Our students learn classical techniques using salt, fat, cream and butter. Of course, that food tastes great. But you can't cook that way all the time. You must learn how to modify classical techniques to serve health-conscious guests," Wook, a certified food and beverage executive and a master certified food executive, explains.

Wook believes that patrons should be able to create a balanced meal from the menu, which is why menu planners should have a solid under-standing of nutrition standards. "Most people know what's 'good' for them, but they want a choice," Wook explains. "Chefs need to know how to preserve flavors when improving the nutrition profile of a dish. Ingredients will affect flavor and so will technique. You have to look for all the different places in a recipe where you can make a change to create a healthier result more in line with today's guidelines – and also flavorful. The more informed you are, the better."

Asian Ratatouille

Chef Wook Kang, Instructor, Le Cordon Bleu College of Culinary Arts, Chicago, Illinois

Yield: 8 cups
12 servings – ¾ cup

This very versatile side dish or delicious appetizer is also excellent served in small phyllo cups as an hors d´oeuvre.

Peanut oil, divided	3	tablespoons
Japanese eggplant, ½ inch dice	2	pounds
Red bell pepper, ½ inch dice	1	pound
Green bell pepper, ½ inch dice	8	ounces
Zucchini, ½ inch dice	1	pound
Onion, chopped	8	ounces
Ginger, minced fresh	1	tablespoon
Garlic, minced	2	cloves
Plum tomatoes, diced	4	ounces
Chinese oyster sauce	1	tablespoon
Chinese hoisin sauce	1	tablespoon
Rice vinegar	2	teaspoons
Japanese mirin	1	tablespoon
Chinese or Japanese sesame oil	1 ½	teaspoons
Salt	½	teaspoon
Black pepper, freshly ground	½	teaspoon
Scallions, finely chopped	3	
Cilantro leaves, finely chopped	2	tablespoons
Thai basil, finely shredded	1	tablespoon

1. Heat 2 tablespoons peanut oil in a large skillet. Saute the eggplant, peppers and zucchini until browned. Remove them from the pan and reserve.
2. In the same pan, add remaining oil. Sauté the onion, ginger and garlic, and cook over medium-low heat until they are tender.
3. Add the reserved vegetables and the tomato, and cook about 5 minutes, stirring often. Add the oyster sauce, hoisin sauce, rice vinegar, mirin and sesame oil.
4. Cook, stirring, a few minutes longer.
5. Season to taste with salt and pepper.
6. Fold in the scallions.
7. Sprinkle with cilantro and Thai basil. Serve hot or at room temperature.

Per Serving

Calories	110	Cholesterol	5	mg
Fat	5	g	Sodium	200	mg
Saturated Fat	1	g	Carbohydrates	15	mg
Trans Fat	0	g	Dietary Fiber	4	mg
Sugar	8	g	Protein	3	g

Opportunities for Chefs

The cornerstones of a healthy diet are adequacy, balance, moderation and variety. Various nutrition standards, such as the *Dietary Guidelines for Americans 2010* and *MyPlate*, are built on that foundation. The *Dietary Guidelines* and *MyPlate* should be used for the basis of menu planning and recipe development for healthful meals. Nutrition tools such as food labeling and food rating systems based on nutrient density are used to communicate healthy diet principles to consumers. While it is not necessary for chefs to know the specific amounts needed for every nutrient, it is helpful to understand the tools developed to implement national health policy and to consider how menus and recipes might better fulfill nutrition recommendations. As people seek more healthful food in restaurants and other foodservice settings, the chef who understands how the cornerstones of nutrition are reflected in current standards and tools will have a head start in meeting consumer demands.

Learning Activities

1. Choose food labels from two similar items (cereal, condiments, etc.) and compare the Nutrition Facts panel of each food item.

2. Visit *MyPlate* at www.choosemyplate.gov and create your personalized plan. Use your *MyPlate* plan to design a healthful menu.

3. Find food labels that make different legal health claims.

4. From each food group, identify a core, healthful option and a food from that same group that is a high-fat or high-sugar choice. Compare calories and nutrient contributions of each pair.

For More Information

- Claims That Can Be Made for Conventional Foods and Dietary Supplements, http://fnic.nal.usda.gov/nal_display/index.php?info_center=4&tax_level=3&tax_subject=256&topic_id=1342&level3_id=5140

- Dietary Reference Intakes, http://fnic.nal.usda.gov/nal_display/index.php?info_center=4&tax_level=3&tax_subject=256&topic_id=1342&level3_id=5140

- How to Understand and Use the Food Label, www.fda.gov/food/labelingnutrition/consumerinformation/ucm078889.htm

- *MyPlate*, www.choosemyplate.gov

- *Dietary Guidelines for Americans 2010*, www.dietaryguidelines.gov

CHAPTER 3

Carbohydrates

LEARNING OBJECTIVES

After completing this chapter, you should be able to:

- Describe how the body uses carbohydrates

- Distinguish between simple carbohydrates and complex carbohydrates and list examples of the foods that contain them

- Explain the importance of fiber in the diet and identify the differences between insoluble and soluble fiber

- List the recommendations of *Dietary Guidelines for Americans* related to sugar, refined grains and fiber

- Identify common and uncommon whole grains and give examples of how to increase their use in menu planning

- Explain the functions of sugar in food preparation and discuss how to decrease the amount of sugar used while maintaining texture and flavor

- Compare and contrast caloric sweeteners (sugars) with non-nutritive sweeteners (sugar substitutes)

Carbohydrates, often called the "ideal fuel," provide energy for the body. The *Dietary Guidelines for Americans* suggest eating plenty of whole-grain complex carbohydrates that are high in vitamins, minerals and fiber, and lots of nutrient-rich fruits and vegetables, while limiting added sugars, which provide little more than calories, as well as refined grains.

Carbohydrates are typically grouped as starches, which are complex carbohydrates, and simple sugars or simple carbohydrates. Complex carbohydrates are made of long chains of simple sugar units. They are found in grains, breads, cereals, pasta, dried peas and beans, and starchy vegetables like potatoes and corn. Naturally occurring simple sugars (one or two sugar units) are found in fruit, milk, honey and syrups. Simple sugars are added in food preparation and processing in the form of table sugar, corn syrup, high-fructose corn syrup and other sugars.

Many carbohydrates also contain fiber, which is chemically similar to starch. Fiber is an indigestible carbohydrate that contains chemical bonds that cannot be broken down by enzymes in the human digestive tract.

A common misconception about carbohydrates is that they are fattening. Some carbohydrate intake is necessary for basic bodily functions, but too many calories from any energy source will convert to body fat and cause weight gain. One gram of carbohydrate, simple or complex, contains 4 calories – the same number of calories as 1 gram of protein and fewer calories than a gram of either alcohol (7 calories per gram) or fat (9 calories per gram). Carbohydrates become calorically heavy when they are eaten in combination with fat – for example, bread laden with butter, French fries cooked in oil, and potatoes and pastas with rich sauces. Cutting carbohydrates often results in cutting fat calories, too. It is important to read labels to identify calories, fat and carbohydrate. Some low-fat foods, such as salad dressings, remove fat and add sugar with little reduction in calories.

More complex carbohydrate-based dishes and whole grains with reasonable amounts of healthy fat used in preparation or plating would be a great improvement in the typical person's diet.

Nutrition Science

How the Body Uses Carbohydrates

Carbohydrates have three main functions in the body: to provide energy, assist in fat metabolism and spare protein.

Providing energy. Red blood cells, the brain and the nervous system use carbohydrates as their essential fuel. During digestion, the body breaks down or converts all sugars and starches from foods into **glucose**, the smallest sugar unit and the major source of energy for the body's cells.

After digestion, glucose enters the bloodstream ("blood glucose" often known as "blood sugar") providing fuel for cells throughout the body. Some glucose is stored in the liver as **glycogen** to be used when blood sugar gets too low and body cells need fuel. The amount of glycogen is relatively small when compared to stored fat and muscle protein. An adult carries about a half-day's supply of energy as glycogen. In addition, some glycogen is stored in the muscles to be used during exercise. Once glycogen stores are full, the body will convert excess glucose into fat, which is stored as body fat.

Fat metabolism. Breaking down fat requires a small amount of carbohydrates for the chemical reaction to produce energy. If carbohydrates are not available, fat is broken down incompletely, resulting in the accumulation of by-products called ketones that can have toxic effects on the body.

Protein sparing. When carbohydrates from food are low, the body first uses protein from food for energy. When that protein is gone, the body uses protein from lean body tissues (muscle and organ tissue) to produce glucose for brain and nerve functions and for metabolic processes. A minimum of 100 grams, or 400 calories, of carbohydrate is necessary daily to prevent protein from being used as an energy source.

Carbohydrates in Foods

There are two types of carbohydrates – simple (sugars) and complex (starches). Carbohydrate-rich foods also provide varying amounts of fiber and essential vitamins and minerals.

Sugars

Simple carbohydrates include naturally occurring sugars in fruits, vegetables, milk and honey as well as added and processed sugars in soft drinks, candy, baked goods, jams, jellies, syrups, etc. All simple carbohydrates contain small sugar units – **monosaccharides** (one sugar) and **disaccharides** (two sugars) – that are easily broken down and converted to glucose. Fruits contain simple sugars and also contribute fiber, vitamins, minerals and protective phytochemicals. Milk and other dairy products that contain simple carbohydrates also provide calcium, phosphorus, riboflavin, vitamin D and protein. Other simple carbohydrate foods, however, such as table sugar, soft drinks, honey, jams and jellies, are often considered **empty-calorie** foods because they provide few nutrients except carbohydrates. Some call these nutrient-poor foods (or junk) as opposed to nutrient-rich carbohydrate foods.

The human body can't tell the difference between natural and refined sugar. By the time they are absorbed, they are identical. Most natural sugars, however, are in foods that also carry essential protective nutrients. **Table sugar**, on the other hand, is 99% pure sugar and provides 16 calories per teaspoon (4 grams) with virtually no other nutrients.

The U. S. Department of Agriculture estimates that Americans consumed about 79 pounds of caloric sweeteners (primarily cane and beet sugars and high-fructose corn syrup sweeteners in soft drinks) per person in 2011. [1] This number represents about 375 calories per day! The *Dietary Guidelines for Americans*, 2010, report that Americans get 16% of calories from added sugar, primarily from sweetened soda, energy and sports drinks, fruit drinks, desserts and candy. [2]

Types of Sugar and Their Sources

All the chemical names of sugars end in "ose." Glucose and fructose are monosaccharides. Sucrose, maltose and lactose are dissacharides.

Sugars	Common Names	Sources
Glucose	Blood sugar or blood glucose, dextrose	Corn syrup, sugar, fruits, and vegetables such as carrots and beets
Fructose	Fruit sugar	Fruits and juices, honey, table sugar, high fructose corn syrup
Sucrose (glucose+fructose)	Sugar, table sugar or granulated sugar	Sugar, brown sugar, molasses, turbinado, raw sugar, cane sugar, powdered sugar, fruits
Maltose (glucose+glucose)	Malt sugar	Molasses, bread
Lactose (glucose+galactose)	Milk sugar	Milk, dairy products, whey

Sources of Added Sugars on Ingredient Lists

Sugars are added to many foods during processing. The sugar content and type are listed on food labels. Below are various names for sugars found on ingredient lists:

- Brown sugar
- Corn sweetener
- Corn syrup
- Dextrose
- Fructose
- Fruit juice concentrates
- Glucose
- High-fructose corn syrup
- Honey
- Invert sugar
- Lactose
- Maltose
- Malt syrup
- Molasses
- Raw sugar
- Sucrose
- Sugar
- Syrup

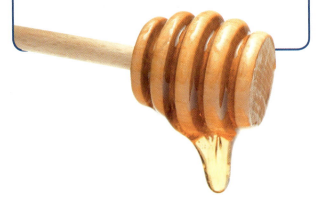

Natural sugars, such as the lactose found in milk and fructose found in fruits, are not limited because the foods they are in typically provide many other nutrients. **Added sugars**, which are incorporated into foods and beverages during processing and production, provide calories with few nutrients. Major sources of added sugar include candy, soft drinks, fruit drinks, pastries, cookies, sweetened cereals and desserts.

Research has shown that the one health problem caused specifically by eating too much sugar is dental caries, also called tooth decay. [3] Cavities are formed when bacteria in the mouth mix with carbohydrates to produce acid, which eats away at teeth and leads to tooth decay. All types of sugars, both naturally occurring and refined, can promote tooth decay, particularly if consumed in sticky foods. Sugary foods eaten between meals are more likely to cause tooth decay than those eaten only at mealtime. Starches also may promote tooth decay if they remain in the mouth and on the teeth for a long enough time.

While the scientific evidence does not support the popular belief that sugar causes hyperactivity in children, there is evidence that eating sweetened foods influences the brain to seek more sugar, which can lead to a habit of eating many sweet foods that are usually not nutrient-rich and can cause weight gain. [4, 5] Some studies connect the growing rate of childhood obesity to high levels of intake caused by the advertising and promotion of sweet foods to America's children. [6] Limiting the amount of soft drinks, sweetened beverages, candy, sugary desserts and highly sweetened breakfast cereals and snacks, especially for children, makes good sense. Although parents and caregivers have the primary role in controlling the diets of children, chefs and the food industry can play an important role by providing healthier options.

In some cases, small amounts of sugar added to nutrient-dense foods, such as breakfast cereals and reduced-fat milk products, may increase intake by enhancing palatability and thus improving nutrient intake without contributing excessive calories or sugars.

Starches

Starches – complex carbohydrates or polysaccharides (many linked sugar units) – are long strands of thousands of glucose units. Because of their length, "complex" starches take longer to break down during digestion. As a result, they enter the bloodstream more slowly than simple sugars.

Starch, which is a plant's form of glucose storage, is found in grains, breads, legumes, cereals and vegetables. Popular examples include pasta, baked beans, polenta, carrots, bagels, tortillas, oatmeal, rice and potatoes. Many complex carbohydrates, particularly whole grains and legumes, also contain fiber, vitamins, minerals and protective phytochemicals. Research has shown that whole grains reduce the risk of heart disease, stroke, cancers of the digestive tract and obesity.

Glycemic Index

Dividing carbohydrates into simple and complex makes sense on a chemical level, but it doesn't do much to explain what happens to different kinds of carbohydrates inside the body. The **glycemic index** is a scale that ranks carbohydrates by how much and how high they raise blood glucose levels compared to pure glucose. The index is sometimes used to evaluate carbohydrate quality. Foods with a high glycemic index, like white bread, cause rapid spikes in blood sugar. Foods with a low glycemic index, like whole oats, are digested more slowly, causing a lower and gentler change in blood sugar.

Some research has linked diets rich in high-glycemic-index foods, which cause quick and strong increases in blood sugar levels, to an increased risk for diabetes, heart disease and obesity. Foods with a low glycemic index have been linked to controlling type 2 diabetes and improved weight loss.

Glycemic Index Levels	
Low	0 – 55
Moderate	56 – 69
High	70 or more

What Health Authorities Say about Added Sugar

One of the key recommendations of *Dietary Guidelines for Americans 2010* is to reduce the intake of calories from added sugars to lower the calorie content of the diet without compromising nutrient adequacy.

The American Heart Association (AHA) recommends a drastic reduction in the consumption of added sugars. AHA suggests that a prudent upper limit of intake is half of the discretionary calorie allowance, which for most American women is no more than 100 calories per day (25 grams) from added sugars and for most American men, no more than 150 calories per day (about 38 grams). Recent evidence suggests that eating excessive amounts of added sugar boosts triglyceride levels, increasing risk of heart disease.

The World Health Organization recommends that less than 10% of calories come from added sugars, defined as "free sugars."

Sources: *Dietary Guidelines for Americans 2010*, www.dietaryguidelines.gov, American Heart Association; www.americanheart.org/presenter.jhtml?identifier=4471; and World Health Organization and the Food Agriculture Organization of the United Nations, www.who.int/hpr/NPH/docs/who_fao_expert_report.pdf

Some guests may be using the glycemic index to control their diets, so chefs should know what it is but are not expected to plan menus using these values.

The index is difficult to use because individual foods have differing scores and effects, thus making a mixed diet almost impossible to evaluate. But eating whole grains, beans, fruits and vegetables – foods with a low glycemic index – is good for many aspects of health.

The amount of grains a person should eat depends on age, sex and level of physical activity. Recommended daily amounts range from 6- to 8-ounce equivalents for adults. Most Americans consume enough grains, but not enough whole grains. At least half of all grains eaten should be whole grains. Serving whole-grain breads, rolls and crackers is a start; whole-grain pastas, pancakes and pizza dough, brown rice, oatmeal and barley are excellent menu additions. The *Dietary Guidelines* suggest that we lower our intake of refined grains and substitute whole grains for them when possible.

A Serving of Grain Is . . .

- ½ cup cooked rice or other grain
- ½ cup cooked pasta
- 1 ounce uncooked pasta, rice or grain
- 1 ounce bread slice
- 1 very small muffin
- 1 ounce ready-to-eat cereal
- ½ cup cooked hot cereal
- 1 4½-inch pancake
- 1 small round or square cracker
- 1 small tortilla

Source: www.choosemyplate.gov

casebycase

'Health Through Food'

At New York's Upper-East-Side, 150-seat Rouge Tomate (www.rougetomatenyc.com), Executive Chef Jeremy Bearman and Culinary Nutritionist Kristy Lambrou, MS, RD, CDN, follow a 90-page charter called SPE®, which stands for Sanitas Per Escam – Latin for Health Through Food. Its primary objective is to enhance the nutritional quality of meals without compromising taste.

The brainchild of Belgian entrepreneur Emmanuel Verstraeten, whose dream was to offer food that is both delicious and nutritious, SPE combines cutting-edge research with international health standards and is kept up to date by a scientific committee of world-renowned nutrition experts and scientists. SPE guidelines revolve around three key elements:

- Sourcing: selecting ingredients seasonally, locally, and with a focus on nutritional characteristics

- Preparation: using specific cooking techniques that preserve the integrity and nutritional qualities of the ingredients

- Enhancement: optimizing nutritional value by the synergy of product combination and menu diversity

Emmanuel Verstraeten created the Rouge Tomate concept in Brussels and exported the concept to New York in 2008, where within months the restaurant was awarded one Michelin star. He recently launched SPE Certified (www.SPEcertified.com), a certification and consulting company dedicated to assisting all foodservice operators (commercial and non-commercial) address consumer concerns about sustainability, nutrition and health. Rouge Tomate and SPE Certified have been featured in Time magazine, in leading business publications and on major television networks.

"Chef Jeremy Bearman and I are a true collaborators," says Kristy. "I not only calculate full nutrition analysis for each dish before it goes on the menu, I am also in the kitchen on a daily basis working side by side with the cooks, giving me a complete understanding of our food preparation from start to finish.

"Our goal is to deliver quality calories in a nutrient-dense, great-tasting meal," Kristy continues. "Our guests get 40% of the daily value for vitamins and minerals and 3 to 4 servings of fruits and vegetables in a 3-to-4 course meal."

All of Rouge Tomate's seafood is sustainable; all meat is grass fed. Whole grains, cruciferous vegetables and a fatty fish are always on the menu. No butter or cream is used in entrees and appetizers and only limited amounts in desserts. The restaurant emphasizes food synergies whereby ingredients eaten together are more powerful than when eaten separately. For example, combining flavonoid-rich foods with other ingredients containing vitamins C and E increases the body's antioxidant capacity, resulting in a nutritionally superior dish.

"For us," Kristy explains, "it's not about what you can't use; it's thinking about what you can use -- about balance, portions and preparation. We look at produce for our inspiration, and then we consider what else to put on the plate to boost nutrient density and maximize taste."

FDA Statement on Whole-Grain Label Claims

The Food and Drug Administration (FDA) is responsible for regulations and activities dealing with the proper labeling of foods, including ingredient statements, nutrient content and health claims. FDA also offers guidance to help manufacturers understand what the agency considers appropriate for statements on food labels, including those related to whole-grain content.

According to the FDA, whole grains are cereal grains that consist of the intact, ground, cracked or flaked kernel, which includes the bran, the germ and the inner most part of the kernel (the endosperm). Some examples of whole grains include whole wheat, oatmeal, whole-grain cornmeal, brown rice, whole-grain barley, whole rye and buckwheat. Spelt, often thought of as a unique whole grain, is actually a member of the wheat family.

When trying to select products that contain whole grains, look for those that show whole grains listed first on the ingredient list. The ingredient list on a food label shows ingredients in the order of the most abundant by weight. For products such as bread or pasta to be labeled whole grain, the grain can be ground, cracked or flaked, but it must retain the same proportions of bran, germ and endosperm as the intact grain.

An Equivalent of 1 Cup of Fruit Is . . .

- 1 cup fruit, raw or cooked
- 1 cup 100% fruit juice
- ½ cup dried fruit
- 1 apple, banana, orange or similar size fruit

Source: www.choosemyplate.gov

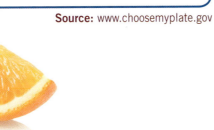

Vegetables

Any vegetable or 100% vegetable juice counts as a serving from the vegetable group. Vegetables may be raw or cooked; fresh, frozen, canned, or dried/dehydrated; and whole, cut-up or mashed. It is best to use healthful cooking techniques to maximize the health benefits of vegetables. Deep-fried vegetables should be limited or used in small amounts as crispy garnishes.

The amount of vegetables a person should eat depends on age, gender and level of physical activity. Recommended total daily intake ranges from 2 ½ to 3 cups for adults. It is wise to eat a wide selection of vegetables regularly; including plenty of dark green and orange varieties as well as dried peas and beans. These vegetables are richest in vitamins, minerals, fiber and protective phytochemicals.

The Equivalent of 1 Cup of Vegetable Is . . .

- 1 cup raw or cooked vegetables
- 1 cup vegetable juice
- 2 cups raw leafy greens

Source: www.choosemyplate.gov

Fruit

Any fruit or 100% fruit juice counts as part of the fruit group. Fruits may be fresh, canned, frozen or dried and may be whole, cut-up or pureed. The amount of fruit a person should eat depends on age, gender and physical activity. Recommended daily intake is 2 cups a day for adults.

Frozen, minimally processed fruits are equal in nutrients and calories to fresh fruits. Fruits canned or bottled in fruit juice or water are also equal to fresh fruit. Fruits canned in light or heavy syrup generally have at least twice the calories and sugar of fresh or frozen fruit.

Dried fruits are more concentrated sources of natural sugars and fiber than fresh varieties because much of the water has been removed. Fruit juices retain the carbohydrate, vitamins and minerals of the fruit, but the pressing or extraction process removes the fruit's fiber and many protective phytochemicals. Thus, from a nutrition perspective, eating a whole or sliced apple is better than drinking apple juice. Fruit drinks do not count as fruit servings as they usually offer little fruit but lots of sugar.

Culinary Applications: Sugar

In addition to improving flavor and texture, sugars help retain moisture, act as a preservative and extend shelf life. As a preservative, sugar increases the firmness of canned fruit, discourages browning and retards flavor loss. Reducing the sugar content of an item causes it to dry out faster and spoil more quickly. When cooking with sugar, consider form (crystal, powder or syrup) as well as sweetening power in order to maximize taste and texture. Heating sugar, which causes caramelization, changes flavor and texture.

Types of sugar include:

- **Table sugar** (sucrose), which is produced by concentrating sugar cane or beet juice, is composed of joined molecules of fructose and glucose.

- **Confectioner's sugar** (powdered sugar), also a sucrose product, is finely ground to a powder and mixed with some cornstarch, which prevents it from caking and makes it easy to incorporate into cooking mixtures. A light sprinkling of confectioner's sugar (and perhaps a few berries) over a dessert makes an attractive garnish.

- **Superfine sugar**, another sucrose product, is ground fine but not powdered. It dissolves quickly and is useful in batters, meringues and for sweetening beverages.

- **Brown sugar** is the sugar crystals of molasses syrup.

- **Fructose** is light syrup or crystals made from cornstarch or the simple sugar found in fresh fruits. For most food applications, fructose provides 1.2 times the sweetness of table sugar.

- **Turbinado** sugar is raw sugar that has been partially refined and washed. Raw sugar is processed from cane sugar and retains some of the cane sugar molasses. It can also contain contaminants such as molds, fibers and waxes. Raw sugar should not be given to infants.

Sweeteners also come in the form of syrups. Syrups are useful in cooking when a smooth glaze is desired.

Flavor variations can be achieved by using a variety of syrups:

- **Honey** is a natural mixture of fructose and glucose. It is made by bees from nectar and stored in hives as food. Honey comes in different flavors based on the plant providing the nectar. Thus, chestnut honey will have a flavor different from orange blossom honey. Regardless of the source, honey is a more concentrated source of carbohydrate than sugar and has about 25% more calories than an equal measure of sugar. Both provide only calories and no other nutrient in significant amounts. Honey can carry bacteria and should not be given to babies or those with a poor immune response.

- **Molasses** is syrup produced when sugar is extracted from sugar cane. It is deep brown and has a distinctive flavor. Molasses is the only sweetener with some iron, calcium and potassium, but because the amount used in a serving of prepared food is usually very small, its nutrient value is not significant.

- **Maple syrup** is made from a reduction of the sap flow of sugar maple trees and is mainly composed of sucrose, fructose and glucose. Often maple syrup is replaced by pancake syrup, which is sugar syrup with maple flavoring.

- **Corn syrup**, a liquid made from cornstarch, is composed of maltose, fructose and glucose.

- **High-fructose corn syrup** (HFCS) is corn syrup treated with enzymes to change about half of the glucose into fructose, which makes it super-sweet.

- **Agave nectar** composition varies, but typically is primarily fructose. It has about the same amount of calories as sugar, but some say its sweeter flavor (up to 1.4 to 1.6 times sweeter than sugar) means less is needed, saving calories. Agave nectar is often substituted for sugar or honey in recipes. Because agave is primarily fructose, it takes longer to influence blood sugar levels. Some people with diabetes use agave as a sweetener. Vegans commonly use agave nectar to replace honey in recipes.

High-Fructose Corn Syrup

High-fructose corn syrup (HFCS) is a group of corn syrups that have undergone enzymatic processing to convert some of their glucose into fructose. The fructose is then mixed with pure corn syrup (100% glucose). Because of traditional agricultural subsidies for corn and taxes on imported sugar, HFCS is less expensive than sugar and, as a liquid, is easier to blend and transport.

Use of HFCS has expanded greatly since the Food and Drug Administration granted it generally recognized as safe (GRAS) status in 1983. Soft drinks are a major source of high-fructose corn syrup in the diets of many Americans. The ingredient is also used in many other processed foods such as yogurt, cookies, salad dressing, cereals, jams, sauces, tomato soup, and even peanut butter and processed meats. Check the ingredient list on food labels.

Studies suggest that high rates of obesity parallel the rise in consumption of HFCS and that larger quantities of fructose stimulate the triglyceride formation and insulin resistance that contribute to diabetes. The Corn Refiners Association and other industry organizations have launched aggressive campaigns to position HFCS as natural and argue that it is safe and equal to sugar in health effects. The bottom line is that most people eat too much added sugar, whatever the form. Nevertheless, many consumers prefer products that say "no high-fructose corn syrup" and prefer to purchase products with other sweeteners or no sweeteners.

Functions of Sugar in Cooking

- **Adds sweetness**. The main characteristic of most cakes and pastries is their sweetness; thus, sugar is the defining ingredient in most baked goods.

- **Aids in the creaming process**. The crystalline structure of granulated sugar makes it an effective agent for the incorporation of air into batters mixed by the creaming method. Fat, which is the other main ingredient in creaming, holds the air introduced by the sugar.

- **Creates softening of spreading action**. By interacting with the starch component of flour to delay its gelatinization, sugar causes batters and cookie dough to stay softer longer and spread out over a greater area before setting.

- **Promotes good grain and texture**. Sugar has a denaturing effect on the gluten in flour. Along with the delay in gelatinization, this effect produces a softer crumb and finer grain in breads and cakes.

- **Retains moisture and prolongs freshness**. Sugar absorbs moisture from other ingredients as well as from the atmosphere, thus keeping a finished product moist.

- **Imparts crust color**. Sugar caramelizes and helps form a browner, firmer, crisper crust during baking.

- **Aids in fermentation of yeast**. Sugar supplies a source of food for yeast; the amount of sugar in a recipe can control the rate of fermentation.

- **Balances acidity**. Foods containing vinegar, tomatoes and other acidic ingredients have a more balanced and pleasing flavor profile if a small amount of sugar is added.

Most fats in food and in the bloodstream are in the form of **triglyceride**, three fatty acids linked together. Fats can have three of the same or three different fatty acids forming the triglyceride. When food fat comes from saturated fat, the body tends to make more triglyceride, thus elevating fats in the bloodstream.

Realistically, if you are eating a mixed diet including baked goods, meat, and dairy products, you can't avoid eating some saturated fats. The *Dietary Guidelines* advise replacing saturated fat in the diet with monounsaturated and polyunsaturated ones as much as possible. Government advice is to consume less than 10% of total calories from saturated fats, and lowering levels to 7% of calories reduces cardiovascular risk even more. Major sources of saturated fat include regular full-fat cheeses, pizza, grain-based desserts, dairy-based desserts, chicken dishes, franks, sausages, bacon and ribs, burgers, tortillas, burritos, and tacos. Several saturated-fat sources, particularly processed meats, sausages and bacon, have been linked to increased risk of colorectal cancer as well as cardiovascular disease.

Research in the last decade suggests that **stearic acid**, one of the shorter-chain saturated fatty acids, which is found in butter, meat and chocolate, does not have a cholesterol-raising effect in the body. Stearic acid can be converted in the body to oleic acid, a monounsaturated fatty acid with heart-healthy benefits.

Monounsaturated fat contains a carbon chain with one point of unsaturation. The structure contains one ("mono") double bond where the carbon molecule is not saturated with hydrogen. Food sources include olives, peanuts, avocados, almonds and their corresponding oils as well as canola, grapeseed and hazelnut oils. Monounsaturated fats are typically flavorful, with the exception of canola and grapeseed oils, which are bland.

Monounsaturates are generally considered the healthiest form of fat because they do not elevate LDL cholesterol levels and do not lower protective HDL cholesterol. When possible, substituting monounsaturated fats for saturated ones is a heart-healthy choice. Because all fats have lots of calories, substituting with monounsaturated fat is better adding it.

Polyunsaturated fat refers to a carbon chain with two or more ("poly") double bonds or two or more points of unsaturation. These fats tend to be of plant origin and are generally flavorless. Food sources include soybean, corn, sunflower, sesame, safflower and walnut oils. Sesame oil is often toasted to create a unique flavor. Mustard oil also contains polyunsaturates but is always used sparingly because of its intense flavor.

All food fats are really a mixture of the three types of fatty acids, but different fats vary in the amount of each type of fatty acid they contain (see table below, *Composition of Dietary Fats*). The type of fatty acids consumed is now thought to be very important in influencing the risk of cardiovascular disease. Although all food fats contain some of each type of fatty acid, foods are categorized by the type that is present in the greatest amount. Olive oil is called a monounsaturated fat (73% monounsaturated, 14% saturated, 11% polyunsaturated), while butter is called saturated (actually 63% unsaturated, 26% monounsaturated, 4% polyunsaturated). Sesame oil is sometimes categorized as a polyunsaturated fat and sometimes as a monounsaturated fat. It has 42% polyunsaturated, 40% monounsaturated fat and 14% saturated fat.

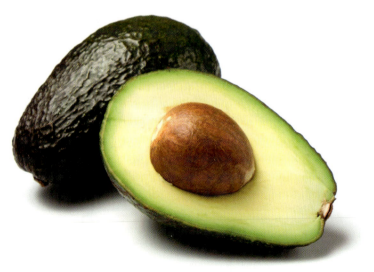

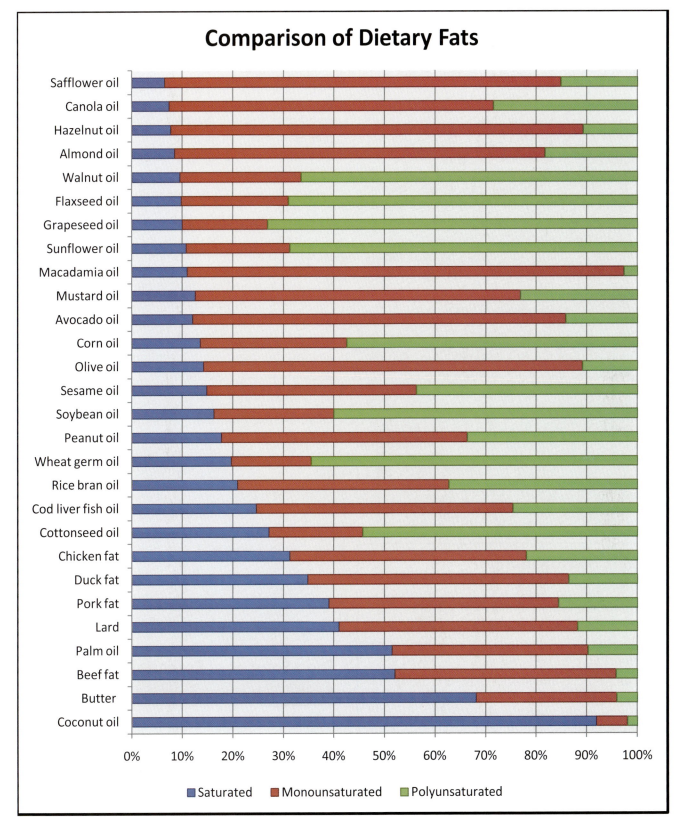

Comparison of Dietary Fats

Safflower oil
Canola oil
Hazelnut oil
Almond oil
Walnut oil
Flaxseed oil
Grapeseed oil
Sunflower oil
Macadamia oil
Mustard oil
Avocado oil
Corn oil
Olive oil
Sesame oil
Soybean oil
Peanut oil
Wheat germ oil
Rice bran oil
Cod liver fish oil
Cottonseed oil
Chicken fat
Duck fat
Pork fat
Lard
Palm oil
Beef fat
Butter
Coconut oil

0% 10% 20% 30% 40% 50% 60% 70% 80% 90% 100%

■ Saturated ■ Monounsaturated ■ Polyunsaturated

Adapted from: U.S. Department of Agriculture, Agricultural Research Service. 2009. USDA National Nutrient Database for Standard Reference, Release 24. Nutrient Data Laboratory, www.ars.usda.gov/services/docs.htm?docid=8964

Trans Fatty Acids

When liquid oil is turned into a solid through the process of hydrogenation, some of its fatty acids, particularly those that are monounsaturated, are transformed and trans fatty acids are created. **Trans fatty acids** contribute to the stability of hydrogenated fats, helping them stay fresh, prolonging the shelf life of processed foods and baked goods, and keeping snacks, cookies and crackers crisp.

Although trans fats make up a very small portion of total dietary fat intake in the United States (approximately 2% to 6%), they are even more harmful to heart health than saturated fat. Medical research has indicated that trans fats should be reduced or eliminated because they can raise the level of LDL (bad) cholesterol while simultaneously lowering the levels of HDL (good) cholesterol.

Most trans fats are added during food manufacturing. In January 2006, the Food and Drug Administration began requiring that the Nutrition Facts panel on food labels list trans fat content. Mandatory disclosure has prompted food manufacturers to reduce sources of trans fat. Some cities have public health laws that ban the use of trans fat by restaurants. According to the law, food products can list zero grams of trans fat if the food contains less than 0.5 grams per serving. If you typically consume several servings of a food that has .49 grams of trans fat per serving then you could be consuming several grams of trans fats daily. Check the ingredient list for partially hydrogenated oils that are a clue to the presence of trans fat.

Very small amounts of trans fats are produced naturally by grazing animals, so tiny amounts can be found in meat, milk and dairy products. Because these foods contain such small amounts of trans fat and since they contribute greatly to meeting total nutrient needs, elimination of these foods is not recommended by *Dietary Guidelines for Americans*.

Essential Fatty Acids

A few fatty acids are essential, meaning they must be supplied by the diet because the body needs them but cannot make them. Also other fatty acids can be made from them by the body. These **essential fatty acids** (EFA) – linoleic and alpha-linolenic – help keep cell walls flexible and protect against hardening of the arteries and high blood pressure. All essential fatty acids are polyunsaturated.

Research has shown that certain types of essential fatty acids are particularly important to health.

- **Alpha-linolenic acid** is the important member of the **omega-3 fatty acids** family. This fatty acid has been researched the most and has been found to reduce the risk of cardiovascular disease, reduce blood clotting, promote eye health and improve autoimmune diseases such as arthritis. The best sources of omega-3 fatty acids are fatty fish such as herring, salmon, mackerel, trout, sardines, anchovies and oil-packed tuna. Grass-fed meats are also a good source. The American Heart Association recommends at least 2 weekly servings of fish, preferably omega-3-rich choices.

What Is Hydrogenation?

To transform liquid vegetable oil into a solid or spreadable form – for example, margarine or solid shortening – the oil must be hydrogenated. Hydrogenation is a commercial process by which hydrogen molecules are forced under pressure through the oil. In addition to hardening the fat, hydrogenation increases its stability and prolongs its shelf life and the shelf life of products made with it. During this process, the molecular structure of the oil is changed and the result is a partially saturated fat. The more an oil is hydrogenated, the greater the change and the more solid the final product. Sometimes the structure of the fat is changed and trans fats are formed. Squeeze bottle or soft tub margarines are less hydrogenated than hard stick margarines.

Food Sources of Essential Fatty Acids

Fatty Acid	Food Source
Linoleic acid	Green leafy vegetables, seeds, nuts, grains, vegetable oils (corn, safflower, sesame, soybean, sunflower)
Alpha-linolenic acid	Oils (canola, flaxseed, soybean, walnut, wheat germ), nuts and seeds (flaxseeds, walnuts, soybeans), fish, grass-fed beef and lamb, soybeans, tofu

Plant sources include walnuts, ground flaxseed, flaxseed oil, canola oil, soybean oil, pine nuts, wheat germ, purslane and other leafy green vegetables. Some foods, such as eggs, milk, soft or liquid margarine, salad dressings and some cereals, have been modified to have more omega-3s. Read labels to identify these foods. The body does not use omega-3s from plant sources as well as omega-3s from fish.

- *Linoleic acid* is the important member of the *omega-6 fatty acids*. This fat is necessary to maintain healthy cell membranes, particularly to avoid skin disorders. Omega-6 fatty acids can stimulate inflammation and raise blood pressure. Food sources are primarily safflower, sunflower, grapeseed, walnut, corn and soybean oils and green leafy vegetables. Most Americas get plenty of omega-6s from oils.

- *Omega-9 fatty acids* are being used to develop heart-healthy cooking oils that have no trans fat or cholesterol, are low in saturated fat and rich in monounsaturated oleic acid. These branded oils are available to the food service industry.

Fun Fact

Oil packed tuna has more healthful fats than water packed tuna. Some of the health-promoting fats from the tuna go into water that is usually discarded. But drain oil packed tuna to avoid excess calories. Save the oil from oil-packed fish to use as the oil in salad dressings or cooking when "tuna" will add to flavor.

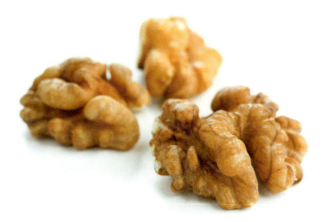

What's That Smell?

Free fatty acids, by-products of fat digestion or breakdown, are single fatty acids unbound to other substances. They are formed when a fat or oil spoils and turns rancid. They are easily noticed because they smell bad. Discard old or improperly stored butter and nut and vegetable oils that have an off odor. They should not be eaten.

Ratio of Omega-3 to Omega-6 Fatty Acids

Optimum balance between omega-3 and omega-6 fatty acids is important. Current thinking is that there is probably too much omega-6 and not enough omega-3 in most American diets. The popularity of French fries and processed foods has made over-consumption of omega-6 fatty acid a concern.

Cholesterol and Lipoproteins

Cholesterol is a wax-like substance produced by animals and humans and is essential to life. It is part of the outer membranes of cells, provides a fatty protective jacket around nerve fibers in the body and brain cells, and serves as a building block for certain hormones. The cholesterol molecule is also part of the structure of *bile acids*, which are produced in the liver, stored in the gallbladder and later involved in the digestion and absorption of fat in the digestive tract. In the skin, cholesterol is transformed into vitamin D with the aid of sunlight.

Most cholesterol is made in the body (endogenous). There is also cholesterol in many common foods (exogenous). Endogenous cholesterol is made by the liver and in other body cells. The amount of cholesterol a person makes is largely determined by genetics but also is influenced by the type of fat eaten. Research has found that the most influential components affecting blood cholesterol levels are total dietary fat, saturated fat and trans fatty acids.

Dietary recommendations suggest that dietary cholesterol intake be limited to less than 300 milligrams daily. Dietary cholesterol is found only in animal products, never in plant products, even if plant products are high in fat.

Cholesterol in the human body is sometimes called serum cholesterol because it is found in the liquid part of blood, not in the red blood cells. Two main types of proteins in blood, high-density lipoproteins (HDL) and low-density lipoproteins (LDL), carry cholesterol. In simple terms, LDL takes cholesterol into the blood stream and HDL clears cholesterol out of the blood stream. Thus they are sometimes called **good cholesterol** and **bad cholesterol**. **Total cholesterol** measured in the blood is a combination of both. High levels of LDL are considered dangerous because LDL acts as the vehicle that helps deposit cholesterol on arterial walls, contributing to the buildup of plaque associated with cardiovascular disease, specifically **atherosclerosis**. LDL cholesterol levels in the blood are increased by saturated fat in the diet.

HDL carries less cholesterol and more protein. As it circulates through the bloodstream, HDL picks up cholesterol in the blood and returns it to the liver to be reprocessed or excreted. HDL cholesterol levels in the blood are decreased by the intake of polyunsaturated fats and remain unchanged with the intake of monounsaturated fats. For good health, it is beneficial to maintain a high level of HDL cholesterol in the blood.

Both endogenous and exogenous cholesterol create total cholesterol, which is measured by testing blood. When the total cholesterol or LDL cholesterol is too high, it becomes a health risk. A person with high cholesterol is usually advised to reduce dietary sources and may be prescribed medication to reduce the absorption or synthesis of cholesterol. Current medical thinking focuses on assessing the ratio of HDL to LDL cholesterol rather than total cholesterol, which combines both HDL and LDL. If the ratio is good, the risk of heart disease is of less concern so treatment may not be necessary.

Some people make excessive good or bad cholesterol independent of food intake because of genetics. Adults are typically advised to have their cholesterol and other blood fats checked every five years and

Food High in Dietary Cholesterol

Food	Cholesterol (milligrams per 3 ½-ounce portion)
Organ meats	
Beef brains	3,010 mg
Goose or duck liver	515 mg
Lamb sweetbreads	400 mg
Chicken liver	345 mg
Turkey giblets	282 mg
Beef liver	275 mg
Egg yolks	185 mg per egg
Shrimp	195 mg
Red meats	60 - 80 mg
Poultry	60 - 70 mg
Seafood	90 - 120 mg
Fish	40 - 60 mg
Butter	33 mg/tablespoon

make dietary modifications or take medications if total cholesterol, LDL cholesterol levels, or other blood fats are too high.

Current thinking is that the type of fat consumed is as important, or more important, than the amount of dietary cholesterol eaten. Consuming less than 300 mg per day of cholesterol can help maintain normal blood cholesterol levels. Currently dietary cholesterol intake by men averages about 350 mg per day, exceeding the recommended level, while average cholesterol intake by women is 240 mg per day.

The major sources of cholesterol in American diets include eggs, chicken, meat and burgers. All of the cholesterol is in the egg yolk; egg whites do not contain any cholesterol. Years ago, common dietary advice was to severely limit eggs. Some scientific evidence now suggests that one egg per day, including the yolk, does not result in increased blood cholesterol levels and does not increase the risk of cardiovascular disease in healthy people. Eggs are an excellent and economical source of protein and many other nutrients. Fat becomes a problem if eggs are served with bacon, sausage or with Hollandaise or other rich sauces. And while liver and organ meats have very high levels of cholesterol, as you will see on the chart, they are not eaten regularly or in large amounts by most Americans.

Dietary Fat and Heart Health

Heart disease is the number one killer of men and women in America. Prevention of heart disease is a critical public health goal. Many Americans have elevated blood cholesterol levels, a key risk factor for heart disease and stroke. Both are caused by deposits of cholesterol-rich plaque in blood vessel linings. Over time, the vessels become hardened and narrow (atherosclerosis), and blood flow to the heart or brain is slowed down or blocked, causing a heart attack or stroke. Heart disease can begin in childhood, so heart health should be a consideration in planning and preparing food for children as well as adults.

Many factors, such as smoking, body weight, genetics and stress, are involved in elevating blood cholesterol levels. All fats, including the most heart-healthy varieties, have lots of calories; too many calories cause weight gain, which leads to a variety of health risks. As rates of overweight and obesity soar in both adults and children, every chef should be knowledgeable about fats for personal health and for the health of customers.

The American Heart Association made the following recommendations for controlling fat and boosting heart health years ago:

- Choose lean meats and poultry without skin and prepare them without added saturated and trans fat.

- Select fat-free, 1% fat and low-fat dairy products.

- Cut back on foods containing partially hydrogenated vegetable oils to reduce or eliminate trans fat in the diet.

- Cut back on foods high in dietary cholesterol.

- Aim to eat less than 300 milligrams of cholesterol each day.

These recommendations have been incorporated into the current *Dietary Guidelines*. For chefs this means replacing butter, lard and shortening with vegetable oils, replacing some meat with seafood, reducing the availability and portions of fried foods, trimming fat from meat, choosing cheeses with less fat, and using fat free milk and lower fat dairy products.

Dietary Fat and Cancer

Cancer is the second leading cause of death in America, right after heart disease. Research suggests that dietary fat may be involved in the development of some forms of cancer, particularly prostate cancer. In breast, colon and many other cancers, increased risk is associated with obesity. Since fat contributes many of the additional calories that lead to overweight, fat calories should be controlled to avoid obesity. The American Cancer Society's recommendations for cancer prevention include tracking body mass index (BMI), a statistical measurement indicating body fat through a ratio of weight and height. The ideal BMI is below 25. A BMI chart is found in Appendix E.

Shellfish and Cholesterol

Shellfish, like shrimp and crayfish, are moderately high in cholesterol. The form of cholesterol in shellfish, however, does not seem to elevate serum cholesterol levels. The American Heart Association says that shellfish do not need to be limited on heart-healthy diets, assuming they are not deep-fried or eaten with lots of butter. Shellfish are an excellent source of protein, low in fat and saturated fat, a good source of omega-3 fatty acids, and high in the minerals selenium, copper, zinc and iodine.

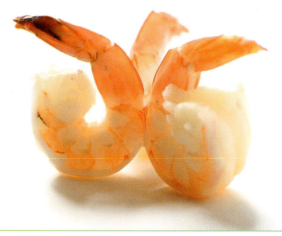

Fats Used in Cooking

Vegetable Oils

All liquid oils have almost the same caloric content, about 125 calories and 14 grams of fat per tablespoon. Oils contain primarily unsaturated fats and are predominantly of vegetable origin (although fish oil is also unsaturated). Vegetable oils contain different amounts of mono- and polyunsaturated fatty acids. Oils high in polyunsaturates include safflower, sunflower, corn, soybean and cottonseed. Oils high in monounsaturates include canola oil, peanut and other nut oils, and olive oil. The most highly praised member of this family is olive oil, which is 77% monounsaturated fat. In taste test comparisons, with few exceptions, monounsaturated fats are more flavorful than polyunsaturated fats. This factor is important for the cook who needs to create the greatest flavor from a minimum of fat.

Some manufacturers are now making blends from oils that are thought to be heart healthy, often with added vitamins, antioxidants and other protective substances.

Olive Oil

Widely promoted as a heart-healthy monounsaturated fat, olive oil is always cholesterol free and is the primary fat used in Mediterranean cuisine. Italian law defines types of olive oil based on pressing, flavor and acidity; olive oils from other countries generally use the same terminology. Olive oils differ in intensity of color, flavor and fruitiness. Some have a strong olive flavor while others are very mild (light in color and flavor). From a nutritional perspective, however, calories per tablespoon remain the same. When an olive oil is labeled "*refined*," it means the oil has been filtered; it does not mean the olives are top quality or first pressed.

Olive oil is an excellent choice for salad dressings, drizzles and marinades. Pure olive oil is fine for sauteing and cooking; extra virgin olive oil is more flavorful and better for other uses. The smoke point of olive oil is fairly low, so it is not very good for frying. Very mild olive oil can be used in baking or when you want an oil without much flavor.

Seed and Nut Oils

Peanut, canola, almond, mustard seed and hazelnut oils are like olive oil in that they are primarily monounsaturated. Safflower, sesame, sunflower and walnut oils are rich in polyunsaturated fats. Chinese peanut oil, dark sesame oil, macadamia nut oil and walnut oils have very distinct nutty flavors, so just a little has a full-flavor impact. Most light-colored oils are much milder in flavor.

Flax oil and wheat germ oil have robust flavors but are heat sensitive and fragile in chemical structure. They are usually used as food supplements rather than cooking ingredients but can be added to finished dishes in small amounts, particularly in spa cooking.

Tropical Oils

Coconut, palm and palm kernel oils are unique in that they are vegetable oils that are very high in saturated fat. Traditional nutritional advice is to avoid these oils, but they are found in many processed foods because they increase stability and shelf life and are relatively inexpensive. Usage has gone down as mandatory labeling has made consumers more aware of saturated fat content.

Some research, however, suggests that coconut oil may not be as unhealthy as once thought. Coconut oil is composed of mostly medium-chain fatty acids, which are metabolized differently from long-chain fatty acids. They tend to be used for energy rather than stored as fat, and they have antimicrobial and antiviral properties. Thus, foods with coconut oil may be useful for those with HIV or stomach ulcers caused by pylori bacteria and for individuals with low immunity.

Chefs should not be particularly concerned about using small amounts of shredded coconut in cooking or as a garnish; it's not the same as deep-frying in coconut oil. A tablespoon of dried, shredded coconut has 33 calories, 3.2 grams of fat and 2.9 grams of saturated fat.

Vegetable Oil Spray

Non-stick vegetable oil cooking sprays are an excellent way to grease pans for cooking while using a minimum amount of fat. Choose brands that leave no unpleasant aftertaste on delicate cakes and other foods. Non-stick spray oils contain lecithin (a fat-related substance), which is added as a release agent so that cakes and muffins can be easily removed from their pans. Parchment paper or foil pan liners are not required when these sprays are used. Coating a pan with cooking spray (or brushing it with oil) and then dusting the pan with flour helps with removing certain types of cakes. A light vegetable oil (canola, safflower or corn, for example) brushed onto the pan with a pastry brush or sprayed from a pump-spray bottle also works. Commercial oil can be purchased in either aerosol-spray or pump-spray forms.

For those with ecological concerns, the Aerosol Education Bureau confirms that since 1978, nearly all United States aerosol manufacturers have stopped using chlorofluorocarbon propellants (CFCs), which are thought to injure the ozone layer. This move is in compliance with bans by the Environmental Protection Agency, Food and Drug Administration, and Consumer Product Safety Commission. Most commercial oil spray products use a hydrocarbon propellant blending propane, isobutane and ebutane, all gases that are environmentally safe.

casebycase

'Farm to Fork' Rules in New Haven's Schools

Timothy Cipriano, executive director of Food Services for the New Haven, Connecticut, Public Schools, oversees breakfast, lunch and summer programs in 45 schools. On an average day, 17,000 of the 20,000 students in New Haven's K–12 system eat a meal – or two – at school. During the summer months, the school district's food truck sets up shop at seven different sites in the city.

"About 80% of our kids qualify for a free or reduced-price meal through the federal Child Nutrition Program," Timothy explains. "But this is the city that is also home to Yale University, so we have a very affluent and outspoken population that supports a progressive food system with community gardens, an emphasis on organic foods, and a strong desire to avoid ingredients like dyes and artificial sweeteners."

When Timothy left the world of commercial foodservice a decade ago, he wanted to use his expertise to make a difference in the lives of school children. "I thought, 'How can I serve these kids good, fresh food. There's got to be a way to do more farm-to-fork preparation.' " And Timothy found it.

Four years ago, the New Haven Schools used 80,000 pounds of locally grown food per year. Now that number is up to 160,000 pounds. "At our central kitchen, we cook as much from the raw state as we can," Timothy says. "We choose locally grown foods first when they are competitive with the open market. And we work closely with the state of Connecticut and our major suppliers to limit the processing of the commodity foods we receive from the government. All of our chicken is not processed into nuggets; all of our potatoes are not processed into instant."

Timothy credits the district's registered dietitian, Sarah Maver, with keeping his operation on the straight and narrow when it comes to federal regulations. "The new meal patterns introduced in 2012 are great – more vegetables, less fat and sodium – but they create a huge math problem," he says. "And frankly, they may lead schools to use more processed foods because it's easier. We are fortunate to have Sarah, who helps us use local, fresh foods to the best advantage for our kids."

Nuts

While nuts are high in fat, most of the fat is the heart-healthy monounsaturated type. Eating unsalted peanuts and tree nuts, specifically walnuts, almonds and pistachios, can reduce cardiovascular disease risk and lower LDL cholesterol levels. The Food and Drug Administration has also recognized the potential heart-health benefit of nuts and allows a qualified health claim that states that most nuts may reduce the risk of heart disease.

Nuts may also aid weight loss and weight control. The fat, protein and fiber in nuts help people feel full longer, so they may eat less during the day. But nuts should be consumed in small portions. They are high in calories and also can contribute to weight gain.

Butter

More than 120 different flavors contribute to butter's unique taste. In many cuisines, butter is considered the best-tasting fat for both cooking and baking. Most chefs prefer unsalted butter. Salt can be added to butter for flavor and to prolong shelf life; it often masks "off" flavors in older butter. Butter is made from pasteurized sweet cream. It is an animal fat that contains cholesterol (33 milligrams per tablespoon) and a solid fat that contains saturated fat (7.1 grams per tablespoon). By law, the minimum fat content of butter is 80%; premium and European-style butters have 82% to 88% fat. Water content varies from 10% to 18%, plus 2% milk solids. Whipped butter can be used as a spread to reduce fat and calories per tablespoon but can't be used reliably in cooking or baking. The culinarian should consider butter a luxury to be used moderately and enjoyed wholly.

Nutrient Content of Various Nuts (per ounce)

Nuts (amount per 1 ounce)	Calories	Protein (g)	Carbs (g)	Total Fat (g)	Saturated Fat (g)	Monounsaturated Fat (g)	Polyunsaturated Fat (g)
Almonds, 24	160	6	6	14	1	9	3.5
Brazil, 6	190	4	3	19	4.5	7	6
Cashews, 16	160	5	9	12	2	7	2
Chestnuts, 3	60	1	14	0	0	0	0
Hazelnuts or filberts, 21	180	4	5	17	1.5	13	2
Macadamia, 11	200	2	4	21	3.5	17	0
Peanuts, 32	160	7	5	14	2	7	4.5
Pecans, 20 halves	200	3	4	20	2	12	6
Pine nuts, pignoli, 167	190	4	4	19	1.5	5	10
Pistachio, 49	160	6	8	13	1.5	7	4
Walnuts, English, 14 halves	190	4	4	18	2	2.5	13
Walnuts, black, 14 halves	180	7	3	17	1	4.5	10

Source: U.S. Department of Agriculture, Agricultural Research Service. 2009. USDA National Nutrient Database for Standard Reference, Release 24. Nutrient Data Laboratory, www.ars.usda.gov/services/docs.htm?docid=8964

Margarine

A French chemist invented margarine during the late 19th century as an inexpensive butter substitute for the army of Napoleon III. **Margarine** is a blend of oils and solid fats that is heated and combined with water, milk or milk solids, emulsifying agents, flavorings, preservatives, coloring and vitamins. Margarine is partially hydrogenated to make it firm and spreadable. Solid (stick) margarine looks like butter.

Although margarine was once considered the perfect alternative to butter because it has no cholesterol, it is now under scrutiny along with other hydrogenated products because of the presence of trans fatty acids. The Nutrition Facts label on margarine lists the amount of total fat, saturated fat and trans fat per tablespoon.

Soft (tub) margarine spreads contain water and air and about 60% fat. Diet imitation margarine and reduced-fat spreads can contain about 40% fat and at least 50% water. These products, as well as soft-tub margarine, are unreliable for baking and cooking. When heated, their chemistry changes and water is released.

While it lacks the unique taste of butter, solid, **stick margarine** has roughly the same fat content – approximately 80% – but it is much lower in cholesterol. In fact, most brands contain no cholesterol. To satisfy kosher dietary laws (separating meat from dairy products), select margarine made without milk solids or animal fats for cooking or serving with most meals. Check the label for ingredients. Such margarines are labeled Kosher or Pareve. Select a margarine whose first ingredient is liquid oil high in polyunsaturates (such as liquid safflower oil); avoid products that have hydrogenated or partially hydrogenated oil as the first ingredient.

Several currently available margarines have added plant stanols. These margarines are called functional foods or **nutraceuticals** – that is, foods with ingredients specifically added for health effects. In this case, the plant **stanols** in the margarine can lower blood cholesterol levels if eaten regularly and in quite large quantities.

Solid Shortening

Most **shortening** is made of highly polyunsaturated vegetable oil and contains about half the saturated fat of butter. Solid shortening is designed to go in, not on, food. Because it does not have to taste good or feel good in the mouth, it can contain a generous quantity of emulsifiers to preserve the suspension of the fat in liquid, to hold more air and to stabilize the moisture content of batter. One popular shortening contains 80% liquid soybean oil suspended in a honeycomb matrix of 20% hardened (hydrogenated) oil. It is 100% fat, contains no water and has high levels of emulsifiers added to stabilize the structure of baked goods and increase their absorption of moisture. Recently, many shortenings and cooking fats have been reformulated to remove trans fats.

Lard and Bacon Fat

Lard is rendered pork fat, plus a very small amount of water. It is 100% animal fat and has 14 milligrams of cholesterol per tablespoon. It is 39.2% saturated fat – not as much as one might think. Lard seems to be less harmful to the diet than previously believed; nevertheless, it is not really an option in low-fat cooking because of calories and amounts usually used. Lard is often used in piecrusts and baked goods to impart flakiness and tenderness. It is also a primary cooking fat in cuisines where pork is widely used. Bacon grease (fat released when bacon is cooked) can be used in small amounts to add a distinct flavor. **Bacon fat** is nutritionally similar to lard but contains more sodium. Bacon fat, like lard, has slightly more unsaturated fat than saturated fat but does contain almost 40% saturated fatty acids and is not a great choice. One tablespoon of bacon fat has about 115 calories, 13 grams of fat, 12 milligrams of cholesterol and 20 milligrams of sodium.

Schmaltz

Schmaltz is rendered chicken, goose or duck fat. In kosher cooking, chicken fat is commonly used in cooking meals with meat when dairy products such as butter cannot be used. Goose fat is traditional in cassoulet; duck fat is often used, especially in French cuisine, for frying potatoes. Duck fat has a particularly high smoke point and crisps fried foods especially well.

Each of these poultry fats imparts a unique flavor. While traditional dietary guidance suggests removing the skin from chicken because of its fat, chicken fat is primarily monounsaturated. There is little point in removing chicken skin if one must add more fat or oil to cook skinless chicken. As with many fats, the issue is not so much type of fat but rather the amount used.

Cream and Sour Cream

Types of **cream** are grouped by fat content. By law, heavy cream, also called whipping cream, must have at least 36% milk fat; light whipping cream, 30% to 36% milk fat; light cream (coffee cream), 18% to 30% milk fat; half-and-half, 10.5% to 18%. Two exceptions to the regulations are fat-free half-and-half and whipped cream in a squirt can. Fat-free half-and-half is usually a blend of nonfat milk, sweeteners, thickeners, artificial colors and flavors, preservatives, and added vitamins. Typically, it is used to lighten coffee, but it can be substituted for half-and-half in recipes to reduce fat content and calories. Squirt-can "whipped creams" have widely varying amounts of fat; some have no fat at all.

Sour cream is generally light cream soured with lactic acid bacteria and then homogenized until smooth and pasteurized. Light sour cream with reduced fat is also available. Nonfat sour cream is an emulsion of nonfat milk solids, thickeners and stabilizers. While this version does cut calories and fats, it does not usually impart the flavor, mouth feel and richness of sour cream. Sometimes a better substitution is Greek-style yogurt, another yogurt product or silken tofu.

Should You Use Butter, Margarine, Solid Shortening or Oil?

Butter tastes great, but contains cholesterol and saturated fat. Margarine lacks butter's flavor and contains some saturated fat – slightly less than one-third that of butter. Margarines may have some trans fat but no cholesterol. You can bake with margarine. Solid shortening has a neutral (or an artificial butter) taste, is reliable for achieving certain qualities in baked goods and has about half the saturated fat of butter. Solid shortening has no cholesterol, but some brands contain trans fats. Because both margarine and shortening are hydrogenated, vegetable oil plus a small amount of butter is sometimes a good alternative. For many uses and in many cuisines, olive and other vegetable oils – with varying flavors and levels of mono- and polyunsaturated fats, but little saturated fat and no cholesterol – are the best choice for healthful cooking.

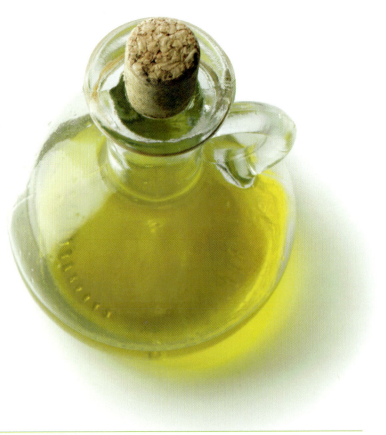

Nutrient Content of Dairy Products and Dairy Substitutes
All values are for 1 cup.

Item name	Calories	Protein (g)	Fat (g)	Saturated Fat (g)	Cholesterol (mg)	Calcium (mg)
Milk, nonfat	80	8	0	0	5	299
Milk, evaporated skim	200	19	1	0	10	740
Buttermilk, low-fat	100	8	2	2	10	284
Milk, low-fat, 1% fat	100	8	3	2	10	305
Milk, 2% fat	120	8	5	3	20	293
Milk, whole, 3.25% fat	150	8	8	5	25	276
Milk, evaporated	340	17	19	12	75	658
Half-and-half	310	7	28	17	90	252
Light cream	700	5	74	46	265	166
Heavy cream	830	5	89	55	330	156
Yogurt, plain, skim	140	14	0	0	5	488
Yogurt, plain, low-fat	150	13	4	3	15	448
Yogurt, plain, whole-milk	150	9	8	5	30	296
Yogurt, Greek, 0%	120	20	0	0	0	150
Yogurt, Greek, 2%	150	19	5	3	15	150
Kefir	150	8	8	--	--	--
Sour cream, light	320	8	24	15	80	340
Sour cream	440	5	45	26	120	253
Cottage cheese, nonfat	100	15	0	0	10	125
Cottage cheese, 1% fat	160	28	3	2	10	138
Cottage cheese, 2% fat	190	27	6	2	25	206
Cottage cheese, 4% fat	240	24	10	6	50	160
Cheese, ricotta, part-skim	340	28	20	12	76	670
Cheese, ricotta, whole-milk	430	28	32	21	125	510
Goat milk	170	9	10	7	25	327
Buffalo milk	240	9	17	11	45	412
Sheep milk	260	15	17	11	65	473
Rice milk	110	1	3	0	0	283
Soy milk	130	8	5	0	0	61

-- denotes value is not available

Source: U.S. Department of Agriculture, Agricultural Research Service. 2009. USDA National Nutrient Database for Standard Reference, Release 24. Nutrient Data Laboratory, www.ars.usda.gov/services/docs.htm?docid=8964

Nutrient Content of Various Cheeses

All values are for 1 ounce. The cheeses listed are among the most commonly used cheeses. Check food labels of other cheeses used in cooking or served.

Item name	Calories	Protein (g)	Fat (g)	Saturated Fat (g)	Cholesterol (mg)	Calcium (mg)
Cream cheese, fat-free	30	4	0	0	5	100
Cream cheese, low-fat	60	2	5	3	15	42
Cream cheese	100	2	10	5	30	28
Mexican queso fresco	40	3	3	2	10	81
Mozzarella, part-skim	70	7	5	3	20	222
Mozzarella, whole-milk	90	6	6	4	20	143
Feta	70	4	6	4	25	140
Goat cheese, soft	80	5	6	4	15	40
Brie	90	6	8	5	30	52
Camembert	90	6	7	5	20	110
Asiago	100	7	8	5	25	202
Provolone	100	7	8	5	20	214
Blue	100	6	8	5	20	150
Gouda	100	7	8	5	30	198
Gorgonzola	100	6	9	6	25	150
Muenster	100	7	9	5	25	203
Edam	100	7	8	5	25	207
American	110	6	9	6	25	175
Cheddar cheese	110	7	9	6	30	204
Cheddar cheese, reduced-fat	80	8	5	4	15	257
Swiss	110	8	8	5	25	224
Monterey jack	110	7	9	5	25	211
Fontina	110	7	9	5	35	156
Colby	110	7	9	6	25	194
Mascarpone	120	2	13	7	35	40
Havarti	120	5	10	7	25	202
Parmesan	120	11	8	5	25	314
Gruyere	120	8	9	5	30	287

Source: U.S. Department of Agriculture, Agricultural Research Service. 2009. USDA National Nutrient Database for Standard Reference, Release 24. Nutrient Data Laboratory, www.ars.usda.gov/services/docs.htm?docid=8964

Storing Fats

Fats have a tendency to absorb strong odors, so they should be stored covered or well wrapped and away from strong-scented ingredients. Take special care to prevent rancidity, which alters taste and is potentially toxic as well. Rancidity can result when fats are exposed to air and combined with oxygen and water. Research shows that by-products of rancid fats can cause damage to the lining of blood vessels, which may lead to cardiovascular disease.

In general, unsaturated fats (oils) have a less stable molecular structure than saturated (solid) fats. They are more vulnerable to changes from exposure to heat, light and moisture. Oils should be stored in opaque containers in a cool, dark location or should be refrigerated. Cold temperatures sometimes turn oil cloudy. This cloudiness is not harmful; clarity returns as the oil reaches room temperature. Dark-colored specialty oils, such as walnut and hazelnut, are the least stable. Once opened, they should be refrigerated. Their shelf life is from 4 to 6 months. Refined vegetable oils (such as canola, safflower and corn) should be stored in a cool, dry location away from air, heat and light. They generally stay fresh for 6 to 10 months. Many vegetable oils naturally contain vitamin E or similar antioxidants that will help prevent rancidity. Safflower oil is an exception and must always be refrigerated.

Saturated fats such as butter and cream contain enzymes that can affect and accelerate rancidity. It is best to use unsalted butter because salt may mask the smell of rancidity. Butter and margarine should be refrigerated or frozen for short-term use; for long-term storage, they should be frozen.

Tips for Reducing the Fat in Recipes

When cooking with fat, chefs need to choose the right fats and oils and use the correct temperature and cooking techniques. The special qualities of fat are hard to replicate. Successful substitutions, especially in low-fat and low-calorie baked goods, are tricky. Generally, when you cut back or cut out fat, you also must adjust a whole range of carefully balanced components in the recipe. Enhance flavors by increasing or adding agents such as citrus zests, various extracts and, sometimes, sugar. To maintain the desired texture in baked goods, you will need a suitably viscous aerating and moisture-holding fat substitute such as fruit purees (prune, apple or banana), corn syrup, various vegetable oils, whole eggs or stiffly whipped egg whites. Sometimes, adding a little butter will help achieve the proper taste.

To restore the tenderness when fat is removed, try cake flour instead of higher-protein all-purpose flour. Since cake flour absorbs a different quantity of moisture, you must adjust liquids as well. Try acidic dairy products such as yogurt or buttermilk; they inhibit gluten development so that the item remains tender. Sometimes when acids are added, they can be balanced with some neutralizing baking soda.

Fat not only carries flavor but also helps to blend flavors and soften or mute strong or harsh flavors and sweetness. When fat is reduced, other flavors might have to be toned down to prevent them from becoming overpowering. High-fat recipes are more forgiving of mediocre ingredients because of the softening and blending properties of the fat. Thus, when fat is at a minimum, ingredients of the highest quality become even more important. Fat also stabilizes flavors. A lean sauce may taste fine one day but not so good the next.

When reducing the fat in a recipe, think of fat as a limited resource. The more you use in some menu items, the less available for others. Identify which fat or fats will contribute the most to the recipe and get the most flavor and function from the fat used.

More Healthful Cooking Tips

- Choose low-fat dairy products, such as non-fat yogurt, part-skim ricotta cheese, part-skim mozzarella cheese, buttermilk and evaporated skim milk. For example, using canned evaporated skim milk as an alternative to cream can help create a low-fat sauce that still feels "rich."

- For sauces, concentrate flavors through reductions of stocks and vegetable or fruit juices.

- Rather than a roux, use fruit and vegetable puree or pure starch (arrowroot or cornstarch), gelatin, potato flakes or tapioca as a thickening agent for a sauce or soup.

- Bread and butter on the table can be made more interesting by supplying a variety of tasty whole-grain breads with alternative spreads such as olive oil, fruit butters and chutneys, vegetable pâtés, or bean purees. Consider adding red pepper, fresh herbs or a variety of spices to the bread itself (either before or after baking).

- Replace some or all of the saturated fat (butter, cream, etc.) in a recipe with healthier fats such as olive, nut, canola or avocado oil.

- Certain foods require a lot of fat to create the flavor and texture people expect and want. For these foods, consider reducing the portion size or change plate presentation to provide a smaller amount of the "real thing."

- Test fat-free half-and-half, evaporated skim milk, Greek yogurt or reduced-fat sour cream as a replacement for some of the cream or sour cream in a recipe. Adjust seasonings and add thickeners if necessary.

- Add some brewed tea, vegetable stock or fruit juice to salad dressings to increase volume and decrease calories per tablespoon.

- Use small amounts of toasted nuts or some nut oil in salads to increase monounsaturated fat and create interesting flavors and textures.

- Shift the balance of entree plates by increasing low-fat vegetables and whole grains and serving smaller portions of high-fat meats or cheeses.

- Use a small amount of strong-flavored cheeses that pack a punch rather than milder high-fat cheeses that melt well. Use cheese on top rather than mixed in dishes to create more visual and taste impact with less cheese (and fat).

- Use buttermilk in some soups and salad dressings to provide creamy texture and interesting flavor without fat.

- A little sesame oil mixed with rice vinegar makes a fine Chinese-style slaw or chicken salad dressing.

- Experiment with pureed potato or potato flakes as a thickener to replace some or all of the cream in some soups.

- Check out eggs that have more omega-3 fat and less cholesterol. Specific branded eggs are from chickens fed special feeds to change the fat and cholesterol content of their eggs.

- Try some of the butter and fat replacers available to the food service industry. Some oils are useful for frying and are altered to provide fewer calories per gram. A variety of fat replacers, including some fruit purees, can be used in place of some of the fat in baked goods that are supposed to be soft and chewy.

- Commonly used food substitution charts often create culinary failures. Real fat provides flavors and textures that are not easily replicated. The same recipe with fat-free yogurt substituted for sour cream will be different. Test, taste and adjust as necessary to create healthful foods to meet your culinary standards and goals. Healthful food must be delicious as well as nutritious.

Reading the Label

The Food and Drug Administration and the Department of Agriculture have set specific regulations on allowable product descriptions. The following claims apply to 1 serving.

Fat Free	less than 0.5 grams of fat
Low Fat	3 grams or less of fat
Reduced or Less Fat	at least 25% less fat than the usual product
Light	one-third fewer calories or 50% less fat than the usual product

A Word from the Chef
What's Cooking in the Community?

When the Association of Black Cardiologists (ABC) approached Chicago's Washburne Culinary Institute to partner in an educational initiative, Provost William Reynolds (now retired) was eager to help. "Washburne is located on Chicago's South Side where many African Americans live," Bill explains. "This population is at high risk for heart disease, so we were happy to demonstrate how to make some traditional food favorites more heart healthy while preserving classic tastes and textures."

ABC asked Bill and his team to improve the nutrition profile of the typical Sunday dinner enjoyed by the African American community – fried chicken, macaroni and cheese and collard greens. Washburne served lower-fat versions of these favorite foods one Sunday at a neighborhood church.

"All told, we fed about 300 people in three shifts," Bill recalls. "Each time, we explained how, working together, our chefs and dietitians had adjusted the traditional recipes to be lower in fat, especially saturated fat." Overall, the healthier fare was well accepted.

"We were encouraged to see leaders in the African American community such as pastors and physicians becoming more aware of nutrition and reaching out for assistance," Bill notes. "Following the ABC event, for example, a local physician asked us to help him develop some healthful cooking materials for his African American patients. 'I just don't have anything to work with,' he told us. Building relationships with trusted local leaders is an effective way for culinarians and dietitians to reach vulnerable populations. "Washburne," Bill says, "is working hard to educate its students and the community."

Oven-Crisp Chicken

William Reynolds, Retired Provost, Washburne Culinary Institute, Chicago, Illinois **Yield: 10 servings**

This recipe was developed at the Washburne Culinary Institute as a healthful and delicious alternative to fried chicken. It can also be made with chicken thighs. You can use canola oil (1½ tablespoons.) in a spray bottle or canned non-stick canola spray.

Skinless, boneless chicken breasts	10	half breasts, (about 5 - ounces each)
Panko bread crumbs	2	cups
Sesame seeds	1 ½	tablespoons
Sweet paprika	1	teaspoon
Kosher salt	1	teaspoon
Onion powder	½	teaspoon
Pepper	¼	teaspoon
Egg whites	2	each
Canola oil spray		

1. Preheat oven to 450° F. Place a wire cooling rack over a sheet pan. Spray the rack with canola oil

2. Mix panko crumbs, sesame seeds, paprika, onion powder, salt and pepper in a bowl.

3. Beat egg whites until very foamy in another bowl.

4. Roll each chicken breast in egg whites. Then roll each in panko mixture. Press with your fingers if necessary so crumbs cover all surfaces.

5. Spray each piece with canola spray on both sides and place on prepared rack.

6. Bake chicken until surface is crisp and golden brown, about 15-20 minutes. Allow chicken to rest 5 minutes and serve warm.

Per Serving

Calories	240	Cholesterol	85	mg
Fat	6 g	Sodium	320	mg
Saturated Fat	1.5 g	Carbohydrates	9	mg
Trans Fat	0 g	Dietary Fiber	1	mg
Sugar	0 g	Protein	34	g

Spinach Salad with Green Goddess Dressing

Brent Ruggles, CEC, Regional Executive Chef,
Las Colinas Country Club, Irving, Texas

Serves: 10

Selecting a healthful fat or oil and moderating the amount of fat used are two goals in healthful cooking. This recipe does both! The salad dressing combines the healthful fat of a creamy avocado for texture with a low-fat sour cream and mayonnaise and nonfat buttermilk. The smoked almonds in the spinach salad are reminiscent of a smoky bacon but substitute a healthier fat.

Green Goddess Dressing — Yield 5 cups

Mayonnaise, low-fat . . . . 2 cups	
Sour cream, low-fat. . . . . 1 cup	
Chives or scallions, fresh, minced . . . . ½ cup	
Parsley, fresh, minced . . . . ½ cup	
Lemon juice, fresh . . . . 1 ½ ounces	
Vinegar, white wine . . . . 1 ½ ounces	
Worcestershire sauce . . . . 1 ounce	
Avocado, fresh, peeled and seeded . . . . 2 each	
Buttermilk . . . . 2 ounces	

1. Place all ingredients in bowl of food processor fitted with metal blade.
2. Pulse for 6-8 seconds, 4 or 6 times or until well blended.
3. Taste and adjust seasonings as necessary.
4. Use immediately or cover and refrigerate.
5. Use 2 tablespoons of dressing for each salad. Reserve remaining for additional use.

Per Serving

Calories	70	Cholesterol	5	mg
Fat	6 g	Sodium	95	mg
Saturated Fat	1.5 g	Carbohydrates	3	mg
Trans Fat	0 g	Dietary Fiber	1	mg
Sugar	1 g	Protein	1	g

Spinach Salad with Green Goddess Dressing and Smoked Almond Garnish — Serves 10

Baby spinach, washed well . . . . 1 pound 4 ounces	
Green Goddess salad dressing . . . . 10 ounces	
Red onions, fresh, peeled and sliced into thin rings . . . . 5 ounces	
Smoked almonds, whole . . . . 10 tablespoons	
Tomatoes, currant or grape . . . . 10 ounces	
Pepper, freshly cracked or coarsely ground . . . . ¼ teaspoon	

1. Place spinach on a chilled plate. Drizzle with green goddess dressing (or serve dressing on side if guest prefers).
2. Garnish salad with 3 thin red onion rings, 1 tablespoon smoked almonds, tomatoes.
3. Sprinkle cracked black pepper over top of salad at service.

Per Serving

Calories	150	Cholesterol	5	mg
Fat	11 g	Sodium	230	mg
Saturated Fat	1.5 g	Carbohydrates	13	mg
Trans Fat	0 g	Dietary Fiber	5	mg
Sugar	2 g	Protein	4	g

Fats at-a-glance

Type of Fats	Characteristics	Sources	Health Effect
Saturated Fats	Solid at room temperature (usually) Carbon chain is saturated with hydrogen	Mostly animal fats Tropical oils (coconut, palm)	Raise LDL cholesterol Raise total blood cholesterol
Trans Fats	Most formed during hydrogenation of oils and used in food processing	Partially hydrogenated oils	Raise LDL (bad) cholesterol May lower HDL (good) cholesterol
Monounsaturated Fats	Liquid One double bond on carbon chain	Olives, peanuts, avocados, almonds, canola oil, grapeseed oil, hazelnut, pecans, pumpkin seeds, sesame seeds	Improve blood cholesterol levels Reduces LDL (bad) cholesterol
Polyunsaturated Fats	Liquid Two or more double bond on carbon chain Types: Linoleic acid Omega-6 fatty acids Linolenic acid Omega-3 fatty acids	**Omega-6** Polyunsaturated Fats Soybean, corn, safflower **Omega-3** Polyunsaturated Fats Soybean oil, canola oil, walnuts, flaxseed, Fatty fish (trout, herring, salmon, tuna, mackerel, sardines)	Improve blood cholesterol levels Reduces LDL (bad) cholesterol

Opportunities for Chefs

Fats and oils are part of a healthful diet, but the type and total amount of fat used in food preparation are very important considerations in healthful menu planning. Dietary recommendations suggest that fat be limited to less than 35% of total calories. All fats are concentrated sources of calories, so total fat should be limited to avoid weight gain. Saturated fats, trans fats and dietary cholesterol should be reduced in favor of healthier oils. Fats and oils come from a wide variety of sources. Animal fat is the primary source for saturated fat and cholesterol. Plant oils are generally more heart-healthy options. In general, healthful menus limit fried foods, and ingredients that are high in fat are used in moderate amounts.

Learning Activities

1. Determine the amount of fat and the equivalent in teaspoons of oil for the following foods:
   - 6-ounce filet mignon
   - half rack of pork spare ribs, barbecued
   - 2 pieces of fried chicken
   - 4-ounce grilled pork chop
   - 6 ounces of poached salmon
   - 1 ½ cups macaroni and cheese
   - 1 slice of pepperoni pizza
2. Determine the amount of fat in the following:
   - 12-ounce chocolate milk shake
   - 1 cup vanilla ice cream
   - 1 cup frozen yogurt
   - 1 cup Greek-style yogurt
   - 1 cup tapioca pudding
3. Select your five favorite cheeses and calculate the calories and amount of fat in 2 ounces of each using the chart on page 78 or food labels.

4. Using food labels, identify six foods that contain at least 5 grams of saturated fat, 5 grams of monounsaturated fat or 5 grams polyunsaturated fats.

5. Using the USDA database, figure out the amount of calories, total fat, saturated fat, monosaturated fat, polyunsaturated fat and cholesterol in 1 ounce of chicken skin. Is using boneless, skinless chicken breast or thighs better? Why or why not?

For More Information

- American Heart Association, Face the Fats Restaurant Resources, www.heart.org/HEARTORG/GettingHealthy/FatsAndOils/Face-the-Fats-Restaurant-Resources_UCM_303911_Article.jsp

- *Dietary Guidelines for Americans, 2010*, www.dietaryguidlines.gov

- *MyPlate*, www.choosemyplate.gov

- The International Tree Nut Council Nutrition Research & Education Foundation, www.nuthealth.org

- New York City No Trans Fat Help Center, www.nyc.gov/html/doh/html/transfat/english/faqs.html

- Nutrition for Everyone: Dietary Fats. Center for Disease Control and Prevention. www.cdc.gov/nutrition/everyone/basics/fat/index.html

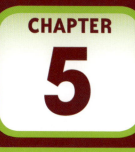

CHAPTER 5

Proteins

LEARNING OBJECTIVES

After completing this chapter, you should be able to:

- Describe the structure and functions of protein
- Explain how the body uses protein
- Discuss the quality and quantity of protein necessary in the diet
- Give examples of complementary proteins
- Describe the unique nutritional benefits of legumes
- Distinguish between animal and plant proteins
- Plan diets with proteins coming from animal and vegetable sources
- Identify appropriate portions of protein foods per serving and for daily consumption

The word "protein" comes from the Greek *proteios*, meaning "of prime importance." Protein is essential for life because it is needed to build and maintain the body. All living cells and most body fluids contain protein. Most Americans, however, eat more protein than the body requires and, along with it, an excess of saturated fat and cholesterol that come from many foods rich in protein.

Functions of Protein

The cells in muscles, organs, blood, bones, nails, hair and skin are made primarily of protein. Worn out cells are replaced constantly in the body so protein is required daily. Proteins in blood help transport iron, fat, minerals and oxygen throughout the body. Antibodies, enzymes and hormones are composed of proteins. Protein is also necessary for blood to clot normally and to maintain the body's acid-base balance.

Like fat and carbohydrates, protein is an energy nutrient. It provides 4 calories per gram. When the diet lacks sufficient calories from carbohydrates and fat, protein that is circulating in the bloodstream will be used for fuel. If more calories are needed, protein will be taken from muscles and other body tissues, which is why people who are dieting may lose lean

Proteins in the Body

Antibodies - Large proteins generally found in the blood that detect and destroy invaders such as bacteria and viruses, thus protecting the body from infection and disease.

Enzymes - Specialized protein substances that help regulate the speed of the many chemical reactions within cells. Enzymes assist in breaking food down during digestion, help build substances such as bone, and help change one substance to another as needed by the body. Although enzymes regulate many reactions, they are not changed in the process. Cells of plants contain enzymes that cause them to grow and ripen.

Hormones - Chemical messenger proteins that regulate body functions to maintain normal levels of essential substances. For example, the hormone insulin regulates blood sugar levels by moving sugar from the blood into and out of cells. Other hormones regulate growth, reproduction and behavior.

tissue as well as body fat. Loss of muscle mass also can occur with prolonged physical activity, high fever, severe burns or in diseases that alter metabolism.

Protein Structure

Amino acids are the building blocks of protein and are linked together in protein strands connected by peptide bonds. *Proteins* are large, complex chemical structures containing many amino acids, each composed of carbon, hydrogen, oxygen and nitrogen. Some amino acids also contain sulfur or phosphorus.

There are 20 distinct amino acids. They are divided into two categories, essential and nonessential. *Essential amino acids* are those that cannot be produced by the body and must be provided by food. *Nonessential amino acids* are those that can be made by the body, primarily in the liver. Histidine is essential for children and pregnant women but is nonessential for all others. Consumption of amino acids as supplements is not required when a variety of foods and adequate calories are included in the diet

Each protein differs in the specific amino acids it contains and the order in which they are linked. Because there are so many ways 20 different amino acids can combine and twist into structures creating protein chains, there is almost an infinite number of possible proteins. Each of the 20 amino acids can appear many times in a protein at various places within the chemical structure. The protein component of hemoglobin, a protein in blood that carries oxygen through the body, contains a total of 574 amino acids; while myosin, a muscle protein, is formed from the linkage of more than 4,500 amino acids. The hormone insulin contains 51 amino acids.

Amino Acids

Essential Amino Acids	Nonessential Amino Acids
Isoleucine	Alanine
Leucine	Arginine
Lysine	Aspargine
Methionine	Aspartic acid
Phenylalanine	Cysteine
Threonine	Glutamic acid
Tryptophan	Glutamine
Valine	Glycine
Histidine *(essential only for children and pregnant women)*	Histidine
	Proline
	Serine
	Tyrosine

Digestion and Metabolism

Because proteins are very large, they must be broken down into smaller units. The process of digestion breaks dietary protein into separate amino acids, which then circulate through the bloodstream and are available to form proteins the body needs. The body does not store amino acids the way it stores fat, so people must eat protein daily or the body will break down muscle tissue to get the protein it needs.

The digestion and metabolism of dietary protein is the ultimate recycling project, creating the approximately 50,000 different proteins the body needs to function properly. Protein beyond the amount needed by the body and any amino acids that do not form complete proteins are used to provide energy.

Protein digestion begins in the stomach where enzymes called **proteases** break the protein's peptide bonds. The enzyme **pepsin** breaks proteins down into smaller chains of amino acids. Protein digestion continues in the small intestine where more proteases break protein down into individual amino acids, which are absorbed through the surface of the intestinal lining. The amino acids are then released into the bloodstream where they are available to be absorbed by various cells to build the many proteins the body needs.

If an essential amino acid is not available to produce a particular protein, the building of that protein will be halted. Because the body cannot make essential amino acids, it is important that the diet supply a variety of protein-rich foods to ensure that all the essential amino acids are available.

Complete or Incomplete Proteins

Sometimes proteins are classified as complete or incomplete. **Complete proteins** are foods that provide all the essential amino acids in sufficient amounts to support the growth and maintenance of body tissues; therefore, complete proteins have what is called **high biological value**. The biological value of protein refers to the amount, type and proportion of amino acids present in a food to meet bodily needs. The egg is used as the standard by which all other protein quality values are based. The egg has a perfect score – a biological value of 100. All the essential amino acids are present in perfect amounts.

Foods that contain complete protein include meat, fish, poultry, cheese, eggs, milk and isolated soy protein. In short, animal and some soy products contain complete proteins. Animal products can also contain abundant amounts of fat, particularly saturated fat, and cholesterol. That is why high-fat, high-cholesterol animal products should be consumed in moderation.

Incomplete proteins lack one or more of the essential amino acids in sufficient quantity to support growth and maintenance of body tissues. Foods that contain incomplete protein provide a lower quality (lower biologic value score) of protein. Examples include grains, legumes, nuts and seeds, and vegetables. Most plant products contain incomplete proteins, which have some, but not all, essential amino acids. Cereal and legume combinations help people around the world meet their protein needs. Plant products are also abundant in fiber, vitamins, minerals and phytochemicals, making them excellent food choices.

While most people choose to include some animal protein in their diets, it is important to note that all of the essential amino acids can be obtained by consuming a variety of plant foods, each with different types and quantities of amino acids. Plant sources of protein can easily meet nutritional needs for protein if a sufficient variety of foods (vegetables, grains, cereals, legumes, nuts and seeds) are included in the diet to provide all the essential amino acids necessary to form complete protein.

Amino acids that are absent or low in number are called **limiting amino acids**, meaning that they limit complete protein formation. By including foods in the diet that complement limiting amino acids, complete proteins are formed. These are called **complementary proteins**, and the process is called mutual supplementation.

Making incomplete proteins complete is as simple as eating a peanut butter sandwich or baked beans and brown bread. For example, bread is rich in the amino acid methionine, but low in lysine. Legumes (peanuts and beans) are rich in lysine, but poor in methionine. When both foods are eaten, they complement each other, together providing the amino acids to form a new complete protein. A small amount of complete protein with a larger amount of incomplete protein will make all of the protein complete. For example, in macaroni and cheese, the cheese completes the amino acids missing in the macaroni, even though there is less cheese than macaroni in the mixture. We used to think that foods with complementary proteins had to be eaten at the same meal. It now appears that all necessary amino acids need to be available in the bloodstream or to cells daily, but that eating them at the same meal is not necessary.

Civilizations throughout history have combined foods to make complete proteins. Examples include rice and beans (Mexican), tofu and rice (Asian), pasta and beans (Italian), corn and lima beans (American Indian), and hummus and pita bread (Middle East). It is interesting to theorize whether this "natural" combining of foods to make complete proteins was by accident, belief or a factor of cultural survival.

Protein Needs

The Food and Nutrition Board of the National Academy of Sciences has established protein requirements based on an individual's age and weight. For adults, the Recommended Dietary Allowance (RDA) is 0.80 grams of protein for each kilogram (2.2 pounds) of body weight. This amount assumes that an individual eats a mixed diet of proteins – some complete, some incomplete. For vegetarians who consume mainly incomplete or plant proteins, protein requirements increase by approximately 15%. Individuals consuming mainly complete or animal proteins actually need about 15% less protein because it is used more efficiently. Most Americans, particularly men, eat more protein than needed, especially if they eat large portions of meat.

Protein requirements increase during pregnancy and lactation, at the onset of certain illness, and while healing or recovering from surgery. Increased exercise may also increase the need for protein. Children under 18 need additional protein to facilitate growth; the younger they are, the more protein they need per pound of body weight.

The World Health Organization has set 40 grams of protein daily as an adequate intake. The *Dietary Guidelines* do not specify an ideal protein intake, but say that 10% to 35% of calories should come from

protein. In the typical American diet, about 20% of calories come from protein. A very high protein intake can decrease calcium absorption and increase the metabolic workload of the liver and the kidneys. The main problem with protein, however, is the company it keeps. Most protein sources also contain fat; consequently, excess protein consumption increases total and saturated fat intake as well. Most sources of animal protein also contain cholesterol.

The *Dietary Guidelines* recommend choosing proteins that are low in total fat and saturated fat. Eating legumes, which contain protein, is encouraged. The availability of protein in legumes, however, is somewhat limited because legumes are not easy to digest. For example, soybeans must be treated to break down their chemical structure. Making soybeans into tofu through the processes of soaking, grinding and fermenting makes the protein more available. Soaking and cooking legumes allows the protein to be digested. Textured vegetable protein and isolated soy protein are also digestible and particularly useful as a protein source for vegans.

Protein and Health

Escalation in portion sizes over the last decade, particularly in casual and fast food restaurants, may have provided dollar value but has not enhanced the health of diners. Oversized portions have contributed to weight gain and various health risks. Downsizing portions, particularly of protein- and fat-rich foods, should be a goal for chefs interested in healthful cooking.

Eating more than the recommended amount of protein has no real health benefits. The fat (particularly saturated fat), cholesterol and calories consumed with fat can raise the risk of heart disease, some cancers and the many diseases associated with obesity. Not many people can sustain high-protein, low-fat diets because there are relatively few foods rich in protein that have no or little fat.

While adequate protein is important for health, a diet very high in protein can cause calcium loss through the kidneys, which can lead to osteoporosis. Regular consumption of fat-free (skim) milk can reduce risk by supplying calcium, but many adults do not get the recommended 3 servings of low-fat milk equivalents daily. When children are given sugary beverages in place of milk, calcium and protein intake is greatly reduced, thus lowering diet quality.

Contrary to wishful thinking and sales pitches, eating excessive protein does not build bigger muscles, increase immunity or make stronger bones. In fact, studies also show that very high-protein diets increase the workload of the kidneys, which must process nitrogen waste. This extra work can worsen problems for individuals with kidney disease.

It is true that a high-protein, low-calorie diet can cause weight loss. Food choices are limited on this regimen so dieters become bored and eat fewer calories. In addition, eliminating carbohydrates (like bread and potatoes) reduces the intake of the fats that accompany them, thus lowering calories (no French fries, no butter, etc.). Much of the "science" of low-carbohydrate (and thus high-protein) diets is based on unproven claims from testimonials and uncontrolled studies rather than from validated scientific research. Not much long-term data exist on safety or adherence to high-protein, low-calorie diets. We do know, however, that these diets are not nutritionally adequate without major supplementation. Many vitamins and minerals, fiber, and phytochemicals come from foods that contain carbohydrates.

Recommended Dietary Allowance for Protein

	Grams of Protein needed Daily
Children ages 1 to 3	13
Children ages 4 to 8	19
Children ages 9 to 13	34
Girls ages 14 to 18	46
Boys ages 14 to 18	52
Women ages 19 to 70 +	46
Men ages 19 to 70 +	56

Source: Center for Disease Control and Prevention. Nutrition for Everyone: Protein. www.cdc.gov/nutrition/everyone/basics/protein.html.

The Scourge of Malnutrition

Economics is an influential factor in food availability and how food choices are made. Protein foods tend to be expensive; many hungry Americans cannot afford enough food, much less costly protein. Experts predict that malnutrition in America will increase; it is not a problem for Third World countries only.

When feeding people with limited funds to buy adequate foods, providing protein is a priority. This is why school lunch, feeding programs for older Americans and other government programs must provide protein foods plus milk at each meal.

Unlike carbohydrates and fat, protein contains nitrogen in its molecular structure. Nitrogen equilibrium – when nitrogen intake equals output – is a measure of protein adequacy. In times of rapid growth, such as infancy, childhood and pregnancy, positive nitrogen balance is desirable so that new tissues can be formed. Negative nitrogen balance, in which loss of protein exceeds intake, can occur in illness, with injury or due to inadequate food intake. A severe protein deficit can lead to protein-calorie malnutrition.

Two diseases are caused by too little protein in the diet. Starving children suffer from *marasmus*, a severe form of protein-calorie malnutrition. *Kwashiorkor* is a disease in which protein is absent but calories, usually from starchy foods, may be adequate. Both of these protein-deficiency diseases are common in developing countries but are also seen in very low-income populations in developed countries. Some individuals who get most of their calories from alcoholic beverages, and generally eat poorly, also develop protein-deficiency diseases.

Protein Is Satisfying

According to a 2007 *Journal of Nutrition* study, when it comes to satiety, protein has more staying power than carbohydrates and fat. Eating a moderately high-protein diet (at least at the Recommended Dietary Allowance) can curb hunger and the body's desire to eat. [1] In addition, a 2004 study in the *Journal of Nutrition* tested a moderately high-protein, low-fat diet compared with a higher-carbohydrate, low-fat diet. Researchers found that those on the moderately high-protein diet did not complain of hunger and were much more satisfied than those on the higher-carbohydrate diet. [2]

Where's the Protein?

Protein is found in meat, poultry, fish, eggs, dairy products, dry beans, nuts, seeds and grains. In general, 1 ounce of meat, poultry or fish, ¼ cup cooked dry beans, 1 egg, 1 tablespoon of peanut butter, or ½ ounce of nuts or seeds can be considered 1 ounce equivalent from the meat and beans group in *MyPlate*.

Slow Roasted Glazed Salmon

Chef Sarah Stegner, Prairie Grass Cafe, Northbrook, Illinois

Yield: 10 servings

Be sure the salmon is well trimmed and free of bones and brown fat. This simple method and presentation requires excellent quality salmon. The butter enhances flavor and texture. Some butter is released on the pan as the salmon roasts. This salmon dish is both very easy and versatile. Serve it hot or chilled atop a spinach salad.

Honey	2	tablespoons
Unsalted butter, at room temperature	2	tablespoons
Lemon zest, grated	1	teaspoon
White pepper	1	teaspoon
Dijon mustard	2	teaspoons
Thyme, fresh, chopped	1	tablespoon
Kosher salt	½	teaspoon
Salmon fillets, skinned, cleaned, boned, ¾ to 1 inch thick	(10) 5 - 6	ounces each

1. Preheat oven to 225° F.
2. In a small bowl combine honey, butter, mustard, lemon zest, white pepper, thyme and salt. Mix well.
3. Arrange salmon on a shallow roasting pan. With the back of a spoon, spread honey-butter mixture to coat the top of each fillet.
4. Slow roast the salmon at 225° F for 25 minutes.
5. Remove any white drippings that may be released from salmon before serving.

Per Serving

Calories	200	Cholesterol	70	mg
Fat	7 g	Sodium	190	mg
Saturated Fat	2.5 g	Carbohydrates	4	mg
Trans Fat	0 g	Dietary Fiber	0	mg
Sugar	3 g	Protein	28	g

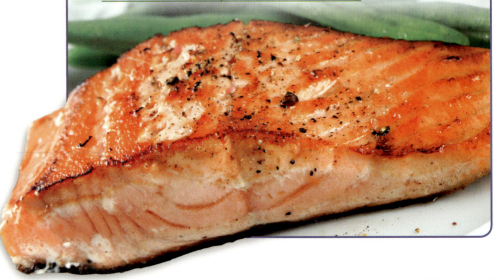

Meat

Meat includes a variety of animals: beef, lamb, pork, veal, goat, bison, buffalo, beefalo, rabbit, venison and other game. The leanest beef cuts include round steaks and roasts (round eye, top round, bottom round, round tip), top loin, top sirloin, and chuck shoulder and arm roasts. The leanest pork choices include pork loin, tenderloin, center loin and ham. In choosing ground meat, the most healthful choice is extra lean ground meat. The label should say at least "90% lean." You may be able to find ground beef that is 93% or 95% lean and ground chicken and turkey that is 97% lean.

Worldwide, goat is the most consumed meat. It is a staple of, among others, Mexican, Indian, Greek, southern Italian, Lebanese, African and Korean cuisines. Sometimes goat meat is called chevon, capretto or cabrito. The meat of a young goat is flavorful and lower in fat than chicken but higher in protein than beef. It is lower in total fat, saturated fat, calories and cholesterol than most meat. Because goat meat is so lean, it requires low-heat slow cookers to preserve tenderness and moisture.

Nutrient Content of Meats

This table lists the nutrient content of commonly eaten meats. All values are for a **3½-ounce cooked edible portion.**

	Calories	Protein (grams)	Fat (grams)	Saturated Fat (grams)	Cholesterol (milligrams)
Beef tenderloin	220	27	11	4	85
Beef, top round steak	210	35	6	2	90
Beefalo	190	30	6	2.5	60
Bison, top round steak	170	30	5	2	85
Buffalo, top round steak	130	26	2	0.5	60
Goat, average of all cuts	124	25	2.6	0.8	64
Ground beef, 20% fat	270	26	18	7	90
Ground lamb, 20% fat	280	25	19	8	95
Ground beef, 10% fat	220	26	12	4.5	85
Ground beef, 15% fat	240	26	14	5	90
Lamb, average of all cuts	175	24	8	3	80
Pork tenderloin	140	26	4	2	60
Pork chop	210	25	11	3.5	75
Pork sausage	230	15	18	6	80
Spare ribs	360	21	31	9	105
Ham	160	16	9	3	60
Rabbit	200	29	8	2.5	80
Veal, average of all cuts	190	32	7	2	115
Venison	160	30	3	1	110

Source: U.S. Department of Agriculture, Agricultural Research Service. 2009. USDA National Nutrient Database for Standard Reference, Release 24. Nutrient Data Laboratory, www.ars.usda.gov/services/docs.htm?docid=8964

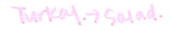
Turkey.→ Salad.

Nutrient Content of Various Cuts of Beef

This table lists the protein and fat content of different cuts of beef from the same animal. All values are for a **3½-ounce cooked edible portion.**

	Calories	Protein (grams)	Fat (grams)	Saturated Fat (grams)	Cholesterol (milligrams)
Flank steak	190	27	8	3.5	80
Strip steak	210	29	9	4	85
Top round steak	190	31	6	2	65
Top sirloin steak	210	29	10	4	90
Tenderloin or filet mignon	220	27	11	4.5	85
Ground beef, 10% fat	220	26	12	4.5	85
Ground beef, 15% fat	250	26	16	6	90
Rib eye steak	250	27	15	6	110
T-bone steak	250	24	16	6	60
Ground beef, 20% fat	270	26	18	7	90
Brisket	290	27	19	7	90

Source: U.S. Department of Agriculture, Agricultural Research Service. 2009. USDA National Nutrient Database for Standard Reference, Release 24. Nutrient Data Laboratory, www.ars.usda.gov/services/docs.htm?docid=8964

Poultry

Chicken, turkey, duck, goose, guinea hen, pigeon, partridge, pheasant and quail are common birds used on menus today. Most poultry is high in good-quality protein and low in fat. The lighter meat is lower in fat than the darker meat. Because fat is deposited under the skin of poultry, consuming poultry without the skin will lower the fat by about 5 grams per 3½-ounce serving. The fat content of the meat is similar whether the skin is removed before or after cooking, as long as the skin is not eaten.

Nutrient Comparison of Poultry

This table lists the nutrient content of various poultry. All values are for a **3½-ounce cooked edible portion.**

	Calories	Protein (grams)	Fat (grams)	Saturated Fat (grams)	Cholesterol (milligrams)
Turkey breast, w/o skin, roasted	135	30	0.5	0.5	85
Guinea hen, w/o skin, raw	110	21	2.5	0.5	65
Duck breast, w/o skin, broiled	140	28	2.5	1.0	145
Emu, full rump, broiled	170	34	2.5	1.0	130
Chicken breast, w/o skin, roasted	165	31	3.5	1.0	85
Chicken thigh, w/o skin, roasted	180	24	8	2.5	135
Cornish game hen, w/o skin, roasted	130	23	4.0	1.0	105
Ostrich, top loin, cooked	150	28	4.0	1.5	95
Pheasant, cooked	240	32	12.0	4.0	90
Squab, cooked	210	24	13.0	3.5	115
Goose, w/o skin, roasted	240	29	13.0	4.5	95
Quail, cooked, with skin	230	25	14.0	4.0	85

Source: U.S. Department of Agriculture, Agricultural Research Service. 2009. USDA National Nutrient Database for Standard Reference, Release 24. Nutrient Data Laboratory, www.ars.usda.gov/services/docs.htm?docid=8964

Words Used to Describe Chicken

Understanding the labeling used on chicken can be confusing because processors use different terms.

Free Range: The animals were given access to a fenced area or pen outside the chicken house. Chickens often stay close to the water and chicken feed, which is usually located within the house, so they may or may not utilize the pen.

Organic: The Department of Agriculture (USDA) defines organic production and prohibits the use of antibiotics in feed or treatment of animals. Feed must be made from organic ingredients, so no pesticides or chemical fertilizers can be used on the corn and soybeans used to make poultry feed. There are other requirements as well.

Retained Water: A "retained water" statement, such as "May contain up to 6% retained water," is found on most packages of fresh poultry. This statement indicates the amount of water retained in the product as a result of essential food safety procedures, such as chilling processed chickens in ice-cold water to reduce their temperature and retard the growth of spoilage bacteria and other microorganisms. Single-ingredient chicken is not allowed to retain any water beyond the minimum required by these essential food safety procedures.

Farm-Raised: All chickens are raised on farms. So the label "farm-raised" can refer to any chicken. When this term is used on menus, it usually means chickens were raised on a local farm.

Natural: Under USDA regulations, a "natural" product has no artificial ingredients, coloring ingredients or chemical preservatives and is processed just enough to get it ready to be cooked. Most ready-to-cook chicken can be labeled "natural," if processors choose to do so.

Produced without Hormones: Food and Drug Administration regulations prohibit the use of artificial or added hormones in the production of poultry in the United States.

Raised without Antibiotics or **Antibiotic-Free:** The flock was raised without the use of products classified as antibiotics for animal health maintenance, disease prevention or treatment of disease. "Antibiotic free" is not allowed to be used on a label but is sometimes found in marketing materials not regulated by the USDA.

Enhanced Chicken Products: Some uncooked chicken products are enhanced with chicken broth or a similar solution. The presence and amount of broth or other solution must be stated clearly and the actual ingredients used in the enhancing solution must be listed on the label. Salt is used in some enhanced products.

Fresh: Use of the word "fresh" on a label indicates that the product has never been chilled – that is, cooled or held below 26° F.

Kosher: Chicken have been killed and processed according to kosher food rules, which require salting plus supervision by rabbis.

Source: National Chicken Council, www.nationalchickencouncil.com

Seafood

Fish and shellfish are valuable sources of high-quality protein. Most seafood is also low in fat. Some fish, such as salmon, trout and herring, are high in omega-3 fatty acids. The specific omega-3 fatty acids in fish are commonly called EPA and DHA. Eating fish rich in EPA and DHA may reduce the risks for cardiovascular disease. The current *Dietary Guidelines* recommend at least 2 servings of fish per week.

Nutrient Comparison of Various Seafood

This table lists the nutrient content of various types of seafood. All values are for a **3½-ounce cooked (baked, broiled or steamed) edible portion**.

	Calories	Protein (grams)	Fat (grams)	Saturated Fat (grams)	Cholesterol (milligrams)
Cod, Atlantic	100	23	1	0	55
Flounder	90	16	2.5	0.5	55
Haddock	90	20	0.5	0	65
Halibut	110	23	2	0	60
Snapper	130	26	1.5	0	45
Salmon, coho	180	27	7.5	1.5	55
Salmon, Atlantic	180	25	8	1	70
Salmon, chinook	180	20	10	3	50
Salmon, sockeye	170	25	7	1	65
Mackerel, Atlantic	260	24	18	4	75
Shad, American	250	22	18	--	95
Trout, mixed species	190	26	8	1.5	75
Walleye	110	24	1.5	0	90
Catfish, farmed	150	19	8	1.5	65
Shrimp	120	23	2	0.5	210
Lobster	90	20	1	0	140
Crab, Alaska king	100	19	1.5	0	55
Crab, blue	90	18	1	0	100
Crab, Dungeness	110	22	1	0	75
Clams, mixed species	150	25	2	0	65
Oysters	80	7	2	0.5	40
Mussels	170	24	4.5	1	55
Squid	170	18	7.5	2	260
Octopus	160	30	2	0	95

-- denotes value is not available

Source: U.S. Department of Agriculture, Agricultural Research Service. 2009. USDA National Nutrient Database for Standard Reference, Release 24. Nutrient Data Laboratory, www.ars.usda.gov/services/docs.htm?docid=8964

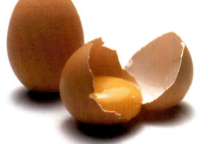

Eggs

Few ingredients are as useful and versatile as eggs. Even though they are part of the same package, egg whites and yolks are very different. The yolk contains some protein and all of the fat and cholesterol. Egg whites are mainly protein. The protein in eggs is of excellent quality.

Nutrient Comparison of Eggs

This table lists the nutrient content of various eggs. **All values are for a 3½-ounce (100 grams) edible portion**. Egg sizes vary according to the bird. The color of the shell does not influence nutrient values.

	Calories	Protein (grams)	Fat (grams)	Saturated Fat (grams)	Cholesterol (milligrams)
Chicken eggs, whole (1 large egg = 50 grams)	140	12	10	3	420
Chicken egg yolks	310	16	26	9	1225
Chicken egg whites	50	11	0	0	0
Duck eggs (1 egg = 70 grams)	180	13	14	3.5	875
Goose eggs (1 egg = 144 grams)	180	14	13	3.5	845
Quail eggs (1 egg = 9 grams)	160	13	11	3.5	835
Turkey eggs (1 egg = 79 grams)	170	14	12	3.5	925

Source: U.S. Department of Agriculture, Agricultural Research Service. 2009. USDA National Nutrient Database for Standard Reference, Release 24. Nutrient Data Laboratory, www.ars.usda.gov/services/docs.htm?docid=8964

The Incredible Egg

Eggs are excellent sources of protein, versatile and easily digested. For many years, mainstream advice was that eggs contained a lot of cholesterol and should be limited to promote heart health. Thirty years of research have shown, however, that eating an egg a day does not significantly impact the LDL-HDL cholesterol ratio that is a predictor of heart disease. Current American Heart Association guidelines and *Dietary Guidelines for Americans* 2010 allow 1 egg a day rather than limiting eggs to 3 to 4 a week as previously advised. This recommendation is for people without cardiovascular disease, congestive heart failure or diabetes. For people with these conditions, egg yolk consumption should be limited to 2 per week. Foodservice operators may want to offer egg white omelets with vegetable fillings.

Part of the issue with eggs is the company they keep. Eggs are frequently served with bacon, sausage, cheese and other high-fat, high-cholesterol foods. While eggs themselves are high in cholesterol (a large egg contains about 185 milligrams of cholesterol in the yolk), they are also a very rich source of protein and many vitamins and minerals. Some chickens are given special feeds that make their eggs rich in omega-3 fatty acids and lower in cholesterol than other eggs.

Eggs also provide lecithin, a fatty molecule that transports and metabolizes fats in the body. As one of the least expensive sources of high-quality protein and other nutrients, eggs also help to control food costs.

Unfortunately, the nutrients that make eggs a high quality food for humans are also a good growth medium for salmonella bacteria. Fortunately, however, on average across the United States, only one of every 20,000 eggs might contain the bacteria. You can reduce this risk by proper chilling and eliminate it by proper cooking. The potential for salmonella is present only with raw or partially cooked eggs that may be used in Caesar salad dressings, soft-cooked eggs, eggnogs, soft meringues, etc. Pasteurized-in-the-shell as well as pasteurized liquid eggs are available. Both are very useful because they pose no threat of salmonella. These eggs are well worth the extra cost when making food that will be held over a period of time or when feeding vulnerable individuals.

Source: American Egg Board. Eggs & Food Safety, www.incredibleegg.org/egg-facts/egg-safety/eggs-and-food-safety#2

Legumes (Dry Beans and Peas)

All varieties of beans are rich sources of fiber, vitamins, minerals and protein, including the essential amino acid lysine, but most are low in the amino acid methionine. Lysine is missing from most grains, which is why the combination "rice and beans" makes a complete protein. The *Dietary Guidelines* suggest a shift in food-intake patterns toward a more plant-based diet that emphasizes cooked dry beans and peas, among other plant foods.

Nutrient Comparison of Cooked Dry Beans and Forms of Soybeans

This table lists the nutrient content of various cooked dry beans and soybeans. All values are for a **1-cup cooked edible portion**. Beans contain no cholesterol and are an excellent source of fiber.

	Calories (grams)	Protein (grams)	Fat (grams)	Carbohydrate (grams)	Fiber (grams)
Adzuki beans	290	17	0	57	17
Baby lima beans	190	12	0.5	35	11
Black beans	230	15	1	41	15
Black-eyed peas	200	13	1	36	11
Butter beans	200	10	0	36	8
Cranberry beans	240	17	1	43	18
Edamame, shelled	200	16	6	18	8
Fava beans	180	14	0.5	32	9
Garbanzo beans	270	15	4	45	12
Great northern beans	210	15	1	37	12
Kidney beans	220	15	1	40	11
Lentils	230	18	1	40	16
Lentils, black beluga	200	12	0	32	8
Navy beans	250	15	1	47	19
Pinto beans	240	15	1	45	15
Scarlet runner beans	200	12	0	40	14
Split green peas	230	16	1	41	16
Tempeh	320	31	18	16	--
Tofu, firm	180	21	11	4	2
Trout beans	200	14	0	36	12

-- denotes value is not available

Source: U.S. Department of Agriculture, Agricultural Research Service. USDA National Nutrient Database for Standard Reference, Release 24. Nutrient Data Laboratory, www.ars.usda.gov/services/docs.htm?docid=8964

Nuts and Seeds

Nuts, nut butters and seeds are a good source of plant protein, providing approximately 10 to 20 grams of protein per 100 grams, with almonds and pistachios providing the highest levels of protein among tree nuts. Peanuts are used as nuts but are really legumes. Dry-roasted, oil-roasted and raw peanuts have similar nutrient values. Nuts rich in monounsaturated fats include macadamias, cashews, almonds, pistachios and pecans. Walnuts, pecans, pine nuts and Brazil nuts are rich in polyunsaturated fats. Some nuts and seeds (flax, walnuts) are excellent sources of essential fatty acids, and some (sunflower seeds, almonds, hazelnuts) are good sources of vitamin E.

Nutrient Comparison of Nuts and Seeds per Ounce

This table lists the nutrient content of various nuts and seeds. All values are for a **1-ounce edible portion**. Nuts and seeds contain no cholesterol and are a good source of fiber. Two tablespoons of peanut butter is about 1 ounce; three tablespoons of flax seeds is about 1 ounce.

	Calories (grams)	Protein (grams)	Fat (grams)	Carbohydrate (grams)	Fiber (grams)
Almond butter	180	4	17	6	1
Brazil nut butter	170	4	17	4	2
Cashew butter	170	5	14	8	1
Hazelnut butter	160	4	14	4	4
Peanut butter	190	8	16	6	2
Sesame seed butter	170	5	15	6	1
Soy nut butter	170	8	13	5	4
Sunflower seed butter	160	6	14	8	4
Walnut butter	180	4	18	4	2
Almonds	160	6	14	6	3
Brazil nuts	190	4	19	3	2
Cashews	160	5	12	9	1
Chestnuts	60	0	0	13	--
Hazelnuts or filberts	180	4	17	5	3
Macadamia nuts	200	2	21	4	2
Peanuts	160	7	14	5	2
Pecans	200	3	20	4	3
Pine nuts or pignolia	190	4	19	4	1
Pistachio	160	6	13	8	3
Walnuts, English	190	4	18	4	2
Walnuts, black	180	7	17	3	2
Sunflower seeds	170	6	15	6	2
Sesame seeds	160	5	14	7	3
Flax seeds	150	5	12	8	8
Pumpkin seeds	160	9	14	3	2

-- denotes value is not available

Source: U.S. Department of Agriculture, Agricultural Research Service. USDA National Nutrient Database for Standard Reference, Release 24. Nutrient Data Laboratory, www.ars.usda.gov/services/docs.htm?docid=8964

Grains

Grains provide protein, carbohydrate and fiber, in addition to vitamins, minerals and phytochemicals. Most grains, including rice and wheat, are deficient in the essential amino acid lysine but provide the amino acid methionine, which legumes lack. That is why in order to get sufficient amino acids to form usable protein, many vegetarians combine grains with legumes. Common examples of such combinations are dal with rice, beans with corn tortillas, tofu with rice, and peanut butter with wheat bread.

Pseudograins are actually seeds that are cooked and used like grains. Quinoa and amaranth are pseudograins. Quinoa, while used like a grain, contains all of the essential amino acids and, like soybeans, is a vegetable source of complete protein.

Nutrient Comparison of Grains and Pseudograins

This table lists the nutrient content of various grains. All values are for a **1-cup cooked edible portion**. Grains contain no cholesterol and are a good source of fiber.

	Calories (grams)	Protein (grams)	Fat (grams)	Carbohydrate (grams)	Fiber (grams)
Amaranth	250	9	4	46	5
Barley, pearled	190	4	0.5	44	6
Bulgur	150	6	0	34	8
Kamut	250	11	1.5	52	7
Millet	210	6	1.5	41	2
Oatmeal	170	6	3.5	28	4
Quinoa	220	8	3.5	39	5
Rice, brown	220	5	2	45	4
Rice, white	210	4	0	45	1
Rice, wild	170	7	0.5	35	3
Teff	250	10	1.5	50	6
Wheat berries	210	8	0.5	45	8

Source: U.S. Department of Agriculture, Agricultural Research Service. USDA National Nutrient Database for Standard Reference, Release 24. Nutrient Data Laboratory, www.ars.usda.gov/services/docs.htm?docid=8964

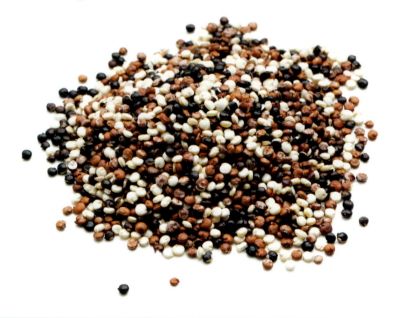

Protein in Cooking

Susceptibility to **denaturation** – changes in the structure by chemical or physical means – is an important characteristic of protein. The most common ways to denature protein are through the addition of salt (as in curing meat), acid (cold poaching as in ceviche), whipping (as in meringues) and heat (as in cooking eggs).

With the application of heat or chemicals, protein strands are broken apart and are then available to link with other protein strands. In this bonding process, known as **coagulation**, protein fragments release water, which is why proteins lose moisture during cooking and when marinated.

Wheat flours contain varying amounts of protein. Hard wheat has a high protein content. When mixed with liquid, the protein in hard wheat forms **gluten**, a firm but elastic substance that affects the texture of baked goods such as bread and pizza dough. Soft wheat flour, such as cake flour, comes from wheat kernels with lower protein content; thus, it produces a product that is more tender and has less gluten.

The food industry uses some amino acids as ingredients. L-glutamic acid and its salt form, monosodium glutamate, are used as flavor enhancers. Aspartame, a food sweetener, is made from the amino acid aspartic acid. Amino acids are sometimes added to processed vegan foods to improve nutrient values. Collagen, a protein component of connective tissue, is used to make gelatin All of these ingredients can be found on ingredient lists of packaged foods.

casebycase

Healthworks at Hallmark

In the wake of health care reform legislation and the influence of various anti-obesity initiatives, increasing numbers of employers are helping their workers pursue healthier lifestyles. There's no better place to begin this effort than in the corporate cafeteria.

In Kansas City, Missouri, Hallmark Cards, Inc., is way ahead of the curve on healthful dining. The company has been providing meals for its employees since 1923 and has had a healthful dining program in place for more than 30 years.

"The program has evolved over time," says Christine Rankin, Hallmark's manager of foodservices, fitness and work-life. "Our employees can choose cafeteria items that help them achieve their personal goals. We also discount the healthiest foods in our foodservice and vending operations by 25%." Over the past two years, Hallmark's Health Rewards program has offered employees an incentive in the form of gift cards or paycheck credits for healthy habits, including healthy dining. "We've had excellent, steadily increasing participation in the program," notes Christine.

Foods such as Asian salmon, grilled vegetable manicotti, and chicken with wine sauce are part of Hallmark's branded menu known as Healthworks. In addition, the company has significantly increased its snack-packs and "grab 'n go" fare, which offer great value and ideal portion sizes.

Healthful dining is part of more than 50 wellness-related programs Hallmark offers its employees. It's no surprise that Business Week has recognized the company for having one of the nation's most innovative corporate cafeterias. In fact, healthful dining is so ingrained in Hallmark's corporate culture that employees don't need signs or table tents to tell them what their best choices are.

"People go through what they know is the 'healthy serving line,' " says Christine, "and they are confident they can find a great-tasting, lower-calorie lunch there. A half-dozen of our chefs are culinary school graduates with restaurant experience. "

Not long ago, Christine doubled the size of the healthy serving line in the Crown Room, the company's largest dining facility. All told, Hallmark's foodservice boasts an 80% to 85% participation rate, meaning that four meals are dished up each day for every five workers in the building.

Turning Dietary Guidance into Meals

Chefs often overemphasize the importance of protein in the diet and make it the central focus of every meal. The *Dietary Guidelines* encourage **lean, low-fat** and **fat-free** choices from the meat and milk groups. Less than 7% of calories should come from saturated fatty acids, and most fat should come from polyunsaturated and monounsaturated sources. For meal planning, this guideline means that protein sources such as fish, legumes and nuts are preferred.

Protein-rich skim or low-fat milk should be available both as a beverage on menus and as an ingredient in cooking. Most Americans do not consume the 3 servings per day of low-fat/non-fat milk products recommended for a nutritionally adequate diet.

MyPlate suggests 5 to 7 ounces of meat equivalents per day. This 5 to 7 ounces is a cooked, edible portion. Assuming people eat three meals per day, food portions from the meat group should be far smaller than typical restaurant portions are today. An entree-sized portion of animal protein of 4 ounces raw weight (100 to 120 grams) and an appetizer-sized protein portion of approximately 2 ounces raw weight (60 grams) are sufficient. The protein can be presented so that a relatively small portion appears larger.

In a restaurant setting, it may be impractical to begin by making such a drastic change in the amount of protein served. Restaurants need to introduce healthier dishes slowly. A restaurant that typically serves a 10-ounce porterhouse steak and decides to change to a 4-ounce sirloin is likely to meet with instant resistance from kitchen personnel as well as customers. It is important to step back and rethink the concept of the main course, shifting the balance on the plate to less meat, fish or poultry and more vegetables and grains.

Old plating methods that place meat at 6 o'clock, vegetable at 10 o'clock and starch at 2 o'clock should be reexamined. When reducing the entree protein portion, the chef needs to find "volume" elsewhere. Whole grains, legumes, vegetables and even fruit can assume a greater supporting role and should be included in the menu description – for example, Caesar Salad with Charred Flank Steak or Shrimp Pad Thai.

It is also important to pay close attention to the quality of ingredients used and to the integrity of the desired product. One cannot expect a 4-ounce portion of meat to hide a plain baked potato and green beans. The same ingredients can be made enjoyable and satisfying. A roasted potato and crisp green bean salad tossed with vinaigrette and served with a 4-ounce portion of sliced grilled beef fanned attractively and garnished with fresh herbs can make a significant difference in quality and presentation, as can thinly sliced grilled marinated lamb mixed with a saute of Vidalia onions and served on a toasted herb roll. The key in these examples is making every ingredient count.

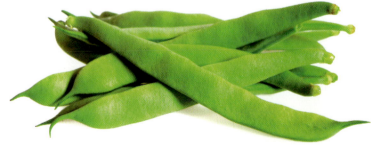

Vegetarian Choices

Many Americans, particularly teens and young adults on college campuses, are choosing to reduce their consumption of animal protein and adopt a vegetarian lifestyle. Some popular books espouse an eating philosophy in which meat is used as a condiment rather than an entree. Vegetarian options should be available on all menus for strict as well as "sometimes" vegetarians. If interesting and delicious, these menu options will be attractive to people who avoid meat for health, environmental or religious reasons. Vegetarian diets typically combine different types of foods and styles of cooking from diverse cultures. (For more information on vegetarianism, see Chapter 12.)

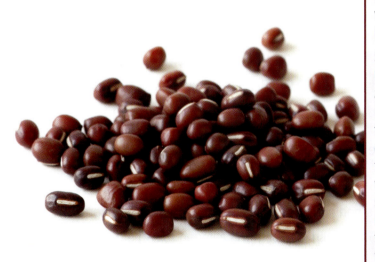

A Word from the Chef

A Healthy Portion of Local and Sustainable

Two-time James Beard award-winning chef Sarah Stegner is co-owner/chef at suburban Chicago's Prairie Grass Café. Sarah is known for her commitment to local foods and sustainability. "I'm not focused on being nutritious, but I do believe you have to offer choices and be open to serving nutritious food," she says. "It's a skill to take what's in season and showcase it – without relying on a fryer to add flavor.

"Some people think nutrition means no fat, no oil, no flavor. But that's simply not true," Sarah explains. "Nutrition is about balance and moderation. That's a key point for aspiring chefs to understand." Not one to rely on lists of substitutes to make a recipe healthier, Sarah says she makes dishes that are what they are: "You need to preserve the food's integrity."

Sarah's fresh tenderloin, sirloin and meat for ground beef come from 100% grass-fed, hormone- and antibiotic-free cattle. The meat is leaner, higher in protein, and higher in vitamins A and E than grain-fed beef. The fish served at the restaurant is line-caught; no nets catch other sea creatures or disturb the sea floor. In addition, Sarah's restaurant partners with Chicago's Shedd Aquarium in its sustainable seafood program, which promotes making environmentally responsible buying decisions by supporting fish species (like tilapia, salmon, halibut and local whitefish) that are abundant while giving those that aren't a chance to recover.

Sarah is also a fan of small, regional family farms and Chicago's year-round Green City Market, which she helped establish in 1999. "Sustainable, locally raised produce is much more important to me than organic," she explains. "Much of the organic food available here is imported from China. We don't know how fresh it is and how it's been handled." Sarah always has a vegan choice on her menus. "All I ask is that the customer let me prepare it my way – isn't that why they came to my restaurant?"

Dehydration: Signs and Cause

Causes	Signs
• Perspiration • Vomiting • Exercise • Burns • Diarrhea • High fevers • Kidney disease	• Dark yellow urine (the lighter the color, the higher the hydration) • Dry mouth (the last outward sign of dehydration) • Flushed skin • Fatigue • Impaired physical performance • Headache • Non-infectious recurring or chronic pain • Heartburn/stomach ache • Lower back pain • Mental irritation and depression

Safe Water

In the United States, fresh, pure water is taken for granted. The U.S. Environmental Protection Agency (EPA) regulates tap water (also referred to as municipal water or public drinking water). Most municipalities filter water and add small amounts of chlorine and fluoride as a public health measure. Water sources generally meet standards set by the Safe Drinking Water Act (www.epa.gov/ogwdw000/sdwa/basicinformation.html).

Despite these safeguards, however, each year there are thousands of cases of water-borne illness from contamination or improper water treatment techniques. Water contaminants include radon (which makes water radioactive), lead from old pipes, nitrates and pesticides from agricultural contamination of ground water, and chemicals from agricultural wastes. Severe storms can cause flooding that pollutes water systems. Municipal water is usually tested for these elements as well as for biological contaminants such as microscopic parasites that are not destroyed by routine chlorination. Areas that use well water, rather than municipal water, should be monitored carefully for water safety. The United States no longer has cholera or typhoid fever, but hurricanes, tornadoes and flooding are a constant reminder that maintaining a safe water supply is a worldwide concern.

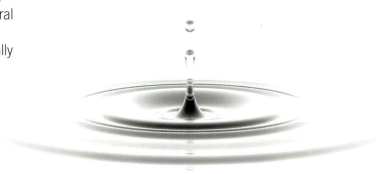

Chlorine and Fluoride

Chlorine is a chemical added in tiny amounts (chlorination) to water as a public health measure to reduce waterborne illness. Chlorine kills micro-organisms such as typhoid and hepatitis.

Fluoride is a substance that contains the mineral fluorine, which is known to strengthen tooth enamel and makes bones stronger. *Fluoridation*, a public health policy for more than 40 years, adjusts the fluoride concentration in drinking water to 1 part fluoride per 1 million parts of water. According to the American Dental Association, tooth decay is reduced by 20% to 40% in fluoridated areas, even when fluoride from other sources – such as fluoride toothpaste, tea, canned salmon and sardines – is widely available. Excessively high fluoride levels, however, may cause spots on (or discolored) teeth.

Source: American Dental Association Fluoridation Facts, www.ada.org/sections/newsAndEvents/pdfs/fluoridation_facts.pdf

The Taste of Water

Minerals, trace elements and carbonation combine to create the taste of water. The most common tastes in tap water come from chlorine (from chemicals used in water treatment), iron (from pipes, storage tanks and nature) and sulfur (usually from natural hot springs). Some natural sources also contain algae, ranging from seaweed to pond scum, which imparts tastes and odors ranging from grassy and musty to spicy and septic.

The taste differences in water are very subtle, especially when compared to wine and other beverages, but they are discernible. A water's unique taste reflects its origin. Geological strata allow water to absorb minerals; each area's mix of minerals contributes to the unique characteristics of a single-source water (water drawn from one location).

Bottled water has varying degrees of minerals that create a range of flavor, mouthfeel and aftertaste, depending on one's sensitivity to taste. Some spring waters contain sodium, magnesium, sulfates, bicarbonates, chromium, copper, calcium and/or zinc. Some spring water also has a natural effervescence, often labeled as *sparkling water*.

How to Conduct a Water Tasting

Conducting a blind water tasting is useful in selecting bottled waters for a foodservice operation. Waters should be judged on the following characteristics:

- **Appearance**: Hold the glass up to the light. A good water will be clear, bright and show no floating particles. Watch out for lint in the glass.

- **Odor**: Sniff the water in the glass. Highest scores are given to those waters with no odor. Some waters will smell of minerals or sulfur.

- **Flavor**: Take a sip of the water and roll it around in your mouth, letting it flow over the tongue. Descriptors for flavor may include: alkaline, bitter, calciferous, cool, flat, fresh, lively, salty/saline, sour, stale or sweet.

- **Mouthfeel**: As you are swirling the water in your mouth, note how your mouth feels. You want a clean edge, a fresh and light texture – nothing flabby, cloying, musty or squeaky. Carbonation, or its absence, together with the size, amount and distribution of bubbles, contributes significantly to the mouthfeel of water.

- **Aftertaste**: After you swallow the water, notice the sensation that remains. Tastelessness, thirst quenching and clean are key qualities.

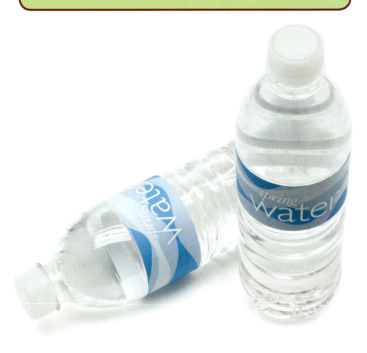

Bottled Water . . . and Water in Bottles

The Food and Drug Administration (FDA) regulates bottled water as a food. FDA established specific regulations for bottled water in Title 21 of the Code of Federal Regulations, including standard of identity, which are regulations that define different types of bottled water and have quality regulations that establish allowable levels for contaminants (chemical, physical, microbial and radiological). Some bottled water producers use municipal water as a source, filtering and removing minerals and chemicals. By FDA definition, **bottled waters** can contain no added ingredients except for antimicrobial agents or fluorides. Most popular brands of bottled water do not contain fluoride, a compound that is important to dental health.

Choose bottled waters from companies that belong to the International Bottled Water Association (www.bottledwater.org), an industry group that requires members to meet health and safety standards higher than federal government standards. NSF certification is also desirable. NSF International, a not-for-profit, non-governmental organization, is the world leader in standards development, product certification, education and risk-management for public health and safety (www.nsf.org).

Water with any added ingredients (other than anti-microbial agents or fluoride) is a multi-component beverage and must bear an ingredient list on the label. Waters with added carbonation (carbon dioxide), soda water (club soda), tonic water and seltzer water are regulated by FDA as soft drinks. Club soda has salt added for flavor. In the United States, carbonated water can be mineral water or processed water. The more carbon dioxide present, the more acidic the taste and the more active the bubbles.

Waters flavored and sweetened with sucrose or high-fructose corn syrup and/or sucralose are basically reduced-calorie fruit drinks. They can condition children to think that all beverages, even water, should be sweet. Other bottled waters have some fruit juice added. Some are flavored with acai, pomegranate, blood orange, red grapefruit or other fruits with antioxidants or phytochemicals. The percentage of juice is always listed on the label. Some have sugar added, but many fruit-flavored sparkling waters have no calories or carbohydrates.

Flavored and/or nutrient-added water beverages are simply bottled water with flavoring. Some may also contain added nutrients such as vitamins, electrolytes (such as sodium and potassium) and amino acids. Ingredients in these flavored and nutrient-added water beverages must meet bottled water requirements if the term "water" is highlighted on the label. In addition, the flavorings and nutrients added to these beverages must comply with all applicable FDA safety requirements and must be identified in the ingredient list on the label.

Water is called **hard** when its mineral content is high, mostly as a result of calcium and magnesium. Because calcium firms the walls of plant cells, cooking with water containing more than 90 milligrams of minerals per liter can affect the texture of foods. For example, dried legumes and vegetables take longer to become tender when cooked in hard water. Coffee and tea made with hard water are weaker brews. **Soft water**, which is high in sodium, softens cell walls faster; vegetables cooked too long in soft water become mushy.

Flowing 'Green'

Bottled waters are not a "green" choice. Environmental awareness is causing some consumers and chefs to take another look at tap water. Some foodservice operations are serving water that has been filtered on-site using a reverse osmosis system. These waters can be offered still or sparkling, with or without ice. LEED (Leadership in Energy & Environmental Design) certification requires an examination of water use. Filtered tap water lessens impact on the environment.

Bottled water is:

- More expensive than tap water
- Uses fossil fuels for manufacture and transport
- Creates a need for glass or plastic bottles, caps and wrapping that produce additional waste, even if recycled

Types of Bottled Water

Type	Definition from Food and Drug Administration Labeling Rules
Artesian water	Water from a well that taps a confined aquifer in which the water level stands above the top of the aquifer
Purified water **Distilled water**	Water produced by distillation, deionization, reverse osmosis or other suitable processes and meeting the definition of "purified water" in the *U.S. Pharmacopeia* (revision 23, January 1, 1995); also may be called "de-mineralized water," "de-ionized water," "distilled water" and "reverse osmosis water"; has virtually no flavor
Sparkling water	Water that, after treatment and possible replacement of carbon dioxide, contains the same amount of carbon dioxide that it had at emergence from the source
Spring water	Water from an underground formation from which water flows naturally to the surface of the earth at an identified location; may be collected at the spring or through a bore-hole tapping the underground formation feeding the spring; may or may not be carbonated or mineral water
Mineral water	Water containing at least 250 parts per million (ppm) total dissolved solids that come from a geologically and physically protected underground water source; minerals must be naturally present

Source: www.fda.gov/downloads/Food/FoodSafety/Product-SpecificInformation/BottledWaterCarbonatedSoftDrinks/ucm077094.pdf

Waters Not Defined by Government Standards

Type	Description
Flavored water	Bottled water with flavoring; must meet bottled water requirements if the term "water" is highlighted on the label; flavorings must comply with all applicable FDA safety requirements and must be identified in the ingredient list on the label
Nutrient-added water	Bottled water that contains added nutrients such as vitamins, electrolytes (sodium and potassium) and amino acids; may also contain flavor extracts and herbal supplements
Fitness water	Water that is lightly flavored to enhance taste; often contains small amounts of vitamins and added oxygen and/or antioxidants

Source: www.fda.gov/Food/ResourcesForYou/Consumers/ucm046894.htm

Coffee

Coffee is a socially acceptable and legal stimulant that helps many people get started and stay energized each day. Contrary to popular wisdom, coffee, the most popular hot drink in the United States, is not made from a bean. Those so called beans are actually seeds of the coffee cherry. High heat used in roasting and processing coffee beans concentrates oils, tannins, tars and other chemicals that provide coffee's essential flavors and create its distinctive aroma. Coffee consumption is increasing annually, and the gourmet coffee trend remains strong. Coffee and its many variations are now sold everywhere. Iced coffee has gained popularity in the past decade, particularly among women and teenage girls. Although "a cup of coffee" is a common idiom, many people drink their coffee from mugs that hold far more than an 8-ounce cup.

Coffee is available in many forms including regular, decaffeinated, light (with half the caffeine), flavored and instant. Pure coffee has very few calories, but many people add milk, cream and/or sugar that alter nutrient value. Instant flavored coffee generally contains substantial amounts of non-fat dry milk, sugar and partially hydrogenated vegetable oil. Many "coffee drinks" contain a significant amount of fat and sugar, and some have 500 or more calories per serving. Lattes and cappuccinos (regular or decaf) contain milk and are an excellent way to boost calcium intake. Both can be a very healthful choice if made with fat-free or low-fat milk.

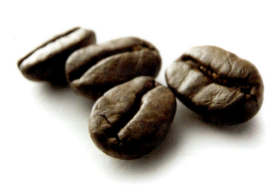

Either chemical solvents or a water process is used to remove the caffeine from coffee. Swiss water-processed decaffeination is currently the safest method. **Chicory**, which has an aroma and flavor similar to coffee but no caffeine, is used as a coffee substitute or is blended with coffee to reduce caffeine content. Scientists at the University of Hawaii and elsewhere are working to create genetically engineered caffeine-free beans by isolating the protein that creates the caffeine gene and then growing plants without that gene.

In addition to caffeine, coffee contains two other stimulants – theophylline and theobromine – which are also present in chocolate, especially dark chocolate, and in tea. The effects of these stimulants is milder than caffeine.

Does Green Coffee Bean Extract Promote Weight Loss?

In January 2012, a very small 22-week study of 16 adults in India who took green coffee bean extract supplements was published and widely reported, raising hopes for a "magic bullet" for weight loss. The theory was that unroasted green coffee beans contain chlorogenic acid, an antioxidant substance that may boost metabolic rate. The extract must be taken as pills or capsules because it is so bitter. The small study was funded by the supplement manufacturer. The study found substantial weight loss among the subjects.

Chefs and others should be wary of publicized health benefits especially when:

- It is a single study

- The research is on only a small number of subjects

- The study is short in duration

- Is in a non-scientific publication or the popular press

- Is presented in a journal that is not peer-reviewed for validity of research methods

- The research is conducted or funded by companies that benefit from the sale of products tested

Source: Vinson, JA, Burnham, BR, Negendran, MV. Randomized, double- blind, placebo-controlled, linear dose, crossover study to evaluate the efficacy and safety of green coffee bean extract in overweight subjects. Diabetes, Metabolic Syndrome and Obesity- Targets and therapy. 2012;2012(5):21-27

Tea

Tea is second only to water as the most consumed beverage in the world. In the United States, people drink much of their tea iced. Like coffee, tea contains no calories unless it is sweetened with sugar, honey or another sweetener with calories. All true tea comes from one plant, *Camellia sinensis*. Teas are made from various parts of the plant and with various processing methods. Varieties include many black, green and oolong teas.

Black tea is the most widely consumed tea in North America, Europe and India. It contains about half as much caffeine as coffee. Actual caffeine content depends on the length of time the tea is steeped and the amount of tea used. The leaves of black tea are oxidized (fermented) before drying, which gives this tea its dark color and full-bodied flavor.

Green tea leaves are processed using heat or steam, which preserves their beneficial phytochemicals. The pale green or yellow liquid is milder than black tea. Green and oolong teas are preferred in Asia.

Oolong tea is a compromise between black tea and green tea. The leaves are briefly oxidized before drying.

Several flavonoids (a type of phytochemical) are found in high amounts in tea. The most important and most studied is **quercetin**. Current thinking is that tea, particularly green tea, may help lower risk of heart disease and some cancers. For maximum health benefits, tea should be steeped about 5 minutes before drinking to allow maximum dispersion of flavonoids into the water. Flavonoids in tea interfere with the body's ability to absorb dietary non-heme (from plant sources) iron. Vegetarians and those who are dependent on iron from non-meat sources should avoid drinking tea with foods high in iron.

The concentration of caffeine and phytochemicals in tea depends on water temperature and length of brewing time. Americans tend to drink weaker tea than do people in many other countries.

Herbal teas and teas flavored with fruits, spices, flowers and nuts are not true tea. Herbal teas are infusions of dried flowers, roots and leaves from various plants. Many herbal teas have properties that relieve or treat health problems. For example, chamomile tea soothes an upset stomach, helps digestion and promotes sleep. Ginger tea relieves nausea. Peppermint tea may relieve bloating or indigestion after a heavy or spicy meal. Most herbal teas have no caffeine. Some contain antioxidant phytochemicals. Some herbal teas can trigger allergic reactions or other side effects; for example, comfrey tea may cause liver damage. In other words, "natural" does not necessarily mean safe.

Caffeine

Caffeine, a chemical with powerful physiologic effects, is present in many beverages, including coffees, teas, cola and other carbonated beverages. Caffeine is also found in herbs, guarana, yerba mate and cola nuts. Other common sources include chocolate, coffee-flavored yogurt and ice cream, and energy bars. Caffeine that is naturally present in food does not require labeling, but some manufacturers list caffeine content voluntarily. If caffeine is added to a food or beverage, it must appear on the list of ingredients.

Caffeine is absorbed rapidly, and its effects last from three to 12 hours. Caffeine has both positive and negative effects that vary from person to person. At one time, caffeine was prohibited for athletes because of its stimulant effects. In 2004, the World Anti-Doping Agency removed caffeine from its list of prohibited substances. [3] The National Collegiate Athletic Association allows minimal amounts of caffeine from food and beverages. [4]

In general, caffeine makes people feel better and more alert and potentially better able to exercise and think. But caffeine should be limited or avoided if there is any evidence of:

- Irregular heart beat or palpitations
- Severe PMS
- Sleep problems
- Bladder problems
- Anxiety or panic attacks

Caffeine: Pros and Cons

The Good	The Bad	The Good and Bad
• Mental stimulant that improves alertness, sharpens thinking and lifts moods • Promotes the release of adrenaline starting at doses lower than 1 cup of coffee, black tea, cola and some soft drinks • Improves muscle coordination and strength if consumed before an athletic event; relaxes muscle tension; can enhance athletic performance of trained athletes • Relaxes the airways of the lungs and eases breathing • Acts as a laxative • 2 - 3 cups/day may lower the incidence of Parkinson's disease • Constricts blood vessels in the brain, easing headache pain for some people	• Increases risk of early miscarriage • May affect fertility in women who drink more than 2-1/2 cups/day • Can cause a brief rise in blood pressure • Can cause irregular or fast heartbeat • Speeds the kidneys' processing of fluid, thus increasing frequency of urination • Can irritate the bladder for those with incontinence • Affects brain chemicals, primarily melatonin, and can interfere with sleep • In high doses, can increase brain chemicals associated with anxiety • Increases production of stomach acid and can affect the valve between the esophagus and stomach that leads to acid reflux and heartburn • Exaggerates attention deficit disorder and hyperactivity • Can increase secretion of stress hormones and hamper the body's ability to regulate blood-sugar levels	• Prevents sleepiness • Does not cause cancer (unless people smoke when they drink coffee) • Does not increase breast cancer but may cause breast tenderness • Can cause drop in calcium if coffee is substituted for milk • Acts as a diuretic and can decrease bloating. Caffeine does not have a diuretic effect in most people unless more than 250 milligrams of caffeine (about 2 cups of coffee) are consumed. The liquid of the coffee adds to fluid intake

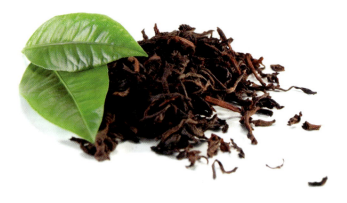

Caffeine Content of Various Beverages

Some typical servings, especially sodas, are more than 8 ounces. FDA limits caffeine in soda to 6 milligrams/ounce.

Beverage	Average caffeine content (milligrams/8 ounces)
Coffee, brewed	95 - 135
Coffee, brewed, decaffeinated	2
Coffee, drip	150
Coffee, drip, decaffeinated	5
Coffee, instant	60 - 75
Coffee, instant, decaffeinated	3
Coffee, espresso (2 ounces)	100 - 130
Coffee, cappuccino	60 - 100
Coffee, latte	60 - 100
Coffee, mocha	60 - 100
Coffee, instant, with chicory	50
Coffee, substitute, cereal grain beverage	0
Black tea	50 - 65
Green tea	30 - 40
Oolong tea	20 - 45
Iced tea	15 - 45
Herbal tea	0
Energy drink	20 - 300
Hot cocoa	5
Soda, cola	20 - 33
Soda, diet cola	20 - 45
Soda, citrus	30 - 37
Soda, pepper	10
Soda, root beer	0
Soda, ginger ale	0

Source: USDA Nutrient Data for Standard Reference, www.nal.usda.gov/fnic/foodcomp/search/

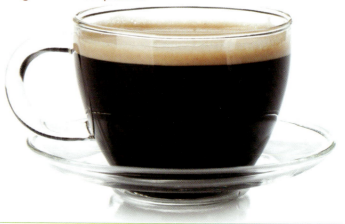

Caffeine Content of Select Foods and Drugs

Product	Serving Size	Caffeine (milligrams)
Over-the-counter drugs		
Excedrin	1 tablet	65
Anacin	1 tablet	32
Dexatrim	1 pill	200
No-Doz	1 pill	100
Vivarin	1 pill	200
Frozen desserts and yogurt		
Ben & Jerry's No-Fat Coffee Fudge Frozen Yogurt	1 cup	85
Ben & Jerry's Fair Trade Coffee Ice Cream	1 cup	70
Häagen-Dazs Coffee Ice Cream	1 cup	58
Breyer's All Natural Coffee Ice Cream	1 cup	30
Dannon Coffee Yogurt	6 ounces	30
Stonyfield Farm Cappuccino Yogurt	8 ounces	0
Chocolates and candies		
Hershey Bar	1 ½ ounces	10
Baking Chocolate	1 ounce	24
Jelly Belly Extreme Sports Beans	1 ounce	50
AMP Energy Gum	Per piece	40
Chunky Bar	1 bar	11.6
Nestle Crunch Bar	1 bar	10
Krackel Bar	1 bar	8.5
Peanut Butter Cup	2 each	5.6
Kit Kat Bar	1 bar	5
Raisinets	10 pieces	2.5
Butterfinger Bar	1 bar	2.4
Baby Ruth Bar	1 bar	2.4
Special Dark Sweet Chocolate Bar	1 bar	31
Chocolate Brownie	1 ¼ ounces	8
Milk Chocolate	1 ounce	1 - 15
Bittersweet Chocolate	1 ounce	5 - 35
After Eight Mint	2 pieces	1.6
Jell-O Pudding Pop Chocolate	1 bar	2

Dairy Drinks

Dairy beverages, which can include milk, kefir, shakes, lattes, lassis and smoothies, are a good way to supply shortfall nutrients such as vitamins A and D, calcium, and phosphorus. Dairy beverages are also an important source of protein. *MyPlate* recommends 3 servings of milk and dairy products daily for children and 2 servings daily for adults, preferably from low-fat sources. To achieve this, it's necessary to eat a dairy product at most meals. To help guests meet this guideline, foodservice operations should offer low-fat milk as a beverage at each meal plus other low-fat dairy options as alternative choices at each meal for those who do not choose milk as a beverage. Milk provides nine essential nutrients – calcium, phosphorus, potassium, protein, vitamins A, D and B_{12}, riboflavin, and niacin – and is one of the most nutrient-rich foods. Milk and milk alternatives are described in Chapter 5.

Federally funded programs such as school lunch and feeding programs for older Americans mandate that milk be served to help these vulnerable groups meet their needs for many key nutrients. Flavored milks, most often chocolate, strawberry, vanilla or banana, may be served in most of these settings. They provide key nutrients but also have added sugar. On average, low-fat chocolate milk contains the equivalent of 4 teaspoons of sugar and 56 calories more than plain low-fat milk. Some feeding programs offer flavored milk with the rationale that it will be more appealing and encourage milk drinking by those who do not like low-fat milk. Other programs do not allow flavored milks with the rationale that they encourage a preference for sweetened foods.

Other beverages such as buttermilk and kefir are generally equivalent in nutritional value to low-fat milk. Low-fat and skim milk can be used in cocoa, hot chocolate, lattes, iced coffee or other beverages to add milk to the diet. Milkshakes also contain dairy products, but the ice cream adds quite a lot of fat and sugar. Smoothies made with yogurt and fruit are a far better choice from a nutritional perspective.

Beverages: Value-Added, High-Profit and Healthful

Italian-style sodas and fruit juices or syrups in carbonated water can be light and healthful. Some restaurants have added bottled artisanal teas, fruit and water beverages or have developed house-made infusions of herbal or citrus sodas, lemonades, root beers, fruit and vegetable juices, herbal beverages, and other drinks that are both popular and profitable. Customers are willing to pay for these types of beverages as long as ingredients are high in quality. Try these ideas or create your own:

Apple ginger sparkler

Aqua fresca

Clementine soda

Fresh kiwi grape juice

Grapefruit sparkler

Hibiscus-honey iced tea

Iced ginger tea

Jasmine spritzer

Lavender spritzer

Lemongrass soda

Mint limeade

Papaya melon citrusade

Peach and rosemary spritzer

Pomegranate-honey cooler

Thai basil soda

Watermelon ginger limeade

Smoothies have become a popular drink, and small meal, as they have grown from a drink for dieters and athletes to a mainstream choice. Smoothies offer lots of creative opportunities, and the combinations and flavors are endless. Many smoothies are fruit drinks, but some contain yogurt or frozen yogurt, thus adding the nutrients that dairy products provide.

Lactose Intolerance

The enzyme lactase is required to break the sugar in milk, lactose, into its two component simple sugars. In some people this enzyme is present in insufficient quantities to digest milk products, so drinking milk can cause discomfort. Lactose intolerance is more common in non-Caucasian populations. The lactase enzyme is available commercially and can be added to dairy products to break down milk sugar. Offering milk with added lactase might be considered when serving populations who have a high incidence of lactose intolerance. Individuals who are lactose intolerant sometimes take lactase enzyme tablets so they can consume small amounts of dairy products.

Juices and Fruit Drinks

One of the main recommendations made by *MyPlate* and the *Dietary Guidelines* is to increase intake of fruits and vegetables. Fruit and vegetable juices are nutrient-rich beverage choices that provide an array of essential vitamins, minerals and protective phytochemicals. Available as single juices, blended or exotic, some juices are also fortified with calcium, fiber and vitamins. Look for 100% pure juice or offer fresh juices and 100% juice combinations. Tomato and vegetable juices are generally lower in calories and higher in nutrients than most fruit juices. Although 100% fruit juice is a good choice, it should be limited to 1 cup per day so that most fruit eaten is whole or cut fruit that retains fiber and other protective substences that are removed when the fruit is juiced.

Citrus, berry, melon and tropical fruit juices are generally rich in vitamins and phytochemicals. Apple and white grape juices are not as high in many nutrients and are more likely to be fortified with added nutrients. Several fruit juices, including orange juice, can be fortified with calcium and are very useful ways for meeting the calcium and vitamin D needs of vegans and lactose-intolerant people. Some juices are fortified with fiber from fruit pulp to replace or exceed the dietary fiber removed when the fruit was juiced. Certainly, whole fruits are richer in fiber than most juices, but fruit juices are a good way to boost fruit and vegetable intake.

Commercial fruit drinks are made with water and fruit juices and are often sweetened with high-fructose corn syrup. They can be lightly carbonated. Some fruit drinks are only 10% fruit juice and are high in calories from sugar but low in nutrients. Because of the added sugar, these juices should be limited in keeping with the *Dietary Guidelines* recommendation to reduce solid fats and added sugars. Fruit drinks made with some fruit juice and carbonated or mineral water with little or no sugar added for flavor are healthier alternatives.

Fruit Smoothies

Smoothies can make a healthy snack or light meal and, when made with the right ingredients, can add valuable nutrients to the diet. Blended and chilled, smoothies can be made from fresh, frozen or canned fruit or vegetables. Smoothies often include ice, yogurt, frozen yogurt or milk. They have a milkshake-like consistency but unlike milkshakes, they usually don't contain ice cream. Many fruit smoothies are combinations of fruits with no dairy component.

Some popular smoothie flavors include:

- Avocado-mango
- Banana, coconut and mango
- Mixed berry
- Carrot-pineapple
- Cherry-almond
- Frosty pine-orange yogurt
- Grape and green tea
- Mango yogurt
- Blueberry-banana
- Sunshine lemon
- Sweet basil
- Vanilla-banana almond

Visit www.3aday.org for creative smoothie recipes.

Coconut Water

Coconut water is one of the fastest-growing new beverages in the United States. Food manufacturers have added it to fruit juices, yogurt, sports drinks and sorbets. Not to be confused with **coconut milk**, which is derived from the meat of mature coconuts, coconut water is the clear liquid found in young coconuts. **Coconut cream** is similar to coconut milk but is made with a higher ratio of coconut to water.

Research on the health benefits of coconut water is limited, and recent claims cannot be substantiated. Compared to many other beverages, however, coconut water can be a healthier option. Like all plant-based foods or beverages, coconut water contains phytochemicals as well as minerals and vitamins. Because it contains electrolytes and minerals, coconut water is often marketed as a sports drink. One cup of coconut water has only 46 calories (less than many other popular beverages) and 9 grams of carbohydrate. It is a good source of fiber, potassium, magnesium and vitamin C. The drawback to coconut water, however, is that it's high in sodium: 252 milligrams per cup.

Soft Drinks

For many Americans, **soft drinks** – called soda pop in some parts of the United States – are a popular beverage. There are hundreds of flavors, sweetening ingredients and levels of sweetness. Soft drinks come in regular, diet, caffeinated and caffeine-free varieties. Some people drink soda pop instead of morning coffee.

While diet soft drinks do not add pounds directly, drinking calorie-free, sweetened beverages alters brain chemistry to seek more sweets. In addition, diet drinks generally replace more nutrient-rich options.

Most regular soft drinks are low in nutrients and high in calories and sugar from high-fructose corn syrup or cane sugar. Regular soft drinks are like liquid candy, often with added chemicals, artificial colors and flavors. Few Americans need these extra calories. By some estimates, 37% of total daily liquid

Functional Beverages

Functional beverages are drinks enhanced with added ingredients to provide specific health benefits beyond general nutrition. Popular ingredients include caffeine, green tea, guarana yerba maté, vitamin C, ginger and ginkgo biloba.

- **Energy drinks** evolved from juice-bar drinks. They are intended to improve stamina and are usually high in carbohydrates and often have caffeine and nutrients added.

- **Sports drinks** are designed to replace fluids lost during physical activity. They are generally high in sodium and potassium.

- **Smart drinks** may contain amino acids and are often herb based. They provide energy with stimulants (often caffeine) without impairing motor functions. There is little scientific evidence supporting increased performance or tied to smart drinks.

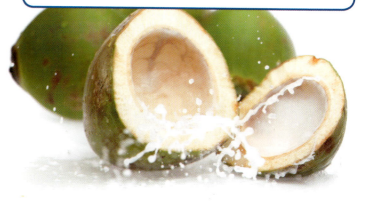

calories come from sugar-sweetened drinks, and consumers don't reduce their food intake when they drink calories from soda and other beverages. [5] Children who consume soft drinks can become accustomed to very sweet flavors, which can cause them to cut back on nutrient-rich beverages such as milk, juice and water. While an occasional soft drink is okay, children should not drink soft drinks regularly. Providing healthful beverages on menus for children is an opportunity for menu development.

Alcoholic Beverages

Unlike other foods for which absorption begins in the small intestine, alcohol is absorbed quickly into the bloodstream through the lining of the stomach and the first part of the intestine. Foods that contain protein or fat slow the absorption and effects of alcohol. Sparkling wines and carbonated mixers stimulate the digestive tract and accelerate alcohol absorption. Once absorbed, 2% to 10% of alcohol is eliminated through the kidneys and lungs; the rest is broken down in the liver. It takes the body about an hour to eliminate 1 ounce of alcohol. Consequently, blood alcohol levels increase steadily when more than 1 drink per hour is consumed.

The health effects of alcohol can be beneficial or harmful, depending on the amount consumed and the age and other characteristics of the drinker. Children, adolescents, and pregnant and nursing women should not drink beverages or eat foods containing alcohol. For people who cannot restrict their alcohol intake, no amount of alcohol is ever safe. People taking medications that interact with alcohol and those who have certain medical conditions should drink alcohol only with the advice of their doctor.

Diners also may choose to avoid alcohol for personal or religious reasons. Thus, any foods containing alcohol should be clearly identified, and beverages without alcohol should be readily available.

Hazards of excessive alcohol consumption include increased risk of liver cirrhosis, cancers of the upper gastrointestinal tract, injury, violence and death. Drinking too much alcohol can raise the levels of triglycerides in the blood and can lead to high blood pressure and heart failure. Consuming too many calories from alcohol can lead to obesity and a higher risk of developing diabetes. Excessive drinking and binge drinking can lead to stroke. Other serious alcohol-related problems include fetal alcohol syndrome and increased risk of birth defects, cardiac arrhythmia and sudden cardiac death.

Beverages containing alcohol supply calories but few essential nutrients. Each gram of alcohol provides 7 calories, almost twice the number of calories in a gram of protein or carbohydrate. Although consuming 1 to 2 drinks per day is not associated with increased nutrient deficiency, heavy drinkers

A Drink Is a Drink Is a Drink

One drink is considered 1.5 ounces of 80-proof liquor or 1 ounce of 100-proof, 12 ounces of beer (5% alcohol), or 5 ounces of wine (12% alcohol). Each of these beverages contains about 1 ounce of pure alcohol per serving. These are quite modest portions and many "single" orders, or drinks, are equivalent to 2 servings of alcohol, especially when drinks are served in oversized glasses.

may be at risk for malnutrition if the calories derived from alcohol are substituted for those from nutrient-rich foods.

Current research suggests that **moderate drinking** – 1 drink for women per day or 2 drinks for men per day – does not endanger health and may promote it. These amounts are primarily based on two assumptions: size and weight (assuming men are larger and have more muscle mass) and the fact that men metabolize alcohol more quickly and efficiently than women. Women metabolize alcohol more slowly than men because they produce less alcohol dehydrogenase, which is an enzyme that breaks down alcohol and helps remove its toxic byproducts from the body. [6]

The National Cancer Institute reports an elevated risk of breast cancer for women who drink alcohol and theorizes that alcohol affects the hormonal levels of older women. Women who drink moderate amounts of alcohol, however, had fewer other cancers, heart disease, stroke, hip fractures and dementia than non-drinkers. [6]

Alcohol and Calories

In mixed drinks, wine and beer, most calories come from the alcohol, but some calories also come from carbohydrates in the grain or fruit used to make the alcohol. When meal planning is done and certain percentages of carbohydrate, protein and fat are recommended, there is usually no provision for additional calories from alcohol because it is not an essential nutrient. When controlling calories, it is important to reduce calories from added sugars and fats in the diet. If a person eats the same amount and adds alcohol-containing beverages, the result will be weight gain. One or 2 drinks each day may be why some people have trouble managing their weight. Care should be taken to reduce added sugars and fats and not skip foods rich in nutrients.

Calories in Alcoholic Beverages

Beverage	Portion	Calories
Beer	12 ounces	150 calories
Light beer	12 ounces	100 calories
White wine	5 ounces	115 calories
Red wine	5 ounces	110 calories
Liquor	1.25 ounces	80 calories

What Is Moderation?

The *Dietary Guidelines* define moderate consumption as 1 drink per day for women and 2 drinks per day for men. Research suggests that this amount provides the most beneficial health effects; greater amounts may increase particular health risks.

Moderate consumption of beer, wine or spirits may have beneficial health effects in some individuals. The pattern of drinking is also important. One or 2 drinks a day maximizes the benefits and minimizes the adverse effects of alcohol. But "saving up" to have 7 or 14 drinks in one or two nights is not a viable option. Binge drinking maximizes the adverse effects and eliminates the positive effects of alcohol consumption.

Over the past several decades, many studies have been published in research journals about how drinking alcohol may be associated with reduced mortality from heart disease. Several studies have shown that moderate amounts of alcohol increase HDL (good) cholesterol. Other studies indicate that drinking moderately lowers risk of dementia and loss of cognitive function in aging adults.

Wine

The health benefits of wine, particularly red wine, have been extolled in the popular press. Evidence continues to mount that regular, moderate wine consumption (1 to 2 glasses daily) helps prevent or delay heart disease, type 2 diabetes, dementia, rheumatoid arthritis and osteoporosis. In the Mediterranean Diet, wine is regularly consumed with meals.

Wine contains the phytochemical ***resveratrol***, which became a household word in 1991 when a *60 Minutes* segment about the French Paradox described it as not only healthful but also a powerful anti-aging agent. Resveratrol, first isolated in the 1960s by Japanese scientists, is the most studied of the phytochemicals known as polyphenols. The compound functions as a plant's defense against damage from bacteria and fungi. It is being studied in clinical trials as a medication, but findings are not yet available. Resveratrol may prevent platelets in the blood from sticking together, which may reduce clot formation and the risk of heart attack and stroke. It also may play a role in reducing LDL cholesterol and slowing the aging process.

Resveratrol is found in the skins of grapes and other fruits. Red wines and red/purple grape juice have more resveratrol than white wine because they are exposed to grape skins for a longer time during fermentation. Red wine and dark grape juices contain many other polyphenols. For example, some researchers believe that polyphenols in the coating of grape seeds are even more potent than resveratrol. Researchers are not sure which of the compounds in red wine provide health benefits but generally agree that a combination of substances in red wine

Wine Headaches

Most people think it is the sulfites in wine that can cause headaches. An allergic reaction to sulfites, however, usually involves breathing trouble and rashes, not headaches.

Sulfites are found not only in wine but also in foods such as dried fruits, baked goods and pickled vegetables. A serving of dried apricots contains almost 10 times the amount of sulfites in a serving of wine.

Research indicates that **tyramine** is the active substance in wine that causes the dilation and contraction of blood vessels that result in headaches. Tyramine is an amino acid by-product produced during fermentation. It is suspected for triggering migraines in up to about 40% of the migraine population. Wine contains several different tyramine compounds. Younger and unfiltered wines contain higher amounts.

Source: The National Headache Foundation, www.headaches.org

provides health benefits. Concord or red grape juice and cherry juice provide similar health benefits.

Red wine also contains the phytochemical **quercetin**, an anti-inflammatory found in fruit and vegetable skins. Quercetin also has antiviral effects that help the body resist flu, infections and lung inflammation and inhibit growth of prostate cancer. [6] More information on phytochemicals is found in Chapter 7.

Beer

Some studies indicate that beer may have the same health benefits as wine. Ales, lagers and stouts in modest amounts (1 glass per day) may reduce the risk of heart attack and stroke, probably because of the presence of phytochemicals known as polyphenols (see Chapter 7). Low-alcohol and non-alcohol beers seem to offer the same heart-protective effects as regular beer. In modest amounts, beer has a relaxing effect on the body, improves blood circulation, reduces stress and promotes urination.

While most calories in beer come from alcohol, beer also contains carbohydrates – about 1 gram per ounce of beer. A 12-ounce glass of beer contains about 150 calories and 13 grams of carbohydrate. Beer also contains some folate, magnesium, niacin and potassium.

In cooking, beer can be used as a marinade to flavor and tenderize meat. It can be used in the batter for some fried foods and, like wine, can be added to gravies or sauces to boost flavor. Beer also can be used in the steaming liquid for sausages and shellfish. Malty beers add a sweet, slightly nutty taste, while lagers add a bitter or herbal flavor. Avoid cooking with beer if food is served to children, pregnant women, or people with alcoholism, liver disease or gout. In excess, beer contributes to all health problems associated with excessive alcohol and/or calorie consumption. Individuals with diabetes should follow their doctor's advice about drinking beer, wine or other alcohol-containing beverages.

Cooking with Alcohol

Like salt, alcohol brings out the flavor of foods and improves flavor perception. In very small amounts, alcohol molecules are volatile and evaporate rapidly. This is why a splash of brandy or liqueur on fruit brings the fruit's aroma to the nostrils and enhances enjoyment. Alcohol also has a unique ability to bond with both fat and water molecules; some alcohol in a marinade will help the marinade and its aromatics permeate the food. When deglazing a pan with wine after searing meat, the browned bits dissolve in the wine and add additional flavor and aroma to a sauce. Other liquids used to deglaze do not offer the same flavor intensity. With almost any use of alcohol in cooking, small amounts of alcohol will create the desired effect. Larger amounts overwhelm flavors and can create unpleasant aromas.

A common misconception is that when alcoholic beverages are used in cooking the alcohol disappears because of the heat. This is not true. Only some alcohol burns away. The amount remaining depends on the temperature and length of cooking. It is important that alcohol not be in foods of people who, for various reasons, should not drink alcohol. If a food contains alcohol, that fact should be in the menu description or mentioned by servers to inform guests who may not want to consume alcohol for religious, health or other reasons.

The amount of alcohol that remains after cooking is listed on the following table.

Preparation	Remaining Alcohol
Immediate consumption	100%
Overnight storage	70%
Stirred into a hot liquid	85%
Flamed	75%

After baking/simmering:
   15 minutes
   30 minutes
   1 hour
   1.5 hour
   2 hours
   2.5 hours
	
	40%
	35%
	25%
	20%
	10%
	5%

Source: USDA Table of Nutrient Retention Factors, Release 6, www.ars.usda.gov/SP2UserFiles/Place/12354500/Data/retn/retn06.pdf

A Word from the Chef
In Your Own Backyard

Phil Papineau, assistant professor in hospitality and service management at the Culinary Institute of America (CIA) in Hyde Park, New York, was instrumental in launching the CIA's award-winning St. Andrew's Café in the late 1980s. St. Andrew's was a trailblazer in healthful fine dining. It continues today as a farm-to-table showcase and a leader in the growing terroir movement; that is, making full use of whatever products are grown in the vicinity in the belief that ecology and social environment shape a food's character – or as Phil sums it up, "Foods produced in an area naturally go with other foods and beverages produced in the same area. In other words, foods that grow together go together."

St. Andrew's Café serves wine and beer and also offers an array of fruit beverages and ciders. "The Hudson River Valley is rich in apples and pears," Phil says. "We use juice products from a radius of about 60 miles. Juices are excellent mixed with sparkling wine or water. We also make no-alcohol mimosas and Bellinis using purees of whole fruit. St Andrew's has offered a local pear wine as well."

In addition, St. Andrew's serves local craft beers. "Craft ales and lagers are flavorful and lower in alcohol than mainstream brews," Phil explains. "They are great with food. We also offer our guests the option of ordering smaller portions of wine rather than a full glass. We try to select wines from biodynamic vineyards." The most advanced form of organic farming, biodynamics, uses the cycles of nature to grow grapes and uses plants and animals to take the place of chemicals and fertilizers – for example, dogs to sniff out diseases and bugs.

"If you know the farm, you know the food," Phil notes. "People are concerned about food safety these days and like the idea of their food not traveling hundreds of miles to get to their plate. And buying local supports the small businesses that are the backbone of the economy. That's good for everyone."

casebycase
'Drink Like You Eat!'

Like his innovative cocktails, Adam Seger, mixologist for IPic Entertainment and founder/creator of Hum Spirits Company, is an unusual combination. As a certified culinary professional and a mixologist, Adam is in the vanguard of a movement stretching the boundaries of the kitchen into the bar.

Having coined the slogan "Drink like you eat," Adam says some of his more unexpected ingredients include roasted West Indian pumpkin puree for a seasonal calabaza eggnog and Iberico ham and manchego cheese infused into Spanish brandy.

Adam personally sources produce from local farmers and has his own bar herb garden at IPic Entertainment's Tanzy Artisanal Italian in Boca Raton, Florida. He uses herbs and local produce to create seasonal drinks in much the same way a chef creates seasonal menus.

Adam seeks out artisan products such as single-farm Michigan sour cherries for his homemade maraschinos and creates his own syrups, including a hot and sweet habanera ginger syrup used in his daiquiris and mojitos. He also makes his own bitters, liqueurs and sweet vermouth. "Use the best ingredients you can afford/obtain, have fun working with them, and cook and mix with love," Adam advises.

Inspired by Paul Prudhomme, from whom he learned to cook by watching television, Seger has introduced his branded bitters, cordials and spirits to market just like chefs bring their branded foods to consumers.

Cucumber Lemon Refresher

Serves: 10

This refreshing beverage can be kept in the cooler both for staff working in the hot kitchen and for guests. It is especially nice served with fresh seafood salads.

Cucumber slices, ⅛ inch thick.	20	each
Lemon slices, ⅛ inch thick.	10	each
Water, hot.	3	quarts

1. Put cucumber, lemon and hot water in a large pitcher or gallon container. Chill overnight or at least 8 hours.
2. Serve cold.

Per Serving

Calories	5	Cholesterol	0	mg
Fat	0 g	Sodium	10	mg
Saturated Fat	0 g	Carbohydrates	1	mg
Trans Fat	0 g	Dietary Fiber	0	mg
Sugar	0 g	Protein	0	g

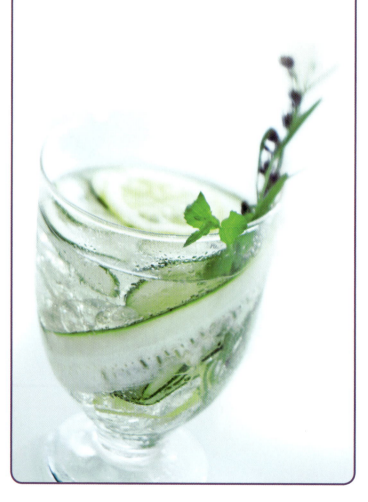

Opportunities for Chefs

Whether it's tap water or bottled sparkling water, fountain drinks or artisanal sodas, "mocktails" or sophisticated beer, wine and cocktails, there should something for everyone on a comprehensive and creative beverage menu. Menus for both children and adults should include fat-free and low-fat dairy options and 100% fruit or vegetable juices should be available. Intakes of both low-fat dairy products and vegetables and fruits are too low in the diets of most Americans. Calorie-free beverages can help meet needs for water without adding sugar or calories.

Learning Activities

1. Conduct a water tasting with various still and sparkling waters. Compare appearance, aroma, taste and mouthfeel.
2. Develop a non-alcoholic beverage menu with selections appropriate for children and adults.
3. Compare labels of three products from each of the following two categories: artisanal sodas and traditional soft drinks.
4. Compare recommended beverage serving sizes with actual serving sizes in a local restaurant or bar.

For More Information

- Bottled Water Basics, Environmental Protection Agency, www.epa.gov/safewater/faq/pdfs/fs_healthseries_bottlewater.pdf

- International Bottled Water Association, www.bottledwater.org

- Preston-Campbell B. *Cool Waters: 50 Refreshing, Healthy, Homemade Thirst Quenchers*. Harvard Common Press: Boston; 2009.

- Safe Drinking Water Hotline, Environmental Protection Agency, 800-426-4791

- Water on Tap, What you need to know, Environmental Protection Agency, www.epa.gov/safewater/wot/pdfs/book_waterontap_full.pdf

CHAPTER 7

Vitamins, Minerals and Phytochemicals

LEARNING OBJECTIVES

After completing this chapter, you should be able to:

- Explain the roles vitamins play in growth and good health
- List and describe the general functions and food sources of fat-soluble vitamins and water-soluble vitamins
- List and describe the functions and food sources of major minerals
- List nutrients of concern that many Americans lack in their diets and foods that are the best sources of these vitamins and minerals
- Identify diseases caused by specific vitamin and mineral deficiencies
- Give tips to ensure that vitamin and mineral intake are sufficient
- Explain what phytochemicals are and give examples
- Identify cooking techniques that promote retention of nutrients and those that cause nutrient loss from foods

Unlike the macronutrients (protein, fat and carbohydrates), vitamins and minerals do not provide energy to fuel the body. Even though the body's need for vitamins and minerals is small enough to be measured in milligrams (1/1000th of a gram) or micrograms (1/1000th of a milligram), these nutrients are vital to maintaining good health.

Thirteen **vitamins** are essential nutrients because they have specific biological functions in the human body and must be obtained through food, either because they are not made in the body or because the body does not make a sufficient amount. All vitamins are organic compounds with carbon in their chemical structure. In some cases, foods provide precursors that are converted in the body to the active form of the vitamin. Absence of a vitamin in the diet causes a specific deficiency disease.

Many minerals exist in nature; 15 of them are considered essential nutrients that must be obtained from food. Unlike vitamins, **minerals** are inorganic substances with no carbon molecules in their chemical structure. Different minerals have different biological functions – for example, as components of body cells, as regulators of metabolic reactions, for growth and development, to produce enzymes and hormones, and to protect cells from damage.

Phytochemicals, also called phytonutrients, are not essential nutrients. They are compounds with biological activity that aid cellular functioning and often protect cells from damage. Their presence in the diet is protective, but specific phytochemicals do not meet the criteria to be essential nutrients. They are discussed in this chapter because, like vitamins and minerals, many phytochemicals work at the cellular level to promote health and reduce risk of disease.

The body of knowledge concerning vitamins and minerals is fairly new, and the science behind phytochemicals is even newer. Our understanding of the delicate balance of vitamins, minerals and phytochemicals and the interaction of all nutrients is becoming clearer each year as research is conducted and reported in medical journals.

Americans consume significantly fewer vegetables, fruits, whole grains, milk and dairy products, and seafood than recommended. These foods provide key nutrients. Consequently American diets are lacking in some nutrients and this is a public health concern. The *Dietary Guidelines for Americans 2010* identifies potassium, dietary fiber, calcium and vitamin D as nutrients of concern. In addition, intake of iron, folate and vitamin B_{12} is of concern for specific population groups. It is recommended that everyone reduce intake of one mineral – sodium. [1]

While all nutrients have important functions, many are easily provided by diets most Americans eat. When a goal is providing healthful foods, increased focus on foods that provide the nutrients most likely to be lacking is a good strategy. This book provides information on many vitamins and minerals so that chefs will have an easy reference as to functions and food sources. Focus should be given to key nutrients, often those that have been identified as nutrients of concern.

Because this book is not intended as a comprehensive medical or nutrition text, it does not provide detailed information about biochemistry, physiology and medical nutrition therapy. That knowledge falls within the purview of the registered dietitian and/or nutrition scientist and is available in nutrition texts and on reputable Internet sites. Chefs and culinary professionals generally do not need to know the specific recommended milligrams or micrograms of particular vitamins or minerals but should know the general functions and best food sources for major vitamins, minerals and phytochemicals.

For vitamins and minerals the Daily Value (the amount designated for food labels) and the DRI (amount recommended for daily intake) for men and women are listed for a point of reference. The foods with the highest amounts of nutrients are on the top of the lists that follow. This knowledge will help guide ingredient selection. With few exceptions, a well-balanced and varied diet can provide all the vitamins and minerals a person needs, without adding supplements. Keep in mind that while providing a wide variety of foods makes vitamins, minerals and phytochemicals available, food storage and cooking techniques affect the final nutrient composition of any food served.

Nutrients of Concern

Because many Americans consume large amounts of *empty-calorie food* (food with calories but few nutrients), getting adequate amounts of essential vitamins and minerals can be a challenge. It is important to select nutrient-dense or nutrient-rich foods. *Nutrient-dense foods* provide vitamins, minerals and other substances that have positive health effects, with relatively few calories. They are lean or low in solid fats, added sugars and sodium.

According to the *Dietary Guidelines for Americans*, intake levels of certain nutrients are of concern for specific groups. Four under-consumed nutrients of public health concern are vitamin D, calcium, potassium and dietary fiber. These four shortfall nutrients are clearly linked to nutrient inadequacy and disease prevention.

Additional shortfall nutrients include vitamins A, C, D, E; choline, magnesium and phosphorus; iron and folate for women of childbearing age; and vitamin B12 for people over age 50. Energy-dense forms of foods, especially foods high in solid fats, sodium and added sugars should be replaced with nutrient-dense forms of vegetables, fruits, whole grains and fluid milk and milk products to increase intakes of shortfall nutrients and nutrients of concern.

Estimated Percentages of Americans with Adequate Nutrient Intakes

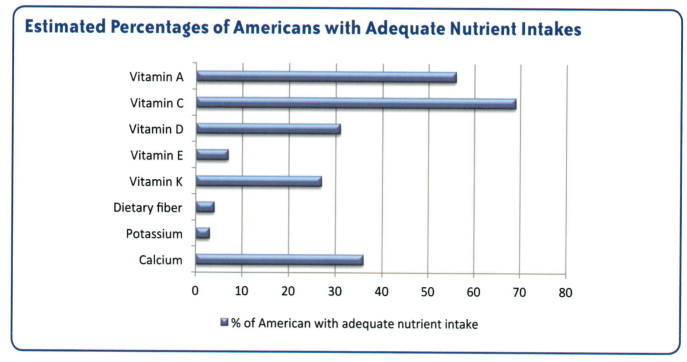

■ % of American with adequate nutrient intake

Sources: Moshfegh A, Goldman J, Cleveland L. *What We Eat in America, NHANES 2001-2002: Usual Nutrient Intakes from Food Compared to Dietary Reference Intakes*. U.S. Department of Agriculture, Agricultural Research Service. 2005, www.ars.usda.gov/ba/bhnrc/fsrg

Moshfegh A, Goldman J, Ahuja J, Rhodes D, LaComb R. *What We Eat in America, NHANES 2005-2006: Usual Nutrient Intakes from Food and Water compared to 1997 Dietary Reference Intakes for Vitamin D, Calcium, Phosphorus and Magnesium*. U.S. Department of Agriculture, Agricultural Research Service. 2009, www.ars.usda.gov/SP2UserFiles/Place/12355000/pdf/0506/usual_nutrient_intake_vitD_ca_phos_mg_2005-06.pdf

Interpreting Nutrient Source Lists

On lists of "excellent" or "good" food sources of specific nutrients, the foods that are considered best sources are found at the top. Some lists provide the grams, milligrams or micrograms for a standard measure of food as typically consumed – for example, 1 cup or 2 tablespoons. When a range is given, such as for the milligrams of a nutrient in ready-to-eat cereal, it is because different brands are fortified at different levels. Other formats list nutrients per 100 grams of food, regardless of the type of food. But some foods that seem to be excellent sources of a particular nutrient per 100 grams might have to be consumed in an unrealistic portion in order to truly qualify as an "excellent source."

For example, 100 grams (3 ½ ounces) of skim milk is less than ½ cup, but 100 grams of cinnamon equals 14 tablespoons. Based on a 100-gram portion, the cinnamon would rank as a terrific source of calcium, providing 1,002 milligrams. The 100 grams of milk provides only 125 milligrams of calcium. The reality is, however, that while one would be very likely to drink 1 cup of skim milk (providing 300 milligrams of calcium), one would eat only a pinch of cinnamon (containing about 5 milligrams of calcium) in a single portion of food. The lesson: Consider the appropriate portion when comparing food sources of any nutrient.

Where to Find Nutrient Content Information

- USDA National Nutrient Database for Standard Reference, www.ndb.nal.usda.gov contains reports on foods by description or food sources by individual nutrients; free of charge

- Commercial nutrient databases

- Bowes & Church's *Food Values of Portions Commonly Used*, 19th edition, or a similar resource book

- The Nutrition Facts portion of the food label, including the percent Daily Value information

- Nutrient information from food manufacturers, distributors or trade organizations

- Smartphone applications that provide nutrient data

Vitamins

Vitamins are essential organic (carbon-containing) substances that the body needs in small amounts. Vitamins facilitate the processes by which other nutrients are digested, absorbed, metabolized or built into body structures.

The absence of a vitamin may cause a nutrient deficiency. Symptoms of that deficiency go away when the vitamin is consumed. For example, inadequate vitamin C causes bleeding gums and easy bruising, which are the initial symptoms of scurvy. When a person with scurvy eats citrus fruits or other foods containing vitamin C, deficiency symptoms stop.

Vitamin Deficiency Diseases

One of the criteria to be a vitamin is that the absence of that substance causes a specific deficiency disease. What are those diseases?

Vitamin C	Scurvy
Vitamin A	Night blindness
Vitamin D	Rickets, osteomalacia
Vitamin E	Hemolytic anemia in infants
Vitamin K	Bleeding
Thiamin	Beriberi, Werneke-Korsakoff Syndrome
Riboflavin	Ariboflavinosis
Niacin	Pellegra
Pantothenic Acid	Parasthesia
Vitamin B$_6$	Anemia, neuropathy
Biotin	Dermatitis, enteritis
Vitamin B$_{12}$	Megaloblastic anemia
Folate	Birth and neural tube defects

There are two categories of vitamins: fat-soluble (A, D, E and K) and water-soluble (thiamin, riboflavin, niacin, folate, vitamin B$_{12}$, vitamin B$_6$, biotin, pantothenic acid and vitamin C).

Fat-Soluble Vitamins

Fat-soluble vitamins are carried in lipids or fats and are stored in fatty tissue and in the liver. They can reach toxic levels if taken in excess over time.

Vitamin A

Vitamin A is an antioxidant and plays important roles in vision, bone and tooth growth, reproduction, cell functions, and the immune system. The active form of vitamin A, *retinol*, is found in animal foods such as liver, egg yolks and dairy products. There are several precursors to retinol; the most active is beta-carotene (12 micrograms of beta-carotene equal 1 microgram or 1 RAE of retinol). *Beta-carotene*, which is converted to vitamin A in the intestine, is a pigment found in fruits and vegetables that are bright orange, yellow and dark green. Beta-carotene's color makes it easy to identify foods high in vitamin A. Because beta-carotene and other vitamin A precursors, known as carotenoids, do not have the same biologic activity as retinols, they must be mathematically converted to retinol activity equivalents (RAE) and international units (IU), an older measurement used in many food composition tables. Human need for vitamin A also is expressed in retinol equivalents (RE).

Inadequate vitamin A intake causes changes in eye tissues that can result in vision problems and blindness as well as changes in the cells that protect organs and skin and act as barriers to bacteria and viruses. Excessive vitamin A over a prolonged period of time can be toxic, causing hair loss, bone pain, fatigue, dry cracked skin, liver damage, high blood pressure, bleeding gums and birth defects. According to recent national consumption studies, more than half of Americans do not consume the recommended daily dietary requirement of vitamin A. Adding more fruits and vegetables to menus is one way to provide vitamins and minerals while controlling calories and is a major recommendation of the *Dietary Guidelines for Americans*. [1]

Vitamin A

Measure	Population	Amount
Daily Value		5,000 international units (IU)
Dietary Reference Intakes (DRI)	Men, ages 14 and above Women, ages 14 and above	900 micrograms RAE 700 micrograms RAE

Note: The Daily Value (DV) was last updated in 1995 when the common measurement for Vitamin A was in international units (IU). The Dietary Reference Intakes (DRI), from the Institute of Medicine, uses retinol activity equivalents (RAE), which is the most recent international standard for measuring vitamin A.

Best Sources of Vitamin A

Deep green and orange vegetables and liver are the best sources.

Food	Serving	Vitamin A (IU)	Vitamin A - RAE (micrograms)
Carrot juice	1 cup	45,133	2,256
Pumpkin, canned	1 cup	38,129	1,906
Sweet potato, cooked	1 potato	28,058	1,403
Carrots, cooked	1 cup	26,571	1,329
Beef liver, cooked	3 ounces	22,175	6,582
Spinach, cooked	1 cup	18,666	1,146
Carrots, raw	1 cup	18,377	919
Kale, cooked	1 cup	17,707	885
Turnip greens, cooked	1 cup	17,655	882
Collards, cooked	1 cup	15,417	771
Chicken liver, cooked	3 ounces	11,329	3,315
Mustard greens, cooked	1 cup	8,852	442
Braunschweiger	2 slices	7,967	2,393
Dandelion greens, cooked	1 cup	7,179	359
Melons, cantaloupe	1 cup	5,411	270
Lettuce, cos or romaine	1 cup	4,878	244
Peppers, sweet, red, raw	1 cup	4,665	234
Lettuce, green leaf, raw	1 cup	4,147	207
Vegetable juice cocktail	1 cup	3,770	189
Papayas	1	3,326	167
Lettuce, butterhead (Boston and bibb types)	1 cup	1,782	93
Cheese, ricotta, whole milk	1 cup	1,095	295
Eggs	2 each	658	178
Milk, nonfat, low-fat, whole, buttermilk	1 cup	500	149
Cereal, ready-to-eat	1 cup	500 - 990	90 - 297

Source: U.S. Department of Agriculture, Agricultural Research Service. 2011. USDA National Nutrient Database for Standard Reference, Release 24. Nutrient Data Laboratory Home Page, www.ars.usda.gov/ba/bhnrc/ndl

A Word from the Chef
Ingredient No. 1: Seasonal, Fresh and Local

"Since the 1970s," notes Sante Fe, New Mexico-based chef, author and educator Deborah Madison, "every decade has had its token vegetarian menu item. In the '70s, it was fat-laden eggplant Parmesan; in the '80s, it was pasta primavera, which usually had little to do with spring vegetables; and in the '90s, it was the ubiquitous Portobello mushroom." Thanks in no small part to Deborah, the multi-award-winning author of 12 books about the glory of local produce, fruits and vegetables are no longer relegated to the side dish, the salad and the single vegetarian menu choice. Her latest book, *Vegetable Literacy*, explores 11 plant families and their edible members that are common in our kitchens.

Seasonality and local sourcing are at the heart of Deborah's approach to food. "Whether you call it fresh or local or seasonal, the concept is the same – fruit and vegetables that have not traveled long distances and have not been stored for long periods of time," she explains. "It's only recently that we have had everything available all the time, but we take this variety for granted. The fact is," she continues, "you can eat seasonally and locally all year – even in the winter. It won't be what you are used to, but it can be done if you rely on local farmers."

Local farmers' traditional planting and growing practices also offer a solution to a problem Deborah refers to as the "elephant in the room" – tired soil. "Plants are only as good as the soil they are grown in," she says. "Plants developed for 'big agriculture' have been hybridized to be in the ground less time than usual in soil that has become little more than planting medium. Fed with fertilizer and watered on demand, they don't develop good, deep roots to absorb nutrients, and with repeated plantings, the soil is not given time to replenish itself."

Deborah notes that the pioneering farm-driven restaurant, Greens in San Francisco, where she was founding chef in the 1970s, was successful from the start in part because they structured their dishes on a meat-as-center-of-the-plate idea – but without the meat. "Our customers never felt like something was missing," Deborah recalls, "because there was always something to focus on, something that assumed the role of meat on the plate."

Looking toward the future, Deborah is concerned about the impact of uneven weather patterns on the food supply. "We have already seen the effect of drought on the price

Sweet Potato and Pineapple Salad

William Reynolds, former Provost, Washburne Culinary Institute, Chicago, Illinois

Yield: 8 cups
Serves: 10, ¾ cup each

This colorful and flavorful salad is a favorite at the restaurant of Washburne Culinary Institute in Chicago. It is a good side dish or accompaniment to chicken or roast pork, an excellent buffet item and good in box lunches.

Dressing:

Canola oil	¼	cup
Lemon juice, fresh	2	tablespoons
Cider vinegar	¼	cup
Salt	½	teaspoon
Pepper	¼	teaspoon
Sugar	1	tablespoon

Sweet potato, peeled, ½ inch dice	2	pounds
Celery, ¼ inch dice	4	ounces (¾ cup)
Red onion, ¼ inch dice	4	ounces (¾ cup)
Pineapple, ¼ inch dice	8	ounces (1 ½ cup)
Dates, chopped	3	ounces (½ cup)
Cashews, coarsely chopped	2	ounces (½ cup)

1. Combine all dressing ingredients and emulsify with a blender or stick blender.
2. Roast sweet potatoes at 350° F for about 30 minutes or until tender.
3. Combine warm potatoes, celery, red onion, pineapple, dates and cashews with dressing and mix gently. Cool before serving.

Per Serving

Calories	210	Cholesterol	0	mg
Fat	9 g	Sodium	190	mg
Saturated Fat	1 g	Carbohydrates	33	mg
Trans Fat	0 g	Dietary Fiber	4	mg
Sugar	14 g	Protein	3	g

of grain and corn and thus livestock," she says. "People are used to buying the most expensive cuts of meat because they are the fastest and easiest to prepare, but those on the economic margins may not be able to afford this anymore. As chefs," Deborah continues, "it's our responsibility to teach people how to choose and prepare alternatives, not only the tougher cuts of meat, but also – and especially – plant foods."

Vitamin D

Vitamin D (calciferol) acts like a hormone to help the body absorb and regulate calcium and phosphorus for strong bones, teeth and muscle. Vitamin D, especially the most active form, *D$_3$ (cholecalciferol),* may provide protection from osteoporosis, hypertension (high blood pressure), cancer and several autoimmune diseases. Vitamin D is also available as *D$_2$ (ergocalciferol).*

Vitamin D is made in the body when a cholesterol-like compound in skin is activated by ultraviolet light and converted to a precursor of vitamin D, which is then converted to its active form by enzymes of the liver and kidneys. People who have little exposure to sunlight because they keep their skin covered or who are seldom outside need more vitamin D in their diet. People who are lactose intolerant and avoid milk should seek non-dairy sources.

Vitamin D deficiency can contribute to fragile bones (osteoporosis), which is a major problem among older Americans, and *osteomalacia* (soft painful bones). Although uncommon in the United States, vitamin D deficiency in children causes soft bones resulting in *rickets*. Low levels of vitamin D in the body may increase the risk of breast, colon and prostate cancers; depressed mood, poor brain functions and more severe dementia in older adults; and bacterial infections and gum disease. There is a significant amount of current research related to vitamin D beyond the long-known functions of building bones and teeth. In great excess, vitamin D can be toxic, causing nausea, fatigue and calcium deposits in organs.

The mineral calcium needs vitamin D to form bone cells, which is why milk is fortified with vitamin D. In addition to fortified milk and cereals, food sources of vitamin D include fatty fish, egg yolks, butter, liver, shrimp and shiitake mushrooms. Cheese and yogurt are usually not fortified with vitamin D; be sure to check the label. One microgram of vitamin D$_3$ is equal to 40 IU (international units) of vitamin D.

Vitamin D

Measure	Population	Amount
Daily Value		400 international units (IU)
Dietary Reference Intakes (DRI)	Men, ages 9 to 70 Women, ages 9 to 70	15 micrograms 15 micrograms

Best Sources of Vitamin D

Fatty fish and fortified milk are the best sources of vitamin D.

Food	Serving		Vitamin D (IU)
Herring, pickled	3	ounces	1,384
Cod liver oil	1	tablespoon	1,350
Halibut, cooked	3	ounces	510
Catfish, cooked	3	ounces	425
Salmon, canned	3	ounces	390
Mackerel, cooked	3	ounces	306
Sardines, canned	1.75	ounces	250
Tuna, canned	3	ounces	200
Milk, nonfat, low-fat, whole, buttermilk	1	cup	100
Egg yolk	1	yolk	20
Beef liver, cooked	3	ounces	15
Orange juice, vitamin D fortified	½	cup	68
Butter	1	tablespoon	9
Cheddar cheese	1	ounce	7
Cereal, ready-to-eat	1	cup	0.6 - 2.9

Source: U.S. Department of Agriculture, Agricultural Research Service. 2011. USDA National Nutrient Database for Standard Reference, Release 24. Nutrient Data Laboratory Home Page, www.ars.usda.gov/ba/bhnrc/ndl

Vitamin E

Vitamin E (tocopherol) acts as an antioxidant in cell membranes and is especially important for the stability of cells that are constantly exposed to high levels of oxygen – particularly lung, brain and blood cells. Vitamin E protects the polyunsaturated fats and other fat-soluble substances in cells from cellular changes thought to contribute to cardio-vascular disease and cancer. Many Americans do not consume adequate vitamin E, which is found in plant foods. There is no evidence of toxicity from the consumption of vitamin E naturally occurring in foods. Toxicity is possible with supplements, causing bleeding problems. Vitamin E is destroyed by high heat.

Vitamin E

Measure	Population	Amount
Daily Value		30 international units (IU)
Dietary Reference Intakes (DRI)	Men, ages 14 and above Women, ages 14 and above	15 milligrams (mg) 15 milligrams (mg)

Best Sources of Vitamin E

All plant foods and salmon are the best sources of vitamin E.

Food	Serving	Vitamin E (IU)	Vitamin E alpha-tocopherol milligrams
Cereal, ready-to-eat	1 cup	2.33 - 28.17	1.26 - 13.5
Sunflower seeds	1 ounce	15.35	7.40
Almonds	1 ounce	11.08	7.43
Sunflower oil	1 tablespoon	8.32	5.59
Safflower oil	1 tablespoon	6.91	4.64
Hazelnuts	1 ounce	6.35	4.26
Spinach, steamed	1 cup	5.35	3.74
Wheat germ	2 tablespoons	4.50	2.28
Turnip greens	1 cup	4.03	2.71
Pumpkin, canned	1 cup	3.87	2.60
Canola oil	1 tablespoon	3.64	2.44
Peanuts	1 ounce	2.93	2.36
Olive oil	1 tablespoon	2.89	1.94
Mango	1 cup	2.75	1.85
Sweet red bell peppers	1 cup	2.17	2.35
Soybean oil	1 tablespoon	1.66	1.10
Sweet potatoes	1	1.21	1.47
Salmon, cooked	3 ounces	1.17	0.69
Avocado	1 ounce	0.89	0.56

Source: U.S. Department of Agriculture, Agricultural Research Service. 2011. USDA National Nutrient Database for Standard Reference, Release 24. Nutrient Data Laboratory Home Page, www.ars.usda.gov/ba/bhnrc/ndl

Vitamin K

Vitamin K (phylloquinone) is necessary to make the proteins involved in blood clotting and also works with vitamin D to help regulate blood calcium levels and form bone. Intestinal bacteria make about half the body's vitamin K; food provides the rest. Green leafy vegetables are a major source. Vitamin K deficiencies are rare. Antibiotics can reduce vitamin K synthesis, thus increasing dietary needs. Individuals on medication to reduce blood clotting may be instructed to avoid foods high in vitamin K.

Vitamin K

Measure	Population	Amount
Daily Value		80 micrograms (µg)
Dietary Reference Intakes (DRI)	Men, ages 19 and above Women, ages 19 and above	120 µg 90 µg

Best Sources of Vitamin K

Green leafy vegetables are the best sources.

Food	Serving	Vitamin K (µg)
Kale, cooked	1 cup	1062.1
Collards, cooked	1 cup	836.0
Spinach, cooked	1 cup	1027.3
Turnip greens, cooked	1 cup	530.0
Beet greens, cooked	1 cup	697.0
Dandelion greens, cooked	1 cup	579.0
Mustard greens, cooked	1 cup	419.3
Broccoli, cooked	1 cup	220.1
Brussels sprouts, cooked	1 cup	163.0
Cabbage, cooked	1 cup	163.1
Spinach, raw	1 cup	144.9
Asparagus, cooked	1 cup	91.0
Endive, raw	1 cup	115.5
Lettuce, green leaf, raw	1 cup	45.5
Broccoli, raw	1 cup	89.4
Lettuce, cos or romaine, raw	1 cup	48.2
Cabbage, raw	1 cup	67.6

Source: U.S. Department of Agriculture, Agricultural Research Service. 2011. USDA National Nutrient Database for Standard Reference, Release 24. Nutrient Data Laboratory Home Page, www.ars.usda.gov/ba/bhnrc/ndl

Water-Soluble Vitamins

Water-soluble vitamins – vitamin C and the B vitamins – should be consumed daily because they are not stored (except for some vitamin B_6 and B_{12}) and are lost through body fluids. Water-soluble vitamins are found in basic foods such as meat, grains, fruits and vegetables. They can be leached out of foods or easily destroyed by incorrect storage or preparation. Excess water-soluble vitamins are generally excreted in the urine, so toxicity from foods is rare. Significant excesses from supplements can be toxic for some B vitamins.

B Vitamins

B vitamins assist the body in making energy from food and help form red blood cells to heal wounds. They are also important for growth and development, proper nerve function and healthy skin, proper digestion, and a healthy appetite. B vitamins are found in proteins such as fish, poultry, meat, eggs and dairy products. Leafy green vegetables, beans and peas also have B vitamins. Many cereals and some breads have added B vitamins through enrichment or fortification. Not getting enough of certain B vitamins can cause deficiency diseases.

Thiamin, riboflavin and niacin are needed as coenzymes for energy metabolism to release energy from carbohydrates, proteins and fats at the cellular level. All three are needed for proper growth. Deficiencies of thiamin, riboflavin and niacin are rare in the United States because many breads and cereals are enriched with these vitamins along with iron and folacin. Alcoholism can create deficiencies, in part because of low food intake.

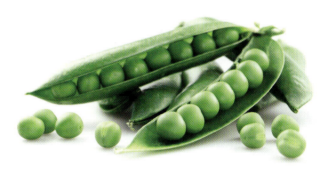

The B Vitamins

Common Names	Also known as
Thiamin	B_1
Riboflavin	B_2
Niacin	B_3
Pantothenic acid	B_5
B_6	Pyridoxine, pyridoxal and pyridoxamine
Biotin	B_7
B_{12}	Cobalamin
Folate	Folic acid and folacin

Thiamin

Thiamin, which is widely available in the diet, plays a critical role in the energy metabolism of all cells and in normal nerve and heart function. Thiamin is sensitive to heat and can be destroyed when food is cooked at temperatures higher than that of boiling water. Thiamin occurs in small amounts in many nutritious foods, especially lean pork and legumes, enriched, fortified or whole-grain products, bread and bread products, mixed foods whose main ingredient is grain, ready-to-eat cereals, and nuts.

Thiamin

Measure	Population	Amount
Daily Value		1.5 milligrams (mg)
Dietary Reference Intakes (DRI)	Men, ages 14 and above Women, ages 19 and above	1.2 mg 1.1 mg

Best Sources of Thiamin

Lean pork is the best source, but thiamin is provided by many food groups.

Food	Serving	Thiamin milligrams
Cereal, ready-to-eat	¾ cup	0.4 - 1.5
Pork loin, cooked	3 ounces	0.53
Ham, cooked	3 ounces	0.58
Edamame	1 cup	0.47
Acorn squash, baked	1 cup	0.34
Long grain white rice, enriched, cooked	1 cup	0.33
Peas, cooked	½ cup	0.21
Long grain brown rice, cooked	1 cup	0.19
Pecans	1 ounce	0.19
Brazil nuts	1 ounce	0.18
Lentils, cooked	½ cup	0.17
White bread, enriched	1 slice	0.11
Whole-wheat bread	1 slice	0.10

Source: U.S. Department of Agriculture, Agricultural Research Service. 2011. USDA National Nutrient Database for Standard Reference, Release 24. Nutrient Data Laboratory Home Page, www.ars.usda.gov/ba/bhnrc/ndl

Riboflavin

Riboflavin is essential for the metabolism of carbohydrates to produce energy and amino acids. It also helps keep mucous membranes (such as those lining the mouth) healthy. Milk and dairy products are major sources of riboflavin and organ meats such as liver are rich in riboflavin. Ultraviolet rays of the sun and fluorescent light can destroy riboflavin, which is why milk should be stored in cardboard or plastic containers in a dark refrigerator.

Riboflavin

Measure	Population	Amount
Daily Value		1.7 milligrams (mg)
Dietary Reference Intakes (DRI)	Men, ages 14 and above Women, ages 19 and above	1.3 mg 1.1 mg

Best Sources of Riboflavin

Food	Serving	Riboflavin milligrams
Beef liver, cooked	3 ounces	2.4
Cereal, ready-to-eat	1 cup	0.4 - 1.7
Chicken livers, cooked	3 ounces	1.7
Yogurt	1 cup	0.35
Milk, nonfat, low-fat, whole, buttermilk	1 cup	0.45
Almonds	1 ounce	0.29
Mushrooms, raw	1 cup	0.28
Edamame	1 cup	0.28
Egg	1 large	0.23
Pork loin, cooked	3 ounces	0.22
Spinach, cooked	½ cup	0.21

Source: U.S. Department of Agriculture, Agricultural Research Service. 2011. USDA National Nutrient Database for Standard Reference, Release 24. Nutrient Data Laboratory Home Page, www.ars.usda.gov/ba/bhnrc/ndl

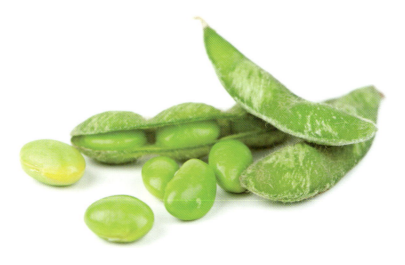

Niacin

Niacin is essential for the metabolism of carbohydrates, fats and many other substances in the body. Protein foods rich in **tryptophan** (an amino acid), such as dairy products, can compensate for not consuming enough niacin in the diet. The body can convert tryptophan to niacin; 60 milligrams of tryptophan can be converted to 1 milligram of niacin. Dietary needs for niacin are stated as niacin equivalents (NE), a measure that takes available tryptophan into account. When large amounts of nicotinic acid, a form of niacin, are taken as a medicine or supplement, itching, flushing, nausea, liver damage and high blood sugar levels can result.

Niacin

Measure	Population	Amount
Daily Value		20 milligrams (mg)
Dietary Reference Intakes (DRI)	Men, ages 14 and above Women, ages 14 and above	16 mg 14 mg

Best Sources of Niacin

Most protein foods provide niacin.

Food	Serving	Niacin milligrams
Beef liver, cooked	3 ounces	14.7
Chicken, light meat, cooked	3 ounces	11.7
Tuna, in water	3 ounces	11.3
Swordfish, cooked	3 ounces	7.9
Salmon, Chinook, cooked	3 ounces	8.5
Turkey, light meat, cooked	3 ounces	5.8
Cereal, ready-to-eat	1 cup	5 - 20
Pork chop, cooked	3 ounces	3.9
Peanuts	1 ounce	3.4
Mushrooms, cooked	½ cup	3.5
Baked potato	1	3.3
Beef, lean, cooked	3 ounces	3.1 - 7.2
Pasta, enriched	1 cup	2.3
Lentils, cooked	1 cup	2.1
Peanut butter	1 tablespoon	2.1

Source: U.S. Department of Agriculture, Agricultural Research Service. 2011. USDA National Nutrient Database for Standard Reference, Release 24. Nutrient Data Laboratory Home Page, www.ars.usda.gov/ba/bhnrc/ndl

Vitamin B₆

Vitamin B₆ (pyridoxine, pyridoxal and pyridoxamine) is part of a coenzyme necessary for metabolism of carbohydrates, fat and especially protein. The nervous and immune systems need vitamin B₆ to function efficiently; it is also needed to convert tryptophan to niacin. The body needs vitamin B₆ to make hemoglobin, which carries oxygen to tissues, and to help regulate blood sugar levels. A vitamin B₆ deficiency can result in a form of anemia that is similar to iron deficiency anemia.

Vitamin B₆

Measure	Population	Amount
Daily Value		2.0 milligrams (mg)
Dietary Reference Intakes (DRI)	Men, ages 14 to 50 Women, ages 19 to 50	1.3 mg 1.3 mg

Best Sources of Vitamin B₆

Food	Serving	Vitamin B₆ milligrams
Tuna, yellowfin, cooked	3 ounces	0.88
Beef liver, cooked	3 ounces	0.87
Potato, baked, with skin	3 ounces	0.70
Banana	1 large	0.5
Garbanzo beans, cooked	½ cup	0.53
Beef, sirloin, cooked	3 ounces	0.52
Chicken, light meat , cooked	3 ounces	0.51
Salmon, wild, cooked	3 ounces	0.48
Spinach, cooked	1 cup	0.44
Turkey, without skin	3 ounces	0.39
Beef, ground, broiled	3 ounces	0.33
Vegetable juice cocktail	6 ounces	0.26
Cereal, ready-to-eat	1 cup	0.5 - 2.5

Source: U.S. Department of Agriculture, Agricultural Research Service. 2011. USDA National Nutrient Database for Standard Reference, Release 24. Nutrient Data Laboratory Home Page, www.ars.usda.gov/ba/bhnrc/ndl

Pantothenic Acid, Biotin and Choline

The B vitamins **pantothenic acid** and **biotin** each act as coenzymes in metabolic processes. Both are available in a wide variety of commonly eaten foods. Deficiencies are uncommon, and toxicities have not been found. Bacteria within the intestine can make some biotin.

Choline was classified as an essential nutrient by the Food and Nutrition Board of the Institute of Medicine in 1998 and is usually grouped with the B vitamins. Despite the fact that humans can synthesize it in small amounts, choline should be consumed in the diet to ensure its availability to make neurotransmitters and lecithin, a substance in cell membranes necessary for fat transport in the blood stream and for cell structure and function. The *Dietary Guidelines* report lists choline as a shortfall nutrient. Food sources include eggs, beef, pork, lamb, salmon, chicken and fish.

Vitamin C

Vitamin C, also called **ascorbic acid**, helps make collagen, which is the structural foundation of cells. Vitamin C helps keep gums and other tissues healthy and aids in the healing of cuts and wounds. It also helps the body absorb iron. Vitamin C is necessary to form thyroxin, the hormone that regulates metabolic rate.

When vitamin C and iron are eaten at the same meal, the body absorbs up to three times more iron from non-meat (non-heme) sources. Iron from meat is well absorbed and does not require vitamin C for absorbtion.

Like vitamin E, vitamin C is a key antioxidant, protecting cells from damage that can increase risk of certain diseases, such as cancer. Vitamin C strengthens the immune system by supporting white blood cells; however, research has not shown that high doses of vitamin C will prevent or cure the common cold. It can, however, lessen symptoms.

Vitamin C has been identified as a shortfall nutrient because many Americans do not eat enough fruits and vegetables, the primary source of vitamin C. Some juices and cereals are fortified with vitamin C. Pregnant and nursing women, those who smoke, and people with injuries, infections or fevers require more vitamin C. Very high doses of vitamin C (more than 2 grams per day) through supplements can cause gastrointestinal symptoms. Deficiencies of vitamin C result in bleeding gums, easy bruising and poor resistance to infection. Severe deficiencies result in scurvy, which is seldom seen except in people who eat virtually no fruits and vegetables. Proper handling and storage of foods high in vitamin C is important because, as the least stable nutrient, vitamin C is easily destroyed by exposure to heat, leaches into water and is lost through evaporation. The amount of loss varies with time and temperature. Serving foods high in vitamin C in the raw state preserves this nutrient.

Vitamin C

Measure	Population	Amount
Daily Value		60 milligrams (mg)
Dietary Reference Intakes (DRI)	Men, ages 19 and above Women, ages 19 and above	90 mg 75 mg

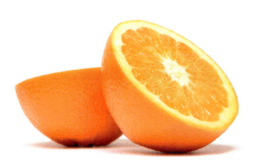

Best Sources of Vitamin C

Fruits and vegetables are the best sources.

Food	Serving	Vitamin C milligrams
Sweet red pepper	½ cup	115
Orange	1 medium	70
Orange juice	½ cup	62
Sweet green pepper	½ cup	60
Broccoli, cooked	½ cup	51
Strawberries	½ cup	49
Grapefruit juice	½ cup	47
Apple juice, with added vitamin C	½ cup	47
Papaya	½ cup	44
Grapefruit	½ medium	44
Brussels sprouts, cooked	½ cup	48
Tomato	1 medium	17
Cereals, ready-to-eat	1 cup	6 - 60

Source: U.S. Department of Agriculture, Agricultural Research Service. 2011. USDA National Nutrient Database for Standard Reference, Release 24. Nutrient Data Laboratory Home Page, www.ars.usda.gov/ba/bhnrc/ndl

Minerals

Minerals are inorganic substances that are essential for good health. They originate in the earth and cannot be produced by living organisms. Most minerals in the diet come directly from plants or indirectly from animal sources that have eaten plants. Minerals are also found in water.

Major minerals are those that the body needs in relatively large amounts (more than 100 milligrams/day). All the major minerals can be found in the body in amounts larger than 5 grams. **Trace minerals** have known biological functions in humans, but are necessary only in tiny amounts (less than 20 milligrams/day). Trace minerals are sometimes called microminerals.

Of the 92 known minerals, at least 21 are necessary for biochemical processes in humans. Minerals differ from other nutrients in that they remain intact during digestion and do not change in structure when performing biologic functions. Some minerals occur as part of the structure of organic compounds, such as hemoglobin and phospholipids in blood. Minerals are stable and not destroyed by heat, light or oxygen.

In general, minerals maintain the body's fluid and acid–base balance; provide structural components for building blood, bone and teeth; and sustain the immune system. Like vitamins, minerals act as cofactors in essential enzyme systems to repair cells and protect them from oxidative changes that cause aging, cardiovascular diseases and cancer. Minerals also participate in metabolic processes, energy production, muscle contraction and transmission of nerve impulses.

Minerals

Major Minerals	Trace Minerals
Calcium	Iodine
Chloride	Iron
Magnesium	Zinc
Phosphorus	Selenium
Potassium	Fluoride
Sodium	Chromium
Sulfur	Copper
	Manganese
	Molybdenum

Phosphorus

Phosphorus is the second most abundant mineral in the body. It helps build and renew bones and teeth. Phosphorus also assists metabolic reactions to produce energy from carbohydrates, protein and fat and helps maintain acid-base balance within body cells. Generally, calcium-rich foods also provide phosphorus. Phosphorus is also found in meats, poultry, fish, eggs and legumes. Phosphorus from nuts, seeds and grains is about 50% less bioavailable than phosphorus from animal sources. Because it is provided by foods from several food groups, inadequate phosphorus intake is rare.

Phosphorus

Measure	Population	Amount
Daily Value		1,000 milligrams (mg)
Dietary Reference Intakes (DRI)	Men, ages 19 and above Women, ages 19 and above	700 mg 700 mg

Best Sources of Phosphorus

Phosphorus is found mostly in animal products and legumes.

Food	Serving	Phosphorus milligrams
Yogurt, plain nonfat	1 cup	356
Fish, salmon, cooked	3 ounces	252
Milk, nonfat, low-fat, whole, buttermilk	1 cup	247
Fish, halibut, cooked	3 ounces	231
Ricotta cheese, part skim	½ cup	225
Beef, sirloin, cooked	3 ounces	200
Cottage cheese	½ cup	179
Lentils, cooked	½ cup	178
Beef, cooked	3 ounces	173
Turkey, cooked	3 ounces	168
Swiss cheese	1 ounce	161
Chicken, cooked	3 ounces	155
Great Northern beans, cooked	½ cup	146
Navy beans, cooked	½ cup	143
Almonds	1 ounce	137
Peanuts	1 ounce	107
Egg	1 large	99

Source: U.S. Department of Agriculture, Agricultural Research Service. 2011. USDA National Nutrient Database for Standard Reference, Release 24. Nutrient Data Laboratory Home Page, www.ars.usda.gov/ba/bhnrc/ndl

Potassium

Potassium plays a major role in maintaining fluid, electrolyte and acid-base balance and cell integrity. It is also critical to the transmission of nerve impulses that maintain blood pressure, bone health and heartbeat. Deficiency, which occurs with dehydration, causes muscular weakness, paralysis and confusion. Long-term low intakes have been linked to hypertension. Potassium has been identified as a nutrient of concern because so many Americans eat less than adequate amounts. In fact, less than 10% of Americans consume adequate potassium. Increasing fruits, vegetables and milk will help meet potassium needs.

Potassium

Measure	Population	Amount
Daily Value		3,500 milligrams (mg)
Dietary Reference Intakes (DRI)	Men, ages 14 and above Women, ages 14 and above	4.7 grams 4.7 grams

Best Sources of Potassium

Mostly in fruits and vegetables and milk.

Food	Serving	Potassium milligrams
Potato, baked with skin	1 large	1,081
Prune juice	1 cup	707
Sweet potato, baked	1 each	542
Beet greens, cooked	½ cup	654
Plums, dried (prunes)	½ cup	637
Raisins	½ cup	618
White beans, cooked	½ cup	414
Tomato juice	1 cup	556
Yogurt	1 cup	531
Orange juice	1 cup	496
Halibut, cooked	3 ounces	421
Lima beans, cooked	½ cup	485
Acorn squash, cooked	½ cup	448
Banana	1 medium	422
Spinach, cooked	½ cup	420
Honeydew melon	1 cup	388
Milk, nonfat, low-fat, whole, buttermilk	1 cup	382
Avocado	½ cup	364
Artichoke, cooked	1 medium	343
Kidney beans, cooked	½ cup	327
Molasses	1 tablespoon	293

Source: U.S. Department of Agriculture, Agricultural Research Service. 2011. USDA National Nutrient Database for Standard Reference, Release 24. Nutrient Data Laboratory Home Page, www.ars.usda.gov/ba/bhnrc/ndl

Sodium

Sodium regulates body fluids, including blood volume. It also regulates acid-base balance, helps nerves and muscles function properly, and helps glucose and amino acids move across cell membranes to be metabolized. Surplus sodium is filtered out of the blood by the kidneys and is excreted in the urine. Sodium is also lost through the skin via sweating.

While dietary guidance recommends increasing or maintaining intakes of most minerals, sodium intake should be limited. In excess, sodium may contribute to hypertension (high blood pressure), which is very common in the United States and is a risk factor for heart attacks, strokes and kidney disease. For reasons that are not clear, some people seem to be "sodium sensitive." For them, there is a direct relationship between salt intake and blood pressure. Elderly individuals, people with diabetes or kidney disease, and African Americans are more sodium sensitive than young Caucasians. Too much sodium also can contribute to fluid retention, weight gain, stomach ulcers, stomach cancer and a form of osteoporosis.

The *Dietary Guidelines* recommend that sodium consumption be limited to less than 2,300 milligrams per day and to 1,500 milligrams per day (less than 1 teaspoon of table salt) for people over age 51, all African-Americans, and those with hypertension, diabetes or kidney disease. Americans typically consume two to three times this amount, about 3,400 milligrams daily. Processed foods – such as canned soups and sauces, cured and deli meats, frozen or packaged meals, condiments (soy sauce, Worcestershire sauce and catsup), salted snacks, pickled foods, seaweed and salad dressings – account for more than 70% of the sodium Americans consume. Trying to reduce sodium in processed foods can be difficult. In many high-sodium foods – for example, breakfast cereals, gelatin desserts and instant puddings – the salty flavor is masked by high sugar content. For information on sodium-restricted diets, see Chapter 13.

Sodium

Measure	Population	Amount
Daily Value		2,400 milligrams (mg)
Dietary Reference Intakes (DRI)	Men, ages 14 to 50 Women, ages 14 to 50	1.5 grams 1.5 grams

Sodium-Rich Ingredients

Sodium is in a variety of compounds used as food ingredients. Sodium both preserves food and enhances flavor. Look for added sodium in ingredient lists. Check labels for sodium content.

Ingredient	Function
Monosodium glutamate (MSG)	Flavor enhancer
Sodium benzoate	Preservative
Sodium caseinate	Thickener and binder
Sodium citrate	Buffer used to control acidity in soft drinks
Sodium nitrite	Curing agent in meat
Sodium phosphate	Emulsifier and stabilizer
Sodium propionate	Mold inhibitor
Sodium saccharin	Artificial sweetener

Humans have a biological preference for sweet and salty flavors. This taste preference plus the wide-spread use of salt and sodium-rich ingredients, particularly in processed foods, creates a challenge for chefs who want to serve healthful foods. Choosing lower-sodium ingredients and reducing the use of salt over time seems to be a good strategy. Techniques for reducing salt and sodium are described in Chapter 9.

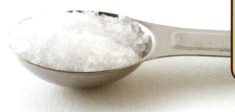

How Much Sodium Is in Table Salt?

Table salt is fine-grained sodium chloride mixed with a trace amount of an anti-caking agent such as calcium silicate. Table salt is 40% sodium by weight and 60% chloride. One gram of salt provides 400 milligrams of sodium. One teaspoon (5.6 grams) of salt will add approximately 2,300 milligrams of sodium to a dish. By weight, all salt contains the same amount of sodium. Teaspoon for teaspoon, however, flaked kosher salt is lighter than table salt and will have somewhat less sodium per teaspoon.

Sodium Content of Common Condiments and Recipe Ingredients

Food	Serving	Sodium milligrams
Table salt	1 tablespoon	6,900
Baking soda	1 tablespoon	3,775
Garlic salt	1 tablespoon	2,880
Baking powder, double-acting, sodium aluminum sulfate	1 tablespoon	1,464
Fish sauce	1 tablespoon	1,389
Tamari sauce	1 tablespoon	1,005
Soy sauce	1 tablespoon	901
Soy sauce, low-sodium	1 tablespoon	533
Dijon mustard	1 tablespoon	360
Hoisin sauce	1 tablespoon	258
Capers	1 tablespoon	254
Catsup	1 tablespoon	167
Anchovies	1 each	146

Source: U.S. Department of Agriculture, Agricultural Research Service. 2011. USDA National Nutrient Database for Standard Reference, Release 24. Nutrient Data Laboratory Home Page, www.ars.usda.gov/ba/bhnrc/ndl

Sodium Contribution of Various Foods

Average intake of sodium is 3,436 milligrams per person per day in the United States.

Food Group	Sodium Contribution to Diet by Rank	Sodium Contribution Diet	Sample Food	Average Sodium Content milligrams
Yeast breads	1	7.3%	White bread 1 slice	170
Chicken and chicken mixed dishes	2	6.8%	Chicken nuggets 3 ½ ounces	608
Pizza	3	6.3%	Pepperoni pizza 1 slice	670
Pasta and pasta dishes	4	5.1%	Macaroni and cheese 1 cup	170
Cold cuts	5	4.5%	Ham 3 ounces	1,128
Condiments	6	4.4%	Catsup 1 tablespoon	167
Mexican mixed dishes	7	4.1%	Taco salad 1 ½ cups	762
Sausage, franks, bacon and ribs	8	4.1%	Hot dog 1 each	461
Regular cheese	9	3.5%	Blue cheese 1 ounce	395
Grain-based desserts	10	3.4%	Cake 1 piece	318
Soups	11	3.3%	Beef noodle soup 1 cup	930
Beef and beef mixed dishes	12	3.3%	Beef stew 1 cup	900
Rice and rice mixed dishes	13	2.6%	White rice, cooked ½ cup	302
Eggs and egg mixed dishes	14	2.6%	Quiche 1 serving	750
Burgers	15	2.4%	Hamburger 1 each	824
Salad dressing	16	2.4%	Italian dressing 1 tablespoon	243
Cereal, ready-to-eat	17	2.0%	Raisin bran 1 cup	354
Potato/corn/other chips	18	1.8%	Potato chips, barbecue 1 ounce	213
Pork and pork mixed dishes	19	1.8%	Pork sausage 1 ounce	202
Quick breads	20	1.7%	Banana bread 1 slice	181

Adapted from: Sources of Sodium Among the US Population, 2005-06. National Cancer Institute, http://riskfactor.cancer.gov/diet/foodsources/sodium

Chloride

Chloride works with sodium to maintain fluid balance, helps transmit nerve impulses and helps regulate acid-base balance. It is also part of hydrochloric acid, a secretion of the stomach that is important to digestion. Americans get plenty of chloride because it is available in foods that contain salt (sodium chloride). It is also found in seaweed, rye, tomatoes, olives, meats and milk. The Daily Value for chloride is 3,400 milligrams.

Magnesium

Magnesium builds and renews bone and teeth and helps muscles and the nervous system work properly. It has a role in regulating blood pressure. It is necessary for carbohydrate, protein and fat metabolism and supports the immune system. According to the *Dietary Guidelines*, many adults do not meet the daily requirements for magnesium. Increasing magnesium and potassium in the diet lowers blood pressure and promotes the relaxation of muscles; thus, these nutrients are considered heart healthy. Magnesium is part of chlorophyll, which makes green leafy vegetables rich in magnesium. Eating vegetables and seafood regularly ensures adequate magnesium intake.

Magnesium deficiency is sometimes seen but is usually associated with disease or medications. People with poorly controlled diabetes or who drink a lot of alcohol secrete magnesium. Signs of magnesium deficiency include muscle twitching or spasms, cramps, weakness and depression. Older adults are at risk of magnesium toxicity if they regularly take antacids or laxatives containing magnesium and do not have good kidney function.

Magnesium

Measure	Population	Amount
Daily Value		400 milligrams (mg)
Dietary Reference Intakes (DRI)	Men, ages 19 to 30 Women, ages 19 to 30	400 mg 310 mg

Best Sources of Magnesium

Food	Serving	Magnesium milligrams
100% Bran cereal	½ cup	121
Halibut, cooked	3 ounces	90
Oysters, steamed	3 ounces	81
Almonds	1 ounce	76
Spinach, cooked	½ cup	78
Swiss chard, cooked	½ cup	75
Lima beans, cooked	½ cup	63
Black beans, cooked	½ cup	60
Edamame	½ cup	54
Beet greens, cooked	½ cup	49
Peanuts	1 ounce	48
Molasses, blackstrap	1 tablespoon	48
Okra, cooked	½ cup	29
Hazelnuts	1 ounce	46
Yogurt	1 cup	29
Rice, brown, cooked	½ cup	42

Source: U.S. Department of Agriculture, Agricultural Research Service. 2011. USDA National Nutrient Database for Standard Reference, Release 24. Nutrient Data Laboratory Home Page, **www.ars.usda.gov/ba/bhnrc/ndl**

Phytochemicals: Potential Health Benefits and Sources

Carotenoids

Carotenoids are fat-soluble phytochemicals with a vitamin-A-like structure. They are the pigments responsible for the colors of many red, green, yellow and orange fruits and vegetables.

Carotenoids have strong antioxidant and other potentially protective properties. Approximately 600 carotenoids have been identified. The table below lists some of the most common.

Carotenoid	Potential Health Benefits	Sources
Beta-carotene	• Slows aging process • Reduces risk of certain types of cancer • Improves lung function • Reduces complications associated with diabetes • Protects eyes	**Yellow-orange** fruits and vegetables such as mangoes, cantaloupe, dried or fresh apricots, papaya, carrots, pumpkins, sweet potatoes, butternut squash, nectarines, and green vegetables such as broccoli, spinach, collard greens and kale
Lutein	• Protects against cataracts and macular degeneration • Promotes eye health • Decreases risk of lung cancer	**Green** and **yellow** vegetables such as broccoli, collard greens, Brussels sprouts, Swiss chard, romaine lettuce, peas, corn, pumpkin and butternut squash
Zeaxanthin	• Protects against cataracts and macular degeneration	**Green** leafy and **orange** vegetables and fruit, especially spinach, green bell peppers, orange peppers, orange juice, oranges, honeydew, peaches, mango, winter squash, corn and egg yolks
Lycopene	• Reduces the risk of prostate cancer and heart disease	**Red** fruits and vegetables such as tomatoes, cooked tomato products, (catsup), red bell peppers, pink or red grapefruit, watermelon and guava

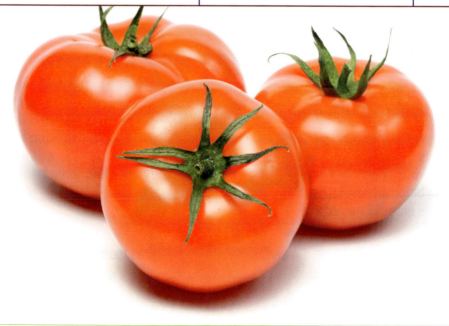

Flavonoids

Flavonoids are among the most potent and abundant antioxidants in the diet. More than 4,000 flavonoids have been identified. Flavonoids, particularly flavanols and proanthocyanidins, have been associated with reduction in the risk of cardiovascular disease.

Potential Health Benefits and Sources of Flavonoids

Flavonoid	Potential Health Benefits	Sources
Anthocyanidins	• Delays diseases associated with aging • Helps prevent urinary tract infections • Aids circulation and nerve function	Purple and red fruits and vegetables, red wine, blueberries, cherries, raspberries, raisins, cranberries, strawberries, red grapes, kiwifruit, plums, red cabbage, kidney beans, beets, pomegranate, acai, tomatoes, eggplant peel, prunes, beets and some ripened olives
Flavonols Quercetin	• Antihistamine • Potent antioxidant • Inhibits the growth of head and neck cancers • Protects lungs from the harmful effects of pollutants and cigarette smoke	Apples, pears, cherries, cranberries, raspberries, grapes, red onions, kale, broccoli, leaf lettuce, garlic, green and black tea, red wine, cauliflower, capers and tomatoes (especially organically grown)
Flavanones Hesperidin	• Protects against heart disease and strengthens blood vessels • Prevents aches and night leg cramps	Citrus fruits and juices, such as oranges and orange juice with pulp, grapefruit and grapefruit juice, tangerines, lemons, limes, mandarins and tangelos
Naringenin	• May help prevent cancers • Potential cholesterol-lowering agent	Citrus peels, fruits and their juices
Flavanols Catechins	• May prevent heart disease and cancer	Green and oolong tea
Proanthocyanidins	• May contribute to maintenance of urinary tract health • May contribute to heart health	Cranberries, apples, red grapes, red wine, berries, chocolate, peanuts and cinnamon

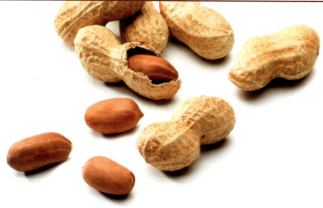

Antioxidant Protection

Although their structures differ, vitamins, minerals and phytochemicals can act as antioxidants, reducing cell damage caused by the oxidation that occurs naturally throughout the body. Antioxidants neutralize or inactivate highly unstable and extremely reactive molecules called *free radicals* that attack the body's cells every day. Free radicals are produced during food metabolism and by other triggers such as air pollution. Experts believe that antioxidants can help prevent free radical damage, which contributes to a variety of conditions, including cancer, heart disease and aging. Some vitamins and minerals and many phytochemicals provide this important biologic function. Examples include:

Vitamin A	Beta-carotene	Lycopene
Vitamin C	Selenium	Resveratrol
Vitamin E	Lutein	

How Much Is Enough? How Much Is Too Much?

The National Research Council sets estimated safe and adequate daily dietary intakes for key vitamins and upper limits above which toxic effects have been reported. More is not better. Vitamins and minerals in amounts found in food are generally safe. Sustained excessive intake of vitamins, particularly fat-soluble vitamins and some minerals (usually from supplements), can be harmful. Although water-soluble vitamins are not stored in the body, they can interfere with medications. And by taking large quantities of water-soluble vitamins, one can develop a physiological reliance on the excessive quantity. For example, people who have taken vitamin C in excessively high doses may have bleeding gums, a symptom of deficiency, after they stop or reduce the dosage. Kidney stones have been reported among those who take mega-doses of vitamin C.

Taking vitamins and minerals in excess is costly, has no physiologic advantage and may create imbalances with other nutrients. Many vitamins and minerals are toxic at high levels. In supplement form, some can interfere with certain clinical laboratory tests and medications and can create stress on the liver and kidneys where they are metabolized.

Enrichment and Fortification

Enrichment restores vitamins and minerals lost during food processing. For example, when wheat is milled and refined into flour, thiamin, riboflavin, niacin and iron are lost. Cornmeal also loses these nutrients in processing. The 1942 Enrichment Act restored the original levels of these four nutrients in flour. More recently, folacin was added at specified levels to enrichment nutrients to protect against birth defects from inadequate folacin. While enrichment has improved the healthfulness of refined flour, many nutrients in whole grains – including fiber, vitamin B_6, magnesium, zinc and other trace minerals – are also removed during milling but are not replaced. Consequently, whole-grain breads and cereals are a better choice because of their more complete nutritional package.

In *fortification*, vitamins and minerals are added to food to boost nutrient levels beyond original values. Most milks and margarines are fortified with vitamins A and D. Some fruit drinks are fortified with vitamin C; soymilk and rice milk are fortified with calcium and vitamin B_{12}; and salt has added iodine. Many breakfast cereals are fortified with a whole day's supply of vitamins and minerals, essentially making them a vitamin/mineral supplement encased in food. Many fortified foods are considered functional foods. See Chapter 8 for more on functional foods.

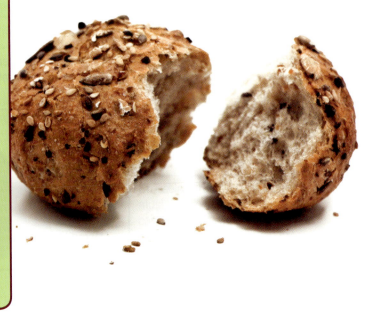

Bioavailability

Just because a food contains certain vitamins, minerals and phytochemcials does not mean the body can use those nutrients effectively. Many factors influence *bioavailability* – that is, the degree to which a nutrient is absorbed and utilized. The human body can adapt to varied levels of vitamin and mineral consumption. A well-functioning digestive tract generally regulates absorption and excretion to meet the body's needs. Ingesting extremely high amounts of specific nutrients overworks the body's ability to regulate. In addition, excessive intake of some minerals can lead to kidney failure and a host of other medical problems.

Nutrient bioavailability is enhanced by:

- Enzymes and bacteria within the digestive tract that can increase the amount of nutrients absorbed

- Vitamin C that boosts the absorption of iron present in plant foods

- Protein and vitamin D that boost calcium utilization

- A small amount of fat or oil that will increase the absorption of fat-soluble vitamins

- The form of a nutrient – for example, vitamin D_3 vs. vitamin D_2

- Fermentation processes, such as those used to make miso and tempeh, that may improve iron bioavailability

- Food preparation techniques, such as soaking and sprouting beans, grains and seeds as well as leavening bread that can reduce binding of zinc by phytic acid and increase zinc bioavailability

- Organic acids, such as citric acid, that can also enhance zinc absorption

Vitamins and minerals also may compete with each other for absorption through the gastrointestinal tract and bloodstream. For example, calcium, magnesium, iron, copper and zinc compete for the same protein carriers for absorption. Thus, too much of one can impede absorption of another.

Some substances bind minerals in the digestive tract, thus reducing the amount absorbed:

- Oxalates in vegetables such as spinach bind calcium so that most of it cannot be absorbed.

- Polyphenols in regular and herbal teas, coffee, and red wine bind iron.

- Phytates in whole grains, legumes and some vegetables bind calcium, iron, phosphorus and zinc.

- Avidin, a protein found in small amounts in raw eggs, will interfere with the absorption of biotin. Avidin is chemically altered with cooking so it is not present in cooked eggs.

On the positive side, cooking can also increase absorption of some vitamins and minerals either by softening cell walls so nutrients can be released or, in the case of legumes, by breaking down bonds between minerals and binders. For example, the vitamin A (beta-carotene) in cooked carrots is more available and absorbable than the vitamin A in raw carrots.

Oxalic and Phytic Acids

Oxalic acid binds some minerals, particularly calcium, so that they cannot be absorbed from the digestive tract. It is found in oranges, spinach, rhubarb, tea, coffee, bananas, ginger and almonds. *Phytic acid* binds some minerals, particularly iron and zinc, so that they cannot be absorbed from the digestive tract. It is found in cereals, nuts, sesame seeds, soybeans, wheat, pumpkin and beans. Thus, the full amount of minerals, as listed in food value tables, is not always available to the body.

The Raw Truth

Is raw food always healthier? Not necessarily. Advocates of raw food diets claim that eating all foods raw (or heated no higher than 115 degrees) increases intake of natural enzymes and that a totally raw diet is healthful. While it is true that many raw foods contain active enzymes, it is unclear if this has much benefit to humans. Certainly, a raw food diet can cause weight loss because many foods are eliminated and total food intake decreases. Providing variety beyond raw fruits and vegetables involves extensive sprouting, soaking and specialized preparation methods.

Cooking destroys pathogens such as *salmonella* and *E. coli* found in some fresh fruits and vegetables. Cooked carrrots supply more beta-carotene than raw carrots. Boiling carrots, however, leads to a loss of polyphenols, an antioxidant. In addition, cooking can destroy some of the vitamin C in fruits and vegetables because vitamin C is highly unstable and easily destroyed when exposed to heat and water. Cooking softens food such as cellulose fiber and meat, allowing for easier digestion. Some foods such as whole grains and legumes are not palatable until cooked.

The bottom line is that eating more fruits and vegetables improves total diet – raw or cooked.

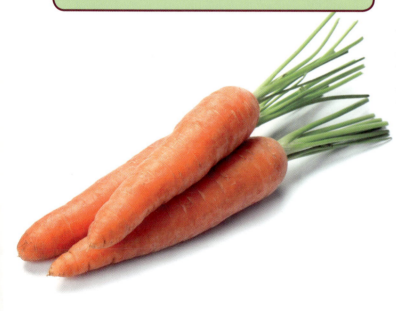

In general, vitamins and minerals are used more fully when they come from food rather than from supplements. When foods are fortified, usually a bio-available form of a nutrient is added. For example, vitamin D in D3 form is added to milk; calcium citrate is added to orange juice. Some fortified breakfast cereals provide significant amounts of vitamins and minerals and can replace a multivitamin/mineral supplement in pill form. Supplements are generally safe in either pill, cereal or health bar form. Problems arise when nutrients taken in excessive amounts create imbalances with other nutrients or become toxic in large quantities. Individuals with allergies, intolerances or aversions to foods may need supplements to replace nutrients they may not get from food. A physician or registered dietitian should evaluate the person's diet and confirm with laboratory tests to ensure the appropriate type and amount of any supplement is taken.

Nutrient Retention

Nutrients in food can be affected by many variables, including nutrients in the soil, degree of maturity at harvest, transportation time, storage, processing and cooking methods. The nutrients from animal foods are influenced by what the animal was fed or ate. Vitamins can be destroyed by exposure to heat, oxygen, light and extremes in pH and moisture. The extent of damage depends on the length of time food is exposed to each element. Careful storage and handling and close attention to proper cooking techniques will help minimize nutrient loss. Minerals are unaffected by high temperatures, but to preserve vitamins, avoid high heat and use the shortest appropriate cooking times. Water-soluble vitamins are particularly vulnerable.

Fresh, whole and minimally processed foods deliver high nutritive value and good appearance, taste and texture. Produce is often harvested unripe so it can withstand shipping. For optimal nutrient value, however, produce should ripen on the plant so the maximum nutrition is gained from the soil and plant. Locally grown produce is more likely to be ripe when picked. To reduce nutrient loss, most produce should be chilled immediately and kept chilled until used. Fruits and vegetables with cut skins should be

'We're Trying to Change the System'

Fletcher Allen Health Care, together with its partners at the University of Vermont College of Medicine and the College of Nursing and Health Sciences, is Vermont's academic medical center. Its mission is to improve the health of the people in the communities it serves by integrating patient care, education and research in a caring environment. Fletcher Allen serves well over 6,000 meals each day; about 1,000 are for patients.

Fletcher Allen purchases local foods, offers organic or fair trade products, has increased its offering of fruit, vegetables and other nutritionally dense foods, and has eliminated deep-fried foods from its menus. In addition, Fletcher Allen has developed strong relationships with the local farming community (including production planning with several farms), started a bee-keeping operation at its Fanny Allen campus and has planted a "healing garden" of herbs and vegetables onsite. The hospital's new radiation oncology facility includes a rooftop fruit and vegetable garden.

"It is our goal to be the most sustainable health care foodservice in the country," explains Diane Imrie, MBA, RD, director of nutrition services. "This passion stems from a simple belief – it's the right thing to do. Better nutrition and a healthier environment result in healthier communities." In keeping with this philosophy,

the hospital was one of the first in the nation to sign Health Care Without Harm's Healthy Food in Health Care Pledge, which promotes sustainable purchasing practices, the inclusion of fresh, local food on hospital menus, and supporting local and regional food producers.

In May 2009, Fletcher Allen opened its new Harvest Café, a sustainably built, energy-efficient cafeteria. Open 22 hours a day, the cafe serves foods such as locally raised ground beef, a line of chicken and turkey raised without non-therapeutic antibiotics, and many vegetarian items. "We support a number of local products," says Diane. "Maple syrup, cheese, rBST-free milk and a variety of local organic vegetables are just a few examples. We also host an on-site farmer's market and support a winter and summer farm share delivered to the hospital."

Upon opening the Harvest Café, Fletcher Allen also announced the establishment of its federally funded Center for Nutrition and Healthy Food Systems, an educational entity that promotes integrating fresh, regional food with patient care. "We have a lot of people to feed everyday," Diane continues. "It's our responsibility to make a change toward better nutrition and a more sustainable food system. We're literally trying to change the system."

covered so that vitamins are not exposed to air. Fruits and vegetables should also be removed from opened cans and covered before storage to avoid bacteria growth and altered flavors.

Frozen fruits and vegetables are equal, and sometimes even better, than fresh varieties because they are picked at flavor peak and quickly frozen after harvest to preserve nutrients. A "fresh" fruit may have spent considerable time in shipping or storage before it gets to your kitchen. Properly stored, frozen fruits and vegetables are not subject to nutrient losses from prolonged shipping or warehouse storage.

Whether or not organically grown produce has a higher vitamin and mineral content than traditionally grown produce depends on variables such as seed variety, soil condition and ripeness at picking. Extensive validated research comparing organic and traditionally grown produce is not yet available. As explained in Chapter 8, there is much conflicting information.

A study from the University of California (UC) at Davis states that some canned foods actually provide higher levels of essential nutrients (in particular, the fat-soluble carotenoids) than similar fresh or frozen items. [4] The canning process locks in nutrients at their peak of freshness and shields them from oxygen. Look for fruits canned in natural juices, rather than heavy syrup, and for low-sodium or unsalted canned vegetables. Canned tomato products are more consistent in quality than their fresh counterparts and will have more lycopene than fresh tomatoes. Canned fruits, vegetables and beans can be a nutritious and convenient alternative to fresh or frozen and more readily available for some foodservice operations. Canned legumes are convenient and save cooking time but can be higher in sodium. Draining and rinsing canned beans will reduce sodium by about 40%.

Additional conclusions drawn from the UC Davis study are:

- **Canned:** Canned foods are packed at their peak of freshness. Due to the absence of oxygen during their storage period, canned fruits and vegetables have a longer shelf life and remain relatively stable up until the time they are consumed.

- **Fresh:** Fresh is best if consumed within a short time after purchasing.

- **Frozen:** Frozen products are packed at their peak of freshness. Frozen fruits and vegetables may be more nutritious if stored for short periods of time under well-controlled temperatures.

- **All Forms:** Fresh, frozen and canned fruits and vegetables contribute to the nation's nutrition and make healthful choices available to everyone, everywhere.

Often, the same steps taken to preserve food quality also retain nutrients. For example, keeping vegetables fresh by washing them whole, covering and refrigerating them will help maintain freshness and nutrient content. Consider whether or not vegetables will be peeled before cooking. Removing the peel exposes more of the vegetable flesh and accelerates nutrient loss. Also, many nutrients are just beneath the peel and are removed during peeling. Edible peels and skins provide valuable fiber and phytochemicals; straining pulp from citrus discards fiber and many phytochemicals and vitamins. Juicing and straining fruits and vegetables extract liquids with many vitamins and minerals but discard the pulp and fiber. American diets need more, not less,

fiber. Purees, coulis and smoothies that incorporate whole fruits and vegetables have broken cell walls that increase nutrient availability; fiber remains in the puree.

When possible, cook vegetables from the raw or frozen state and serve them immediately. To minimize nutrient loss, wash vegetables before cutting them. To cook most vegetables, steam them until just done. If not served immediately, stop the cooking process by plunging the vegetables into ice water, drain thoroughly, wrap and refrigerate until ready to serve. If steaming is not practical, blanch vegetables for a short period in rapidly boiling water. Then follow the necessary steps for maximum nutrient retention. Since water-soluble vitamins are released into cooking liquids, steaming and microwaving cause the least release and most vitamin retention. Reserve nutrient-rich cooking liquids for soups and marinades; to braise or poach meats, poultry and fish; and to cook starches. Note that adding baking soda (alkaline) to maintain a vegetable's color is a popular trick, but doing so changes texture and destroys thiamin and vitamin C.

Avoid frying vegetables. The high heat used in frying, especially deep-frying, creates free radicals in the fat that are unhealthy. Free radicals that contribute to aging, heart disease and cancer risk are produced when oils are continuously oxidized by high temperatures.

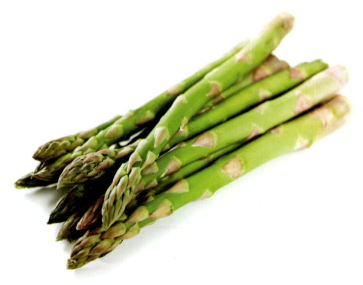

Opportunities for Chefs

Although needed only in small quantities, vitamins, minerals and phytochemicals perform very important functions in the body. Even the root word "vita" indicates the vital nature of these substances. The diets of many Americans are rich in calories, fats, sugars and sodium, but lacking in fiber, essential vitamins, minerals and phytochemicals. Planning, preparing and serving meals that are high in fruits, vegetables, whole grains, lean meats and low-fat dairy products will help guests obtain these important nutrients. Using techniques to preserve nutrients and maximize their absorption adds to the nutrient density of the healthful menu.

Learning Activities

1. Collect 10 food labels. Highlight all ingredients that provide sodium. Identify the amount of sodium in a serving of each food.

2. Select one phytochemical and research its benefits and sources.

3. Review food composition tables or best source of nutrient lists. Identify 10 foods that provide at least 20% of the daily need for five or more vitamins or minerals.

4. Create three recipes that include ingredients rich in at least two nutrients of concern – potassium, dietary fiber, vitamin K, vitamin D, calcium or phosphorus.

For More Information

- American Society for Nutrition, Nutrient Information, http://jn.nutrition.org/nutinfo

- Micronutrient Information Center, Linus Pauling Institute, Oregon State University, http://lpi.oregonstate.edu/infocenter/index.html

- Office of Dietary Supplements, http://ods.od.nih.gov

- Produce for Better Health Foundation, Phytochemical Information Center, http://pbhfoundation.org/pulse/research/pic

- USDA Database for the Flavonoid Content of Selected Foods, Release 2.1, Prepared by the Nutrient Data Laboratory, Food Composition Laboratory, Beltsville Human Nutrition Research Center, Agricultural Research Service, U.S. Department of Agriculture, January 2007, www.ars.usda.gov/SP2UserFiles/Place/12354500/Data/Flav/Flav02-1.pdf

- U.S. Department of Agriculture, Agricultural Research Service. 2011. USDA National Nutrient Database for Standard Reference, Release 24. Nutrient Data Laboratory Home Page, www.ars.usda.gov/ba/bhnrc/ndl

CHAPTER 8

Planning Healthful Menus

LEARNING OBJECTIVES

After completing this chapter, you should be able to:

- Identify current major food trends related to nutrition and health
- Explain how to identify and purchase inherently healthful ingredients
- Describe the impact of the sustainable foods movement on planning healthful menus
- Discuss the benefits and disadvantages of using local and organic foods
- List the benefits of functional foods and give examples
- Create healthful menu items
- Identify ingredients to use and limit when creating healthful foods
- Plan a healthful menu and specify appropriate portion size of each offering

The basic tenets of menu planning focus on balancing colors, textures and shapes, variety of ingredients, cooking methods, food cost, equipment availability, staff abilities, and guests' needs and preferences. *Healthful* menu planning adds careful consideration of total calorie count, type and amount of fat, nutrient density and retention, the amount of added sodium and sugar, and special dietary needs, such as gluten intolerance or food allergies.

The overall success of most menus, however, rests on flavor. No one can sell a healthy product (more than once) if it doesn't taste good. This dimension of menu planning is so important that Chapter 9 is devoted to creating flavorful healthful options.

Fruits, vegetables, whole grains, legumes, fish and seafood, lean meats, healthful oils, and low-fat dairy products are the key ingredients of a healthful menu. While Americans eat enough meat and total grains, studies show that most Americans do not eat enough fruit, vegetables (including legumes), whole grains and low-fat dairy products. Fruits, vegetables and whole grains are rich in vitamins, minerals, phytochemicals and fiber, and are relatively low in calories, fat and sodium.

Focusing on fruits and vegetables makes seasonality an important aspect of menu planning. Generally, produce used in season is at its flavor peak, which allows for simpler preparation. Foods in season are also plentiful and available, which helps control food costs. Patrons look forward to seasonal foods – asparagus and morels in the spring, strawberries bursting with flavor in early summer, juicy tomatoes in late summer, crisp apples in autumn and hearty braised meats with root vegetables in the winter months. While many operations cannot revamp their core menu each season, most can run specials that focus on fresh foods and incorporate seasonal fruits and vegetables into salads, side dishes and desserts.

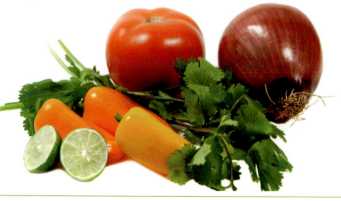

Menu Trends

Food fads come and go, but food trends have more staying power. The trend toward more healthful food preparations has been evolving for several decades. One of the most significant positive nutrition-related trends is serving traditional dishes from ethnic cuisines, such as Mediterranean and Asian, that rely less on meat and more on whole grains and vegetables. Other trends include lighter sauces, smaller meat portions, vegetarian options, small plates, greater emphasis on fruits and vegetables, more whole-grain offerings, and more salads served as main courses.

With the increasing number of overweight and obese Americans, it may seem that the public doesn't care about nutrition. The fact is, however, that healthcare reform and public policies such as calories listed on menus and nutrient disclosure are focusing attention on and making healthful foods and nutrition information more available to all.

Greater emphasis is being placed on menu items that are inherently healthy – that is, foods that are naturally "good for you." According to the market research firm Mintel, inherently healthy menu items are the future of healthy dining. Consumers are looking for foods that include more whole and minimally processed ingredients. [1] While choosing healthful food is ultimately a personal responsibility, the *Dietary Guidelines for Americans* "call to action" asks food producers and retailers (including restaurants) to develop and make available appropriate portions of affordable, nutritious foods in all food establishments. [2]

A National Restaurant Association publication, *Chef Survey: What's Hot in 2012*, showed restaurants can expect to see a growing demand for locally grown and locally sourced products, healthful kids' meals, sustainable seafood, and foods for guests who are gluten-free or allergy conscious and have general concerns about health and nutrition. [3]

Many consumers are seeking foods that reflect their concerns about the environment, energy consumption, social justice, animal welfare and sustainable living. Approximately 30% of U.S. adults fall into a class of consumers who use these values to guide their purchasing decisions. [4]

National Restaurant Association's Chef Survey: What's Hot in 2012

1. Locally sourced meats and seafood
2. Locally grown produce
3. Healthful kids' meals
4. Hyper-local sourcing (e.g., restaurant gardens)
5. Sustainability
6. Children's nutrition
7. Gluten-free/food allergy conscious
8. Locally-produced wine and beer
9. Sustainable seafood
10. Whole grain items in kids' meals
11. Newly fabricated cuts of meat (e.g., Denver steak, pork flat iron, petite tender)
12. Farm/estate-branded ingredients
13. Food trucks/street food
14. Micro-distilled/artisan spirits
15. Artisan/house-made ice cream
16. Health/nutrition
17. Non-traditional fish (e.g., branzino, Arctic char, barramundi)
18. Fruit/vegetable children's side items
19. "Mini meals" (e.g., smaller versions of adult menu items)
20. Culinary cocktails (e.g., savory, fresh ingredients, herb-infused)

Source: National Restaurant Association. Chef Survey: What's Hot in2012. Available at http://www.restaurant.org/pressroom/social-media-releases/images/whatshot2012/What's_Hot_2012.pdf.

Flavor

Healthful flavors are explored fully in the next chapter, but flavor profiling is a significant food trend that must be mentioned here as well. Today's focus on flavor is reflected in customers' growing interest in ethnic cuisines. Many customers seek flavors they have enjoyed while traveling, have read or heard about, or have seen on television food programs. Chefs are cooking with condiments, herbs, spices and unique ingredients from all corners of the world. Various cuisines may fall in and out of favor, but continued public interest in authentic, ethnic flavors remains steady.

The *Dietary Guidelines* recommend significant reductions in sodium (salt), fats and added sugar. All of these components add to flavor. When salt, sugar and fat are limited, chefs have to work harder and are challenged to create alternative flavor enhancers. Salt reduction is discussed in Chapters 9 and 13, fat reduction in Chapters 4 and 13, and sugar reduction in Chapter 3.

Custom Food Preparation

Restaurant customers have always asked for custom food preparation such as degree of doneness for meats and "dressing on the side" with salads. Now there is even more interest in custom food preparation to accommodate individual nutritional needs, especially food intolerances (such as lactose and gluten) and allergies (such as peanuts). Menu items are also customized to meet specific dietary needs including weight loss. These special health considerations are addressed in Chapter 13.

The availability of half portions, fresh vegetables as sides, alternative sweeteners, low-fat salad dressing options, vegetarian entrees, sampler plates, skim milk as a beverage and hummus or olive oil with bread are easy ways to help customers meet their health needs without altering basic menu items or limiting selections.

Starters

Starters, or appetizers, are small portions of savory items served before the main course. Some patrons make a meal by ordering several starters – or "small plates" – rather than an entree. Meze, tapas and dim sum are ethnic variations on the small-plate theme. If a starter must be fried, serve a small portion of the fried component as a part of a dish that includes other foods.

General guidelines for developing healthful starters include:

- Portions should be small to moderate, generally about 8 bites or ½ to ¾ cup.

- Incorporate vegetables, legumes and grains as primary ingredients whenever possible.

- Use endive leaves, mushrooms and cored vegetables to hold fillings for appetizers and hors d'oeuvres.

- Portion meat, fish or poultry at about 2 ounces.

- Use whole grains and legumes creatively.

- Limit high-fat sauces to 1 or 2 ounces.

- Use healthful cooking techniques and heart-healthy fats in preparing starters.

Starters: Guide to Ingredient Choices

Recommended	Limit
<ul><li>All vegetables</li><li>All fruits</li><li>Lean meats</li><li>Poultry</li><li>Seafood, not fried</li><li>Whole grains, such as barley, amaranth, quinoa, bulgur, wheat berries, wild rice, brown rice and farro</li><li>Moderate- or low-fat cheeses</li><li>Beans and other legumes</li><li>Whole-grain breads and pastas</li><li>Small amounts of sauces as garnish and for color, texture and flavor</li></ul>	<ul><li>High-fat meats such as ribs and sausages</li><li>Fried seafood, poultry or vegetables</li><li>Cream</li><li>Patês, sausages and forcemeats</li><li>High-fat cheeses</li><li>Rich sauces</li><li>Nuts and seeds</li><li>Fried garnishes</li></ul>

Soups

Soups can be hot or cold, hearty and filling, brothy and delicate, or creamy and smooth. They can be a start to a meal or a meal in themselves. Soups are inherently a great way to highlight seasonal vegetables and healthful ingredients such as beans and whole grains. When preparing house-made stocks, the chef can control sodium levels. These stocks are generally more flavorful than commercial varieties. Low-sodium stocks – some very high in quality – are available canned, frozen or as concentrates. Chilled soups made from cucumbers, melons or other fruits can be a healthful and interesting option.

Sodium in Chicken Base, Broth and Stock

	Amount	Sodium (milligrams)
Chicken base, standard	¾ teaspoon of base to make 1 cup of broth	704
Reduced-sodium chicken broth	1 cup	554
Low-sodium chicken base	¾ teaspoon of base to make 1 cup of broth	142
Low-sodium chicken broth, canned	1 cup	72
House-made chicken stock, no added salt	1 cup	70

Soup can also be low in calories and play an important role in creating satiety, according to Barbara Rolls, Ph.D., Guthrie Chair of Nutrition at Pennsylvania State University and author of *Volumetrics: Feel Full on Fewer Calories*. Participants in one of Rolls' studies consumed 20% fewer calories when they started their meals with a broth-based, vegetable soup. [5]

General guidelines for developing healthful soups include:

- Portion soups at about 8 ounces.
- Use evaporated skim milk or buttermilk for "creaming."
- Use vegetable purees or instant mashed potatoes as thickeners.
- Use defatted stocks for the foundation of soup.
- Emphasize vegetable-based soups.
- Include legumes and whole grains in soups, especially hearty soups used as a main course.
- Chill cooked soups and remove fat before reheating for serving.
- Use fresh herbs and spices to limit added salt. Turn up the heat with spice.
- Use lemon or flavored vinegars to add flavor and acidity.
- Add a bit of butter, oil or cream just before service for gloss and mouthfeel.

Soups: Guide to Ingredient Choices

Recommended	Limit
<ul><li>Fresh stocks or low-sodium meat, poultry, fish or vegetable commercial stocks and broths</li><li>Evaporated skim milk and buttermilk</li><li>Vegetables of all kinds</li><li>Cornstarch, arrowroot, tapioca or pureed starchy vegetables as thickeners</li><li>Fruits</li><li>Legumes</li><li>Whole grains such as barley and wild rice</li><li>Yogurt</li><li>Lean proteins</li><li>Seafood</li><li>Tomato-based soups and chowders</li></ul>	<ul><li>Cream</li><li>Commercial high-sodium bases</li><li>Roux</li><li>Bacon, sausage</li><li>Cheese</li><li>Fried croutons</li></ul>

Salads and Dressings

Salads can be the most healthful menu items, but add-ons such as cheese, olives, fried croutons and dressings greatly increase calories and fat. For example, a salad at a quick-service chain can sound like a healthful choice but in fact have more than 1,000 calories. A 2-ounce portion of vinaigrette (using a 3:1 ratio of oil to vinegar) can contain 42 grams of oil. At 9 calories per gram of fat, that vinaigrette will have 378 calories just from oil. A creamy (mayonnaise-based) salad dressing is comparable. On the other hand, for an Asian-style salad, cucumbers and other vegetables can be marinated in sweetened mirin or rice wine vinegar, yogurt and fresh herbs with no oil at all.

Calories, Fat and Sodium in 1 Ounce of Salad Dressings

	Calories	Fat (grams)	Sodium (milligrams)
French dressing	130	12.7	240
French dressing, reduced-calorie	55	3.7	285
Ranch dressing	140	14.5	230
Ranch dressing, reduced-fat	55	3.5	260
Blue cheese dressing	135	14.5	265
Blue cheese dressing, low-calorie	30	2.0	340
Italian salad dressing	80	8.0	470
Italian salad dressing, reduced-fat	20	1.8	390
House-made ranch dressing	35	2.5	50
House-made vinaigrette-style dressing	65	7.0	40

General guidelines for developing healthful salads and dressings include:

- Serve 1 to 2 cups of different leafy greens and a variety of fresh, raw, blanched, steamed, roasted or grilled vegetables.

- Choose dark greens most of the time – spinach, baby arugula, romaine, watercress and leaf lettuces – rather than iceberg or pale-colored greens.

- Use plenty of red, orange and yellow fruits and vegetables in salads – sweet potatoes, mangos, oranges, red and yellow peppers, and beets and carrots – for added vitamins and phytochemicals.

- Avocados and nuts provide flavor, texture and healthful fats but should be used in moderation because they are both nutrient dense and calorie dense.

- Use olives and dried fruits in moderation. They are healthful but high in calories.

- Try cut fresh fruits in salads – apples, pears, berries and citrus – or fruit and vegetable combination salads.

- Marinate vegetables, such as artichokes and peppers, in flavored vinegars.

- Limit high-fat garnishes. Use them on top rather than mixed into the salad to control quantity and to have more visual impact.

- Use moderate-fat cheeses like goat, feta, part-skim mozzarella, or reduced-fat cheddar or swiss.

- If crisps or croutons are used, bake, rather than fry them.
- Limit salad dressing to 1 tablespoon for a salad course or 2 tablespoons for an entree salad.
- Use less dressing by tossing greens with the dressing rather than serving it on top or on the side.
- Offer several low-fat dressing options – made from scratch or purchased.
- Have balsamic or wine vinegar and olive oil available for guests who want to mix their own ratio of dressing.
- Use reduced-fat mayonnaise or dressings in tuna, salmon, egg, chicken, pasta, bean and potato salads.
- Use heart-healthy oils – olive, walnut, sesame, canola, safflower, soybean, corn and sunflower – but in moderate amounts. All oils are high in calories.
- Use moderate amounts of egg, cheese, lean meat or seafood in main course salads.

Salads and Dressings: Guide to Ingredient Choices

Recommended	Limit
<ul><li>Fresh vegetables – raw, various cuts, blanched, steamed or roasted</li><li>Fresh fruits</li><li>Dried fruits</li><li>Oils: olive, walnut, sesame, canola, corn, safflower, soybean and sunflower</li><li>Flavored vinegars</li><li>Lemon and citrus juices</li><li>Herbs</li><li>Legumes</li></ul>	<ul><li>Mayonnaise, preferably reduced-fat</li><li>Nuts</li><li>Cheeses</li><li>Eggs</li><li>Meats</li><li>Croutons or crisps</li><li>Dried fruits</li><li>Oils, any</li></ul>

Reduced-Calorie Vinaigrette Dressing Formula

Thicken low-calorie liquids if necessary with cornstarch, arrowroot or xanthan gum. Add appropriate seasonings. Examples are listed below.

Vinaigrette	Low-calorie liquid (2 parts)	Oil (1 part)	Acid (1 part)
Apple-Walnut	Apple juice	Walnut	Apple cider vinegar
Balsamic	Vegetable stock	Olive	Balsamic vinegar
Citrus	Orange juice	Canola	Lime and lemon juice
Asian	Vegetable stock	Sesame	Rice wine vinegar
Vegetable	Tomato juice	Olive	Red wine vinegar
Raspberry	Apple juice	Canola	Raspberry vinegar

Oven Roasted Cod* with Three Colored Peppers & Baby Potatoes

Chef Nora Pouillon, Restaurant Nora,
Washington, DC

Yield: 10 servings each with 1 cup peppers,
1 fish fillet and 2 potatoes

It would be hard to find a better dish that helps diners meet the recommendation for plenty of fish and colorful vegetables. This beautiful and tasty entree is filled with nutrient-rich ingredients.

Olive oil, divided	3	tablespoons
Onions, thinly sliced	2	medium
Garlic, minced	1	tablespoon
Green pepper, seeded and cut in julienne	2	each
Red peppers, seeded and cut in julienne	3	each
Yellow peppers, seeded and cut in julienne	3	each
Chicken stock or white wine	1 ½	cup
Mixed herbs such as thyme, oregano, rosemary, dill or parsley, chopped	⅓	cup
Sea salt	1	teaspoon
Black pepper, freshly ground	½	teaspoon
Cod fillets, cut into 10 portions	3	pounds, 6 ounces
Small bouquet of assorted herbs for garnish		
Baby new potatoes, unpeeled	2	pounds

Rouille: **Yield: ¾ cup**

Red pepper, roasted, pureed	1	
Mayonnaise, light	½	cup
Garlic, minced	2	teaspoons
Saffron (optional)	1	pinch
Cayenne pepper	1	pinch

1. Preheat the oven to 450° F.

2. Heat 1 tablespoon of the olive oil in a large saute pan, add the onion, garlic and peppers and saute for about 5 minutes, stirring frequently. Add the stock or wine, herbs and season with salt and pepper and bring the mixture to a boil. Spoon the pepper mixture into a baking dish large enough to accommodate the fish fillets in one layer.

3. Clean the saute pan and heat until nearly smoking. Add the remaining 2 tablespoons of olive oil and immediately sear the seasoned cod fillets for 1-2 minutes on one side. Remove with spatula and place on top of pepper mixture, seared side up.

4. Bake 5-8 minutes or until desired doneness.

5. Steam the potatoes in a medium saucepan using a collapsible insert or boil them for 10-15 minutes, until a fork can be easily inserted in the potato.

6. Serve fish atop peppers with baby potatoes and a dollop of rouille (2 teaspoons per serving) or aioli (optional) and garnish with fresh herbs.

Rouille:

1. Mix ingredients together in a bowl.

* If Atlantic cod is not available, Alaskan black cod, halibut or any other firm fleshed fish is suitable for this dish.

Per Serving

Calories	300	Cholesterol	70	mg
Fat	10 g	Sodium	420	mg
Saturated Fat	1.5 g	Carbohydrates	23	mg
Trans Fat	0 g	Dietary Fiber	4	mg
Sugar	4 g	Protein	31	g

Sauces

Sauces add flavor, moisture and visual appeal to starters, main courses, vegetables, fruits and desserts. High-fat sauces such as white (Bechamel) sauce, cream sauce and hollandaise sauce should be used in moderation. Salsa, tomato sauce, barbecue sauce and fruit sauces are naturally low in fat and can be used liberally to enhance the appeal and nutrient content of foods.

Most sauces contain a liquid, a thickening agent and other flavorings and seasonings. The liquid base for a sauce is typically:

- Stock
- Milk, yogurt or a dairy product
- Fruit or vegetable juice
- Wine, beer or spirits

The quality of the liquid base determines the quality of the sauce. Stock used for sauce can be made in-house where ingredients, particularly salt, can be controlled. Some high-quality bases and commercially available stocks that are low in sodium can also be used for sauces. Most sauces are thickened with a starchy product, such as flour, cornstarch, arrowroot, breadcrumbs, potato starch (or instant potatoes) or rice flour. Some commercial products use other starches for thickening. The thickening agent affects the appearance of the sauce. For

example, a sauce thickened with flour has an opaque appearance, but when cornstarch is used, the sauce is clear. Servers should know if sauces are thickened with wheat flour or other ingredients containing gluten for those who may ask for gluten-free foods.

General guidelines for developing healthful sauces include:

- Use low-fat ingredients when possible.
- Use reductions for concentrated flavor.
- Reduce the fat in some sauces by replacing a roux thickener with a slurry.
- Use fruit- and vegetable-based sauces when possible. Examples include fruit or vegetable salsas, mango chutney, pureed corn, sweet potato puree, and black bean ragout. These are especially useful in banquet feeding, airline catering, hospitals or anywhere food is held before service. Vegetable and fruit sauces help retain moisture and heat in the main item.
- Yogurt can sometimes be substituted for a higher-fat sour cream in a sauce. Greek yogurts are generally thicker and an excellent substitute. In hot sauces, blend 1 tablespoon of cornstarch into each 1 quart of yogurt and mix well with a wire whisk. This will prevent separation. Yogurt should be added at the end of the cooking process.

Sauces: Guide to Ingredient Choices

Recommended	Limit
<ul><li>Fruit coulis</li><li>Cornstarch/arrowroot thickeners</li><li>Potato starch</li><li>Evaporated skim milk, buttermilk or fat-free half-and-half (for cream)</li><li>Fresh herbs, spices and aromatics</li><li>Natural reductions</li><li>Low-fat milk and yogurt</li><li>Fruit and vegetable juices and purees in sauces</li><li>Meat or poultry stock, reduced</li></ul>	<ul><li>Cheeses</li><li>Cream</li><li>Egg yolks</li><li>Butter</li><li>Oil</li><li>Wine or beer</li></ul>

Side Dishes

Side dishes have evolved from an afterthought in menu planning to an integral component of the main course. Vegetarians and people wanting a light meal may order several side dishes as an entree. Grains, legumes, pastas and vegetables can be prepared in both traditional and innovative ways to create variety and interest.

General guidelines for developing healthful side dishes include:

- Increase the amount and variety of vegetables offered. Serve vegetables that are red, orange, yellow, green, purple and white. Each color group provides different phytochemicals.

- Feature seasonal vegetables steamed, roasted or grilled.

- Limit salt and use herbs, spices, lemon and aromatics to season foods.

- Use flavored salts – sparingly.

- Rinse and drain precooked canned beans to reduce sodium content by about 40%. Packaged dry and fresh legumes are naturally low in sodium.

- Offer side vegetables prepared using different cooking methods, seasonings, and flavors – steamed, roasted, grilled, mashed and sauteed.

- Offer fruit such as grilled pineapple and sauteed apples or pears as side dishes.

- Add interesting color and textures by using wild rice, red rice, black rice, quinoa, millet and nuts.

Side Dishes: Guide to Ingredient Choices

Recommended	Limit
• All vegetables	• Butter
• Fruits	• Cream
• Grains, especially whole grains	• Salt and seasoned salts
• Beans/legumes	• Oil
• Non wheat noodles/pasta (quinoa, rice, buckwheat)	• Bacon and pork fat
• Nuts	
• Seeds	
• Herbs, fresh or dried	
• Vinegars	
• Spices	
• Stocks	
• Salsas	

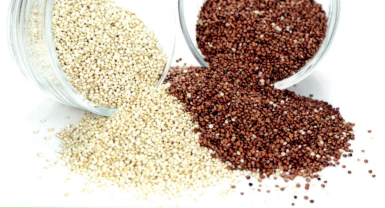

Breads

Both yeast breads and quick breads can be healthful additions to the menu. The *Dietary Guidelines* recommend that at least half of the grains consumed be whole grains. [2] Breads make it easy to achieve that goal. Whole grains contain the entire grain kernel – the bran, germ and endosperm. Examples include whole-wheat flour, bulgur (cracked wheat), oatmeal, whole cornmeal and brown rice.

Look for the Whole Grain Council's product stamp, which indicates that a product contains 16 grams or more of whole grain per serving. The Council's website includes a list of restaurants that offer at least one whole-grain choice at each meal. Restaurants may also use a special symbol on menus to flag items that contain at least a half serving of whole grain.

General guidelines for serving healthful breads include:

- Serve breads in 1- to 2-ounce portions. A 6-ounce muffin is not 1 serving.
- Offer whole-grain and multigrain options.
- White breads should be made with enriched flour.
- Serve small rolls and cut bread into modest portions.
- Use at least 50% whole grain in bread recipes where possible.
- Serve breads with lower-fat spreads such as rosemary white bean spread or hummus. Depending on the operation, olive oil may replace butter as an accompaniment for bread.
- Offer crisp crackers, flatbreads and thin breadsticks.
- Choose options with some seeds, dried fruits and/or nuts for added fiber and nutrients.

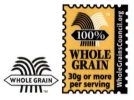

Courtesy Oldways and the Whole Grain Council, **www. wholegrainscouncil.org**

Breads: Guide to Ingredient Choices

Recommended	Limit
• Whole-wheat bread	• Biscuits
• Oatmeal, rye and other whole-grain or multigrain bread	• Croissants
• Italian and French bread	• Bagels, regular or large
• Crisp bread sticks	• Commercial muffins
• Whole-wheat pizza dough	• Cheese breads
• Flatbreads	• Sweet rolls and sweet breads
• Small rye bagels	• Quick breads such as banana bread and pumpkin bread
• Whole-wheat pita	• Corn bread
• Tortillas	• Large sandwich or sub buns
• Whole-wheat English muffins	• Garlic breads or breads with butter or oil toppings
• Seeded and nut breads	• Regular crackers
• Bran and fruit muffins	
• Reduced-fat crackers	

Desserts

Many people enjoy a sweet finish to their meal. Desserts, however, are typically high in sugar and fats. Desserts demand following a philosophy of moderation – a small portion of something sweet and delicious. One of the trend identified in the National Restaurant Association's 2012 survey of chefs is bite-sized and mini-desserts – perfect for health-conscious diners. [3] Another trend is artisan and housemade ice creams – make gelato, it has less fat and calories than traditional ice cream.

General guidelines for adding healthful desserts to the menu include:

- Emphasize fruit – fresh, dried, pureed or frozen.

- Use lower-fat dairy products such as nonfat yogurt, part-skim ricotta cheese and reduced-fat cream cheese.

- Use sweet spices such as ginger, nutmeg or cinnamon.

- Serve a small but satisfying portion. A half-cup of vanilla ice cream has 140 calories; 1 ounce of angel food cake has 75 calories; 2 ounces of chocolate cake has about 200 calories; and ½ cup of rice pudding has about 185 calories.

- Use small (2 ½-inch) cupcake tins and other pans and utensils to make single-serving desserts.

- Use fruit rather than buttercream fillings and frost cakes lightly.

- Serve tarts, crepes and crumbles, and fruit desserts with one crust rather than two or with a nuts-and-oats topping.

- Reduce sugar and other high-calorie sweeteners where possible.

- Serve a small amount of a "rich" dessert with fresh fruit or a fruit sauce to enhance and expand the portion.

- Use small, individual cups, molds or mini-soufflé dishes to control portions and enhance eye appeal.

- Drizzle small amounts of chocolate, fudge, caramel or fruit sauce atop a dessert or to dress the plate, or top desserts with a dusting of confectioner's sugar, only a few calories.

- Include a selection of small amounts of artisanal cheese with some dried fruit and/or nuts. While many of these cheeses are fairly high in fat, they are a nutrient-rich dessert option.

- Enhance desserts with nutrient-rich cherries, berries or other fruits as topping or garnish.

- Substitute finely ground whole-grain or legume flours for all or part of white flour in recipes.

- Eliminate trans fats from partially hydrogenated oils from your kitchen. Minimize saturated fats from butter and cream where possible and substitute with unsaturated plant oils.

- Use butter, where needed for flavor, in moderation.

Desserts: Guide to Ingredient Choices

Recommended	Limit
• Fruit coulis and purees	• Heavy cream and half-and-half
• Fresh cooked fruits such as baked apples, poached pears, roasted apricots, and grilled peaches or figs	• Egg yolks
• Cornstarch/arrowroot thickeners	• Chocolate
• Fruit, berries or sliced melon on the dessert plate for added color, flavor and volume	• Butter
• Grains such as brown rice, oatmeal and cornmeal	• Canned fruits in heavy syrup
• Cocoa powder	• Rich frostings
• Dark chocolate	• Caramel
• Yogurt and Greek yogurt	• Nuts
• Part-skim ricotta cheese	• Ice cream, gelato, frozen yogurt
• Phyllo (or filo) dough baked with little butter	• Sherbet, sorbet, fruit ices
• Chocolate, caramel and other sauces as garnishes or in plate décor (squeeze-bottle technique)	
• Powdered sugar as garnish	
• Egg white soufflés and meringues	
• Finely ground whole-grain flours including whole-grain white flour	
• Nuts, especially walnuts	
• Wheat germ, sesame, poppyseeds and other seeds	
• Sponge cake or angel food cake with fruit toppings	
• Pudding made with low-fat dairy products	
• Gelato made with milk and fruit	
• Dried fruits	

Breakfast

It is true: Breakfast is a very important meal. For example, children who eat breakfast get more important nutrients such as calcium, dietary fiber, folate and protein. [6,7] In addition, children who consume breakfast show improved cognitive function, attention and memory, as well as improved performance on demanding mental tasks and in reaction to frustration. [8]

But children are not the only ones who benefit when they eat breakfast. Adults do, too. Many traditional breakfast items are healthful and, with minor modifications, those that are not so healthful can be given a makeover. General guidelines for developing healthful breakfast items include offering menu items such as:

- Hot and cold whole grains (muesli, steel-cut oats, brown rice, for example) and yogurt bars with various additions such as seeds, nuts and dried and fresh fruits

- Eggs customizable, signature frittata and tofu scramble made with omega-3 eggs

- Housemade chicken sausage patty, turkey bacon, grilled lean ham, Canadian bacon, poached salmon and salmon potato patty

- Nutrient-rich waffles, pancakes or muffins made with whole-grain flour, pumpkin, banana, apple, flaxseed and/or nuts

- Cereal buffet with muesli, assorted whole-grain cereals, fresh fruit and nut options

- Skewers of melon and other cut fruits; baked apples, grilled pineapple, peaches or nectarines

- Reduced-sugar or all-fruit jams

- Breakfast items (omelets or sandwiches) with roasted or grilled vegetables, ratatouille, or vegetable stacks topped with a poached egg

- Egg salad on multigrain toast

- Yogurt, fruits, nuts, seeds, honey for build-your-own yogurt flavors or yogurt parfaits

- Gluten-free menu alternatives such as cornmeal pancakes, buckwheat porridge, rice cereals, crustless quiche, waffles made with cornmeal, amaranth flour and brown rice flour

- Daily specials that include healthful global breakfast small plates with tacos, flatbreads, corn griddle cakes, buckwheat pancakes, crepes, frittatas and panini sandwiches

- Ready-to-eat cereals that are low in sugar (less than 5 grams per serving)

- Whole and cut fruits

- Oatmeal with fresh or dried fruit and nuts

- Cottage cheese or yogurt with fresh fruit

- French toast made with low-fat milk and a minimum of fat, served with fresh berries

- Grilled vegetable and cheese sandwich on whole-grain bread

- Raw vegetable salads to complement breakfast sandwiches and egg dishes

- Poached egg over sauteed spinach on whole-grain English muffin

- Cinnamon toast made with multigrain bread

- Rye bagel with smoked salmon, cucumbers, onions and reduced-fat cream cheese

- Two-egg omelet with spinach and feta cheese or salsa and shredded cheese

Breakfast: Guide to Ingredient Choices

Recommended	Limit
<ul><li>Whole-grain cereals</li><li>Whole-grain breads or rolls</li><li>All fruits and fruit juices</li><li>Vegetables, such as broiled tomatoes, grilled asparagus, grilled onions</li><li>Peanut or nut butter or spreads</li><li>Reduced-fat sausages, turkey bacon, Canadian bacon, lean ham</li><li>Cottage cheese</li><li>Reduced-fat cream cheese</li></ul>	<ul><li>Butter</li><li>Bacon</li><li>Sausage</li><li>Eggs (1 or 2 per portion)</li><li>Sugars and syrups</li><li>Fruit jams</li><li>Cream cheese, sour cream</li></ul>

Beverages

Beverages can be nutrient-rich and low in calories – think vegetable and fruit juices – or they can provide empty calories, such as soda laden with high-fructose corn syrup. Creating flavorful alternatives to alcoholic beverages is a way to showcase creativity and offer lower-calorie beverages to guests. (See Chapter 6 for more on beverages.)

Beverage Trends

Nonalcoholic Beverages

1. House-made soft drinks/soda/pop
2. Specialty iced tea (e.g., Thai-style, Southern/sweet, flavored)
3. Gourmet/house-made lemonade
4. Organic coffee
5. Dairy-free milk (e.g., soy, rice)
6. Agua fresca
7. Flavored/enhanced water
8. Tap water/filtered water
9. Green tea
10. Energy drinks

Alcohol and Cocktails

1. Locally-produced wine and beer
2. Micro-distilled/artisan spirits
3. Culinary cocktails (e.g., savory, fresh ingredients, herb-infused)
4. Food-beer pairings/beer dinners
5. Onsite barrel-aged drinks
6. Bar chefs/mixologists
7. Gluten-free beer
8. Specialty beer (e.g., seasonal, fruit, spiced)
9. Organic wine
10. Craft beer/microbrews

Source: National Restaurant Association. *Chef Survey: What's Hot in 2012.* Available at http://www.restaurant.org/pressroom/social-media-releases/images/whatshot2012/What's_Hot_2012.pdf.

Beverages: Guide to Ingredient Choices

Recommended	Limit
• 100% fruit juice	• Red and white wines
• Fruit juice spritzers	• Spirits
• Seltzer water	• Coconut-based drinks
• Mineral waters	• Salted vegetable juices
• Vegetable juices, low-sodium	• Whole milk
• Nonfat or low-fat milk	• Fruit drinks that often have only 5% to 10% fruit juice and added sugars
• Buttermilk	• Flavored coffee mixes
• Fruit smoothies	• Milk shakes and ice cream beverages
• Kefir	• Beverages made with chocolate or fruit syrups
• Soy, nut or rice milk (for those with dairy intolerance)	• Sweetened soft drinks
• Coffee, regular or decaffeinated	
• Black, herbal and green teas	

Presenting Food: Portioning and Plating

There is sometimes an inherent conflict for restaurants and other places where food is sold when a goal is to limit portions and types of food sold. A restaurant wants to sell food, often in large quantities, and to provide a perception of value to the diner. The suggestion of restraint can impact the bottom line if the only change is reducing portion size. Strategies for success in offering healthier food are described in this chapter. In all types of foodservice operations, from healthcare to college-dining to fine dining, there is value in caring enough about diners to offer foods to keep them healthy and coming back for more from your foodservice operation.

Often it is not the type of food served but rather the quantity served that compromises a healthful menu. Portion sizes have increased over the last 30 years; many items have more than doubled in size – and thus in calories, fat and sugar, too. For example, sodas have grown from a modest 8-ounce serving to 12- and 20-ounce cans to a 64-ounce Double Gulp. Research shows that commonly available portions almost always exceed U.S. Department of Agriculture and Food and Drug Administration standard portions, which are quite modest. For example, cookies, cooked pasta, muffins, steaks, sandwich rolls and bagels generally exceed standards by 200% to 700%. [9, 10] Chefs should know what standard servings are and should know the size of their portions by measuring them.

Since the 1980s, restaurants using oversized dinner plates, bakers using larger muffin tins and fast-food companies using larger drink, sandwich and French fry containers have supported this escalation in portion size. Even home recipes now suggest fewer servings for the same volume of ingredients.

Both larger portions and an increase in away-from-home food consumption have contributed to the weight management challenges so many Americans face. Larger portions provide more calories, encourage overeating and change consumer perception of what a normal, sensible portion looks like. Many experts agree that research on how to stop the obesity epidemic should focus on educating people to expect and eat smaller portions in general – fruits and vegetables being the exceptions to the rule. [9] In a nation that has super-sized almost everything, many people simply don't understand the value of smaller portions. The goal is to right-size; it's healthier and less expensive.

The trick to making healthy indulgences is to provide them in small amounts. It may be time to recalibrate the restaurant kitchen by using scales to evaluate portions, switching to smaller scoops, using more single-serving dishes and bowls, and downsizing dishes, glasses and serving platters. Consider portions carefully. Turn small into an advantage by offering bite-sized desserts, tasting portions, thin crackers and breadsticks. Focus on quality rather than quantity.

Moderating portion sizes and shifting focus from the center-of-the-plate protein require special attention to plating. Enhance the appeal of smaller portions by:

- Slicing meats and fanning (such as a chicken breast or sliced steak on salad greens)
- Using smaller plates to minimize white space
- Using specialty plates that showcase smaller portions
- Offering tasting menus
- Garnishing with fresh fruits and vegetables that complement the dish

Healthful garnishes are a good way to add fruit and vegetables to the plate without extra fat and sugar. Garnishes should bring color, texture, taste and interest to the dish without creating a distraction. Avoid using any item, edible or inedible, that does not contribute to the taste or texture of a dish. Ask yourself, "What purpose does this garnish serve?" Color is not enough. Colorful and healthful garnishes include shredded or finely diced vegetables, sliced or shredded sweet potatoes, carrots, daikon, parsnips, colorful peppers, fresh herbs, relishes, salsas, slaws, legumes, coulis, cooked grains, corn tortilla strips and baked wontons. Drizzle sauces, such as balsamic reduction or raspberry sauce, over food and on plates.

While much of this text has discouraged the use of high-fat ingredients like cheeses, deep-fried ingredients or whipped cream, these items can be effective garnishes to add texture or flavor to a dish. A dollop of whipped cream, a drizzle of fudge sauce, a sprinkling of crispy onion strips or fried sage leaves, or a few candied nuts add richness and visual appeal with just a modest amount of fat. Since the "topping" hits the palate first, it also boosts flavor from the first bite.

Add Texture and Variety with Bread

Pita triangles

Thinly sliced olive bread

Phyllo dough cones or cups

Lavosh, matzoh or flatbreads

Seeded or herbed crisp thin bread sticks

Baked flour tortilla triangles

Baked corn tortilla strips

Baked croutons

Mini-muffins

Bruschetta

Thinly sliced fruit and nut bread or toast

Healthful Plate Enhancers

Add color and textural contrasts that make plates beautiful as well as more nutrient rich.

Apple, fennel and walnut salad

Black beans and corn relish

Carrot sauce

Chimichurri sauce

Dried or fresh cranberry compote

Eggplant caponata

Green tomato chutney

Heirloom tomatoes

Herb pestos

Jicama salad

Mango, papaya, apricot or pineapple chutney

Marinated bean salads

Oranges and Belgian endive

Pickled fruits or vegetables

Pomegranate seeds

Red pepper spread or vinaigrette

Roasted red, yellow and orange peppers

Salsas

Sliced fresh or roasted pears in salad

Sliced roasted beets

Spicy peanut sauce

Winter fruit compote

Children's Menus

According to the National Restaurant Association's 2012 survey of chefs, healthful kids' meals and children's nutrition are top trends. The survey also identified fruit and vegetable side dishes and "mini-meals," smaller versions of adult menu items as trends in kids' meals. [3]

Perspectives on the Children's Menu: Food That Looks Good, Tastes Good and Is Good for You

What Appeals to Children	What Appeals to Adults for Children's Meals
• Small bites or hand-held food items • Identifiable foods or flavors • Foods that can be dipped in appealing sauces • Sweet flavors • Foods that can be customized to the child's preferences • Menu descriptions that let the child know what's in the dish • Interesting shapes • Crunchy textures • Foods similar to the adult menu with minor modifications for the younger palate	• Minimally processed whole foods such as fruits, vegetables, whole grains and lean proteins • Lean meats, preferably in an appropriate size for the child • Accurate food descriptions revealing nuts, dairy, eggs or other common allergens • More grilling, baking and steaming; less frying • "Neat" foods with minimal sauce or sauce as a dip • Bendable straws, lids for beverage containers, small cups for small hands, nonbreakable dishes • Low-fat milk, 100% fruit juice or water • Appropriate portions • Variety to accommodate different age groups and preferences • Appealing presentation of healthful choices • Menu items that make the chef's signature items available to children, too • Menu descriptions that let the parent know what's in the dish

Must-Have Sides

- Fresh fruit – kid-sized pieces, single fruits or fruit medleys, such as orange wedges, apple wedges, melon balls, blueberries, whole strawberries, etc.

- Steamed or stir-fried vegetables – broccoli, asparagus or beans with cheese sauce for dipping, corn on the cob

- Starches – brown rice, mashed sweet potatoes, baked vegetable strips, whole-wheat pasta in interesting shapes

- Carrot sticks or small carrots, red pepper strips, sugar snap peas or peapods

New Ideas and Twists on Old Favorites: Add Some Fun to the Children's Menu

- Quesadilla – whole-grain tortilla with Monterey Jack cheese and salsa

- Turkey mini-wrap – vegetables such as shredded carrots, lettuce and cucumber julienne along with lean turkey breast and cheese filling

- Vegetable mini-wrap – rice paper filled with hummus, julienne vegetables, lettuce and tomatoes; served with selected dipping sauces

- Peanut butter sandwich – on whole-grain bread with banana slices or apple wedges to add to sandwich

- Veggie sticks and ranch dip – red peppers, carrots, celery, cucumbers, jicama, blanched green beans and sugar snap peas standing upright in a container to resemble French fries; served with dipping sauce

- Pot stickers – filled with lean meat and vegetables; served with Asian dipping sauce

- Kid's sushi rolls – filled with raw vegetables, with or without surimi (no raw fish), edamame

- Vietnamese salad rolls – served with dipping sauce

- Guacamole with corn chips – guacamole and salsa with baked chips

- Ham or turkey roll-up – tortilla rolled with turkey or ham, low-fat cheese, lettuce and mayonnaise or mustard

- Burger sliders – made with ground turkey, lean beef, fish or seafood, beans and added vegetables

- Penne pasta – with sauteed broccoli, carrots and peppers

- Macaroni and cheese – with steamed broccoli

- Pasta with tomato or meat sauce – served over whole-wheat pasta or white pasta

- Chicken satay – served with peanut noodles

- Fish taco – served with guacamole

- Tuna melt – on whole-wheat English muffin with low-fat cheese

- Tuna salad cones – low-fat tuna salad scooped into flat-bottom ice cream cones; served with baby carrots

- Chicken fingers – grilled or baked and served with dipping sauces

- Asian treats – edamame, hoisin chicken strips and grilled shrimp

- Shrimp boat – steamed shrimp on romaine lettuce with chili sauce

- Mariner's special – 3 ounces of grilled fish with rice and green beans

- Vegetable stir-fry – with baby shrimp, chicken or beef strips

- Chicken, vegetable or tomato soup – served with whole-grain crackers

- Turkey meatballs and marinara sauce – with whole-grain pasta

- Mini caprese – grape tomatoes with tiny mozzarella balls or cubes; served with basil vinaigrette dressing

- Green eggs and ham – 1 egg scrambled with chopped spinach; served with 2 ounces of grilled ham and whole-wheat toast triangles

- Smashed vegetables – winter squash, sweet potatoes, peas and red skin potatoes

- Waffles with strawberries and blueberries – whole-grain waffles with fruit

- Patriotic oatmeal – small bowl of oatmeal topped with dried red cranberries and blueberries; served with 4 ounces of white, low-fat milk

- Ice cream sandwiches – graham crackers and frozen yogurt

- Fruit and cheese kabobs – cut fruit with cheese cubes

- Fruit smoothies – 6-ounce portion made with frozen fruit and low-fat milk

- Fruit fondue – pineapple, strawberries and banana served with chocolate or raspberry dipping sauce

- Banana split – half banana, sliced and topped with frozen low-fat vanilla and strawberry yogurt, a drizzle of chocolate sauce and a bit of crunchy granola

- Caramel apple slices – sliced apples with caramel dipping sauce

- Berry yogurt parfait – strawberry yogurt layered with sliced strawberries and blueberries; teddy grahams, chocolate covered raisins and sweetened dried cranberries as toppers

- Gelato made with milk and fresh fruit

Selecting Healthful Ingredients

The trend toward using local, organic or sustainable ingredients is important to many guests and chefs. It is useful to remember, however, that including plenty of fruits, vegetables, grains and other inherently healthy products in whatever form – frozen, canned, dried or fresh – is the single most important factor in planning healthful menus. The reality is that many Americans are not particularly interested in nor can they afford to eat "green." In addition, in many operations, the food budget does not allow for organic or other ingredients that are more costly than conventional produce, grain or protein sources. Thus, food-service operations of all types – schools, community feeding programs, college and university, healthcare, nursing homes, quick service, family-style and fine dining – are seeking affordable "green" ingredients. Some restaurants have created their own gardens to provide some ingredients to use and feature.

Heritage and Heirloom Ingredients

Everything old is new again. Heritage meats and heirloom vegetables and fruits are finding a place on contemporary menus. "Heritage" is usually used to describe animals, while "heirloom" refers to plants. These terms describe varieties of animals and crops that have unique genetic traits, were raised many years ago and are typically grown in a sustainable manner.

According to Seed Savers Exchange (www.seedsavers. org), a nonprofit organization dedicated to preserving rare plant varieties, an **heirloom plant** is "any garden plant that has a history of being passed down within a family." While some argue that an heirloom variety must be at least 50 to 100 years old, all agree that heirloom fruits and vegetables are unique plant varieties that are genetically distinct from the commercial varieties popularized by industrial agriculture. Heirloom varieties are less consistent in size, shape and color than commercial varieties but often have more flavor and interesting textures and shapes. Heirloom varieties of beets, beans, carrots,

cucumbers, lettuces, salad greens, spinach, radishes, peas, melons, pumpkins, squash, chard, corn, tomatoes, peppers and eggplant are available. For example, there are 60 varieties of heirloom beans to add interest and variety to the menu.

Seed Savers Exchange members have distributed an estimated 1 million samples of rare garden seeds since the organization was founded nearly 35 years ago. Those seeds now are widely used by small farmers supplying local and regional markets with unique alternatives to commercial produce.

Protecting the Past

Slow Foods (www.slowfoodsusa.org) is a global, grassroots movement with thousands of members around the world. The group links the pleasure of food with a commitment to community and the environment. The Slow Foods USA chapter has created a U.S. Ark of Taste, which catalogs more than 200 foods in danger of extinction. By promoting Ark products, Slow Foods helps ensure they remain in production and available.

The American Livestock Breeds Conservancy (www. albc-usa.org) is a nonprofit membership organization working to protect more than 150 breeds of livestock and poultry from extinction. Founded in 1977, the conservancy is the pioneer organization in the U.S. working to protect historic breeds and genetic diversity in livestock. Heritage varieties include breeds of cattle, sheep, pigs, chickens and turkeys.

Ancient Grains and Pseudograins

As nutrition policymakers and consumers continue to focus on increasing whole-grain consumption, ancient grains have found a place in stuffings, pilafs, crepes, salads, risottos, stir-fries, fritters, bread puddings, garnishes, breading for meats, grits, soups, crusts, pastries and cakes. These grains and grain alternatives can be good alternatives for customers who are sensitive to gluten in wheat, oats, rye and barley.

Pseudograins

Sometimes called grain alternatives, **pseudograins** are foods that are prepared like grains but are actually seeds. Pseudograins are sometimes cooked but also can be ground into flour or used in cereals. Amaranth, millet and quinoa are pseudograins.

Amaranth

Amaranth's tiny beige granules have a nutty flavor and creamy-soft texture. These seeds (not grains) can be used as a breakfast cereal or side dish and make a healthful thickener for soups and stews. Amaranth's broad, leafy greens with red markings can be cooked as a vegetable and taste somewhat like spinach.

Millet

Millet is small and round. It can be white, gray, yellow or red and has a mildly nutty flavor and a soft texture. Millet is popular in Asian and African cooking but has not been fully appreciated in this country. The most widely available form of millet is the pearled, hulled variety. Many multigrain breads contain millet.

Quinoa

Quinoa, pronounced "KEEN-wa," is a seed that has been growing in the rugged highlands of South America for centuries. The small oval granules have a nutty flavor, soft texture and beige hue. Quinoa is particularly high in protein and can be combined with or substituted for rice in pilafs, soups, salads and side dishes. This versatile "mother grain of the Incas" cooks in only 15 to 20 minutes. Red quinoa can be cooked and used to add color, texture and flavor as a garnish or in a sauce. It looks like red caviar.

Spelt

Spelt's "nutty" flavor has long been popular in Europe, where it is also known as farro (Italy) and dinkle (Germany). Spelt is one of the oldest of cultivated grains and is a lesser-known cousin of wheat. It is processed into baking flour, cereals and an assortment of pastas including elbow macaroni, spaghetti and shells.

Kamut® (Khorasan Wheat)

Kamut is an ancient relative of modern durum wheat and is two to three times the size of common wheat with 20% to 40% more protein. It can be substituted for wheat in most products. Kamut is an important crop for sustainable, organic agriculture because of its ability to produce high-quality grain without artificial fertilizers and pesticides.

Teff

Teff was domesticated in Ethiopia between 4000 and 1000 BC. It is grown primarily as a cereal crop. One of the smallest grains in the world, most of a grain of teff consists of bran and germ, the most nutritious parts of any grain. Teff is high in protein, calcium and iron. Teff flour can be used in baked goods and the grains make a good thickener for soups, stews and puddings. Cooked teff can be used as a base to make grain burgers. Teff seeds can also be sprouted and the sprouts used in salads and on sandwiches.

Chefs Collaborative

The foodservice industry is an important participant in the sustainable agriculture movement. From fine dining establishments to college dining rooms, hospitals and schools, foodservice professionals can commit to purchasing, preparing and serving foods grown sustainably. The Chefs Collaborative (www.chefscollaborative.org) is a nonprofit network of chefs that fosters a sustainable food system through advocacy, education and collaboration with the broader food community. The collaborative inspires action by translating information about food into tools for making knowledgeable purchasing decisions that reflect seasonality, preserve diversity and traditional practices, and support local economies.

Chefs Collaborative Statement of Principles

1. Food is fundamental to life, nourishing us in body and soul. The preparation of food strengthens our connection to nature. And the sharing of food immeasurably enriches our sense of community.

2. Good food begins with unpolluted air, land and water, environmentally sustainable farming and fishing and humane animal husbandry.

3. Food choices that emphasize delicious, locally grown, seasonally fresh and whole or minimally processed ingredients are good for us, for local farming communities and for the planet.

4. Cultural and biological diversity are essential for the health of the earth and its inhabitants. Preserving and revitalizing sustainable food, fishing and agricultural traditions strengthen that diversity.

5. By continually educating themselves about sustainable choices, chefs can serve as models to the culinary community and the general public through their purchases of seasonal, sustainable ingredients and their transformation of these ingredients into delicious food.

6. The greater culinary community can be a catalyst for positive change by creating a market for good food and helping preserve local farming and fishing communities.

Sustainable Seafood

Poor fishing practices are destroying not only the population of some fish species, but also those of other marine animals caught and discarded as bycatch, including sea turtles, sharks and many thousands of seabirds. Several organizations monitor local and international waters and share their information with chefs and the public.

- The Smithsonian's National Museum of Natural History maintains a sustainable seafood website (www.mnh.si.edu/seafood) that provides current information on suggested and problematic seafood choices.

- The National Oceanic and Atmospheric Administration (NOAA) maintains FishWatch (www.nmfs.noaa.gov/fishwatch), which reports news on seafood and health.

- The Blue Ocean Institute (www.blueocean.org/seafood-guide) provides seafood and sushi guides.

- The Marine Stewardship Council (www.msc.org) certifies sustainable seafood.

- The Monterey Bay Aquarium Seafood Watch® (www.montereybayaquarium.org/cr/seafoodwatch.aspx) empowers consumers and businesses to make choices for healthy oceans. The aquarium's *Seafood Watch Pocket Guide* assists consumers and foodservice professionals in identifying the most environmentally responsible sources of seafood. The guide is available in a national version as well as in six regional versions. Seafood Watch suggests that food buyers gather details on where fish comes from, whether it was farmed or wild caught, and how it was farmed or caught.

Monterey Bay Aquarium® Seafood Watch®

The Monterey Bay Aquarium Seafood Watch program creates science-based recommendations that help consumers and businesses make ocean-friendly seafood choices. Carry this pocket guide with you and share it with others to help spread the word.

BEST CHOICES

- Arctic Char (farmed)
- Barramundi (US farmed)
- Catfish (US farmed)
- Clams (farmed)
- Cobia (US farmed)
- Cod: Pacific (US non-trawled)
- Crab: Dungeness, Stone
- Halibut: Pacific (US)
- Lobster: California Spiny (US)
- Mussels (farmed)
- Oysters (farmed)
- Sablefish/Black Cod (Alaska & Canada)
- Salmon (Alaska wild)
- Sardines: Pacific (US)
- Scallops (farmed)
- Shrimp: Pink (OR)
- Striped Bass (farmed & wild*)
- Tilapia (US farmed)
- Trout: Rainbow (US farmed)
- Tuna: Albacore (Canada & US Pacific, troll/pole)
- Tuna: Skipjack, Yellowfin (US troll/pole)

GOOD ALTERNATIVES

- Basa/Pangasius/Swai (farmed)
- Caviar, Sturgeon (US farmed)
- Clams (wild)
- Cod: Atlantic (imported)
- Cod: Pacific (US trawled)
- Crab: Blue*, King (US), Snow
- Flounders, Soles (Pacific)
- Flounder: Summer (US Atlantic)*
- Grouper: Black, Red (US Gulf of Mexico)*
- Herring: Atlantic
- Lobster: American/Maine
- Mahi Mahi (US)
- Oysters (wild)
- Pollock: Alaska (US)
- Sablefish/Black Cod (CA, OR, WA)
- Salmon (CA, OR, WA*, wild)
- Scallops (wild)
- Shrimp (US, Canada)
- Squid
- Swordfish (US)*
- Tilapia (Central & South America) (farmed)
- Tuna: Bigeye, Tongol, Yellowfin (troll/pole)

AVOID

- Caviar, Sturgeon* (imported wild)
- Chilean Seabass/Toothfish*
- Cobia (imported farmed)
- Cod: Atlantic (Canada & US)
- Crab: King (imported)
- Flounders, Halibut, Soles (US Atlantic, except Summer Flounder)
- Groupers (US Atlantic)*
- Lobster: Spiny (Brazil)
- Mahi Mahi (imported longline)
- Marlin: Blue, Striped (Pacific)*
- Monkfish
- Orange Roughy*
- Salmon (farmed, including Atlantic)*
- Sharks* & Skates
- Shrimp (imported)
- Snapper: Red (US Gulf of Mexico)
- Swordfish (imported)*
- Tilapia (Asia farmed)
- Tuna: Albacore*, Bigeye*, Skipjack, Tongol, Yellowfin* (except troll/pole)
- Tuna: Bluefin
- Tuna: Canned (except troll/pole)

Support Ocean-Friendly Seafood

Best Choices are abundant, well-managed and caught or farmed in environmentally friendly ways.

Good Alternatives are an option, but there are concerns with how they're caught or farmed – or with the health of their habitat due to other human impacts.

Avoid for now as these items are overfished or caught or farmed in ways that harm other marine life or the environment.

Key

CA = California	OR = Oregon
WA = Washington	

* Limit consumption due to concerns about mercury or other contaminants.
Visit www.edf.org/seafoodhealth
Contaminant information provided by:
ENVIRONMENTAL DEFENSE FUND

Seafood may appear in more than one column

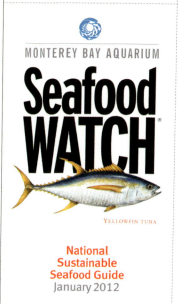

MONTEREY BAY AQUARIUM

Seafood WATCH®

YELLOWFIN TUNA

National Sustainable Seafood Guide
January 2012

Learn More

In addition to the recommendations on this guide, we have hundreds more available from our scientists.

To see the complete and most up-to-date list visit us:
- Online at **seafoodwatch.org**
- On our free app
- On our mobile site
- Or join us on Facebook or Twitter

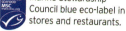

MONTEREY BAY
AQUARIUM®

The seafood recommendations in this guide are credited to the Monterey Bay Aquarium Foundation
©2012. All rights reserved. Printed on recycled paper.

You Can Make A Difference

Support ocean-friendly seafood in three easy steps:

1. Purchase seafood from the green list or, if unavailable, the yellow list. Or look for the Marine Stewardship Council blue eco-label in stores and restaurants.

2. When you buy seafood, ask where your seafood comes from and whether it was farmed or wild-caught.

3. Tell your friends about Seafood Watch. The more people that ask for ocean-friendly seafood, the better!

Why Do Your Seafood Choices Matter?

Worldwide, the demand for seafood is increasing. Yet many populations of the large fish we enjoy eating are over-fished and, in the U.S., we import over 80% of our seafood to meet the demand. Destructive fishing and fish farming practices only add to the problem.

By purchasing fish caught or farmed using environmentally friendly practices, you're supporting healthy, abundant oceans.

Reprinted with permission from Monterey Bay Aquarium, www.seafoodwatch.org or www.montereybayaquarium.org

Salty

Salt (sodium chloride) is one of the most used and, from a health point of view, most overused flavor enhancers. Although salt improves the flavor of food by stimulating the taste buds and by balancing the effects of sweet, sour and bitter, we are becoming increasingly aware of salt's potentially negative effects on health. (See pages 230 to 233 for more information on salt.)

The preference for saltiness in foods, although partially genetic, is strongly influenced by environmental factors and varies a great deal from person to person. In other words, it's an acquired taste. Infants develop a taste for salt at 4 to 6 months of age based on how much salt is in their diet. At any age, however, a gradual reduction in sodium intake over eight to 12 weeks can retrain the palate and increase acceptance of foods with less salt. [6] Supertasters commonly require more salt, not to intensify flavor but to counteract their super- sensitivity to bitter taste.

One way to reduce salt in recipes is to use flavor enhancers such as yeast extracts, yeast-based ingredients or monosodium glutamate (MSG). These ingredients activate taste receptors in the mouth and throat to amplify flavor and compensate for less salt. MSG, for example, contains about one-third the sodium found in salt.

When trying to cut back on salt in your cooking, be aware of salty ingredients already in a recipe such as soy sauce, anchovies, prosciutto, olives, capers, bacon, mustard, oyster sauce and parmesan cheese. Reduced-sodium soy sauce can be substituted for regular soy sauce for a moderate reduction in salt without a significant change in flavor. Rinsing canned vegetables, particularly beans, before adding them to a recipe can reduce sodium content by 40%.

Another approach to reducing sodium is to take advantage of the importance that smell has on flavor by increasing aromatic ingredients and assertive flavors to replace the taste lost when cutting down on salt. Today's diners are receptive to more intense flavors from spices and herbs as well as to the sensation caused by chili peppers.

Unfortunately – from a health point of view – salt also has become a popular addition to many desserts that are already high in fat and sugar, including salted caramel, salted chocolates and salted pralines. Many desserts, however, do have fruit to their credit!

Bitter

Bitter is defined as an acrid, sharp and unpleasant taste. Many people avoid the taste of bitterness. Poisonous foods are often bitter, so from an evolutionary point of view, bitterness helped early humans avoid natural toxins.

The taste of bitterness stimulates the appetite and cuts through the richness of some foods. Chefs typically balance bitterness with salt and sugar or with flavorful sauces and fats. This approach is important because even though many poisonous plants are bitter, other plants that are healthful to eat also have a bitter taste. In fact, many edible plants protect themselves against insects by secreting natural pesticides that are not harmful to humans when consumed in small amounts. Although plants are being engineered to remove these substances through selective breeding, many phytonutrients thought to reduce cancer risk and heart disease are being removed at the same time.

More recently, chefs have been highlighting bitter taste as a way to balance the richness of some foods while cleansing the palate between bites. Small amounts of bitterness can be pleasant and provide flavor contrast. Salads made of bitter greens, such as frisee, endive, watercress, radicchio and arugula, are commonly served with fatty steaks and fish. Cooked collards, Swiss chard, kale and other bitter nutrient-rich vegetables are popular side dishes. Bitterness is sometimes considered a positive attribute in products like coffee, strong tea, beer, wine and many mixed cocktails that contain tonic or bitters as a main ingredient. Although bitterness is not prized in most Western cultures, it is considered a component of a balanced dish in much of India and Asia.

Monosodium Glutamate Explained

Glutamate, or glutamic acid, is one of the most common amino acids. It is found in all proteins and many other foods. In its bound form, glutamate links to other amino acids to make proteins. In its free form, it is a single amino acid that affects the flavor of food. Foods high in free glutamate, such as fermented fish sauces, seaweed products, meat extracts, tomato products and shiitake mushrooms, have been used for centuries to enhance flavor.

Monosodium glutamate (MSG) is a combination of glutamate, sodium and water. It acts like free glutamate and adds umami – a savory, broth-like or meaty taste – to foods. The body metabolizes glutamate, including that in MSG, the same way that it metabolizes glutamate found naturally in foods and the glutamate made in the body.

MSG Benefits

MSG has about one-third as much sodium as salt. MSG contains 12% sodium by weight, while salt contains 40% sodium. Some professionals suggest substituting small amounts of MSG for salt to reduce sodium while preserving a flavoring-enhancing effect. This approach is particularly useful when amplifying flavors for people who have a reduced ability to taste or poor appetite or for those who cannot tolerate large amounts of salt. MSG works by sensitizing taste buds to spread pleasing sensations throughout the mouth and by activating umami sensors.

MSG is most effective in recipes containing meat, poultry, seafood and vegetables and in combined dishes. MSG does not enhance the flavor of highly acidic foods, milk products or sweet foods such as pastries and desserts. It should be added before or during cooking; MSG is not destroyed by heat.

Chinese Restaurant Syndrome

The term *"Chinese restaurant syndrome"* was first used in 1968 in the *New England Journal of Medicine*. The author, a physician, described pain in the back of his neck, heart palpitations and other symptoms after eating in a Chinese restaurant. Others confirmed that they had had similar experiences, and a syndrome was born. While a significant number of Americans report symptoms of what is now called MSG symptom complex, virtually all cases have been anecdotal. Due to public concern that MSG causes headaches, facial flushing, chest tightness, nausea, weakness and neurologic problems and contributes to asthma, it is one of the most studied food additives, The American College of Allergy, Asthma and Immunology states that MSG is not an allergen. The European Union, the United Nations Food and Agriculture Organization, and the World Health Organization place MSG in the safest category of food additives. The Food and Drug Administration lists MSG as Generally Recognized As Safe (GRAS).

What the Research Says

Many well-designed scientific studies have recorded no symptoms when people with reported sensitivities were given MSG under controlled conditions. Some research indicates that individuals who think that they have MSG sensitivity are actually having an allergic reaction to shellfish, soy, peanuts or other ingredients in Chinese cuisine.

Some people may in fact be sensitive to MSG, just as some individuals are sensitive to other foods and food ingredients. They may experience mild, transient symptoms such a facial flushing and rapid heartbeat that do not require treatment. Research continues, but today there is considerable scientific consensus that MSG, as normally used, poses no significant health risk and that MSG in food has no discernible effect on healthy people. Despite this consensus, a number of individuals and advocacy organizations continue to promote the belief that MSG is a dangerous food additive.

According to Food and Drug Administration regulations, when MSG is added to a food, it must be included in the ingredient list. When glutamate-containing ingredients are products components, they are listed by their common name – for example, Parmesan cheese, tomatoes, shiitake mushrooms, Worcestershire sauce, hydrolyzed protein or yeast extract.

Sources:
Federation of American Societies for Experimental Biology. *Executive Summary from the Report: Analysis of Adverse Reactions to Monosodium Glutamate (MSG).* Available at **http://jn.nutrition.org/cgi/reprint/125/11/2891S.pdf**.

Walker R, Lupien JR. The safety evaluation of monosodium glutamate. *J Nutri.*2000;130:1049S-52S Available at **http://jn.nutrition.org/cgi/reprint/130/4/1049S**.

Tarasoff L, Kelly MF. Monosodium L-glutamate: A double-blind study and review. *Food and Chemical Toxicology.*1993;31:1019-35.

Sweet

While our tongues are hard-wired to be cautious of bitter taste, we are born with a strong desire to search out sweet taste. This phenomenon is also thought to be a survival mechanism because sweet foods usually contain energy-rich nutrients. In addition, in response to sweet flavors, the brain releases endorphins, which are neurotransmitters that reduce pain and create a feeling of well being.

Health problems arise when we over-consume refined sugars, which are simple carbohydrates that provide calories but no other nutrients; however, the same calories and carbohydrates are available in nutrient-rich vegetables, whole grains, fruits and beans. (See Chapter 3 for a complete discussion of sugar.)

Some chefs are substituting brown sugar, honey, palm sugar, molasses, agave or maple syrup to add flavor. From a nutrition point of view, however, these sweeteners are no different from refined sugar. Dates and fruit purees are a popular nutrient-rich substitution for sugar. Some spices, such as cinnamon and cardamom, have a sweet note that makes it possible to cut the amount of sugar used.

Sugars are not the only source of sweetness. Sugar alcohols and artificial sweeteners are also available. Some sugar alternatives are available in combination with sugar for use in baking. Diners limiting calories and sugar intake may want "diet" soda as well as **alternative sweeteners** to use in coffee and other beverages. Some alternative sweeteners, often called sugar substitutes, taste sweet at first but have a metallic, licorice-like or chemical aftertaste for certain individuals.

Non-nutritive sweeteners or artificial sweeteners can be used in cooking but generally are not popular with chefs. Although they add sweetness, most don't act like sugar. Non-nutritive sweeteners don't caramelize, add volume, cream well with fat or perform well in baking. Some are not stable when heated. In addition, non-nutritive sweeteners are more expensive than sugar.

Relative Sweetness of Sugars

Sugar sweetness is measured by comparison to the sweetness of sucrose, which is assigned a value of 100.

Sweetener	Sweetness Value
Sucrose (table sugar)	100
High-fructose corn syrup	100 - 130
Fructose	120
Honey, liquid	100
Invert sugar syrup	95
Glucose	70
Dextrose	60 - 70
Maltose	45
Lactose (milk sugar)	40
Corn syrup	30 - 50

Source: Adapted from: McGee H. *On Food and Cooking*. 2nd ed. New York: Scribner; 2004

Relative Sweetness of Sugar Substitutes

The sweetness of sugar substitutes is measured by comparison to the sweetness of table sugar, which is assigned a value of 100.

Sugar Substitute	Sweetness Value
Sucrose (table sugar)	100
Sugar alcohols	
Erythritol (Zsweet®)	70
Sorbitol	60
Mannitol	70
Maltitol	90
Xylitol	100
Aspartame (Equal®, NutraSweet®)	18,000
Acesulfame K (Sunnet®)	20,000
Saccharin (Sweet'N Low®)	30,000
Stevioside (Truvia®, Pure Via®, Sweet Leaf®)	30,000
Sucralose (Splenda®)	60,000
Neotame	800,000

Source: Adapted from: McGee H. *On Food and Cooking*. 2nd ed. New York: Scribner; 2004

Sour

The basic taste of *sour* comes from acidic ingredients. Acidic foods provide bright, sharp flavors that can reduce the need for salt. For example, a small amount of lime juice enhances the flavor of a black bean soup. The most common food group that contains naturally sour foods is fruit, particularly citrus fruits, including lemon, lime, orange, grapefruit, kumquat, tangerine, mandarin, tangelo and Meyer lemon. Vinegars, such as malt, cider, balsamic, champagne, fruit, herb, rice, wine and garlic, also add sourness.

The popularity of international cuisines, particularly Asian cooking, has introduced many new sour ingredients to the chef's pantry – kaffir lime, tamarind, sumac, lemon grass, ponzu, galangal and powdered pomegranate seeds, to name a few.

Just as the American palate embraced the fiery excitement of hot chilies, diners have now turned their attention toward sour taste in food. From green apple martinis to Japanese yuzu to Indian vindaloo, sour is in demand and presents new opportunities for chefs to expand their menus. Sour is a perfect accompaniment to spicy hot food because it cuts the heat and freshens the palate for the next fiery bite.

Americans have a long history of combining sour with sweet as in lemonade and strawberry-rhubarb pie. The growing popularity of a simple squeeze of citrus into soups and salads as well as on grilled meats, seafood and even sweet corn is evidence of a new appreciation of tartness. As diners continue to explore and experience the sour aspect of various cuisines, chefs can use this taste to offer healthier options that cut sodium, sugar and fat from recipes.

Umami

Umami is a Japanese word meaning delicious. Sometimes described as savory, brothy or meaty, the sensation of umami is conveyed by several substances, including the amino acid glutamate. Glutamate is found naturally in many foods, including fish, meat, cheese, tomatoes, mushrooms, peas, corn, seaweed and human milk. Foods that are ripe and at their flavor peak have more umami. Deep red, ripe tomatoes have five times the glutamate

of unripe early tomatoes. Monosodium glutamate (MSG branded as Accent) is often used to enhance and harmonize the flavor of food. Many Asian cuisines routinely use MSG in cooking.

The Monell Chemical Senses Center in Philadelphia specializes in the study of taste and smell and the treatment of taste and smell disorders. Scientists at Monell confirmed the presence of specific taste receptors for umami in 2009. The landmark study found the genes associated with umami perception along with various levels of umami sensitivity. [7]

Taste Interactions

The flavor experience is a mixture of taste, aroma and texture with limitless possibilities. The five basic taste sensations work together to highlight, offset, compliment and balance each other. Desserts taste sweeter with a bitter caffeine beverage than with water; acids taste even more sour with salty foods and cut the fiery effects of hot peppers.

I have a cupboard full of acids! Everyday culture is doing the same thing when it comes to using acid in its food: it is all about enhancing flavor without adding salt. When I lived in England, they joked with me because I would add orange juice to almost everything, especially vinaigrettes. I really like its acidity and the light fruity flavor it adds. On a totally different end of the spectrum is tamarind. We always have tamarind water in our refrigerator and use it to finish sauces. Depending on the country of inspiration, I will use a different acid: for India, tamarind; Japan, ponzu, yuzu; Middle East, sumac, preserved lemon, and yogurt; and for Southeast Asia, lemon, lime and tamarind.

Chef Brad Farmerie
as quoted in Karen Page and Andrew Dornenburg's
The Flavor Bible
Little, Brown and Company, New York 2008

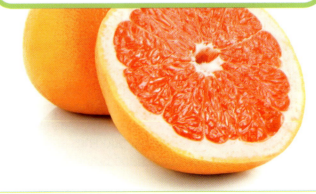

What Makes Us Feel Full?

The main role of food is to satisfy hunger and to provide essential energy, nutrients, and other substances for growth and the maintenance of health. Much of what we choose to eat is influenced by the palatability of foods, including the taste, smell, texture and appearance. Of course, social setting, personal preferences, habits, mood and other environmental factors also influence food intake.

Appetite can be divided into three components: hunger, satiation and satiety. **Hunger** is the sensation that causes us to seek and eat food. As eating proceeds, hunger subsides while satiation, the feeling that governs how much and how long we eat, takes over. Eventually, the feeling of satiation (when hunger ends) ends eating, and a period of not eating begins. **Satiety** refers to the sensations that determine the time between meals. [8] Regulation of appetite – including the hunger, satiation and satiety that influence what we eat – has both a physiological and psychological basis.

Satiety describes the effects of a meal after it has ended. The mechanisms involved in controlling satiety range from those involved with digestion, such as gastric distention and emptying, to more complex hormonal effects. In addition, people do not always eat when they are hungry, possibly due to lack of food or social constraints, and they do not always refrain from eating when satiated, perhaps because of boredom or stress.

The macronutrients – protein, fat and carbohydrates – affect the feeling of satiety. Protein is the most satiating of the three. Increased satiety can come from foods high in fiber or water, too. Fats and carbohydrates are less satiating. It appears that taste, palatability and caloric value greatly influence the degree to which macronutrients promote or reduce appetite. **Palatability**, the measure of a food's pleasantness, and energy-density also influence satiety and therefore hunger. People prefer foods that are energy dense because they are more palatable. Less-caloric foods typically contain more water and less fat. They tend to be more physiologically satiating but generally less palatable. [9]

Barbara Rolls, PhD, a professor at Pennsylvania State University and author of the popular book *Volumetrics* has studied how energy density affects satiety. She states that satiety is the missing ingredient in most weight-loss programs. [10] People need to eat more foods that are higher in water and fiber to create a feeling of fullness. In other words, low-energy dense foods with high palatability mitigate overconsumption and create a high satiety level. These foods include those with protein and fiber, including plenty of fruits, vegetables, whole grains and water. [11]

Flavors Imparted by Cooking

Raw food will taste completely different when cooked, and flavor may vary according to cooking technique. Compare the taste of a raw onion with one that is sauteed or caramelized. Does a hot smoked chicken breast taste different from one that is poached, sauteed or grilled? Think about how simply toasting nuts changes and intensifies their flavors. Heat can enhance or destroy flavor, depending on how it is used. Many flavors can be developed through proper execution of various cooking techniques, often without adding extra calories, fat or salt.

The Heat Is On

A **Maillard reaction** occurs when heat is applied to a food that contains both carbohydrate and protein. This reaction is identified by browning and development of flavor. Examples of the Maillard reaction can be seen in bread crusts and roasted meats.

The browning of sugar is a reaction called **caramelization**. The transformation of sugar results in a rich aroma, color and taste. Caramelizing a simple sweet food can change it into something more complex and rich with a nutty or toasty flavor. Browning onions is an example of caramelization; sauteed, browned onions are more fragrant and sweeter than raw onions.

A Word from the Chef
Going to Great 'Lengths' for Flavor

"My signature flavors are built with a vast palette of vibrant ingredients," says Brad Farmerie, executive chef with the AvroKO Hospitality Group, which includes New York City's PUBLIC (a Michelin star establishment since opening in 2003) and Saxon + Parole as well as the group's newest restaurant, The Thomas, in Napa, California. "I tend to blend richness with spice, all tempered with a decent shot of acidity," Brad explains. "I borrow flavors from all over the globe – miso, soy, mirin, ginger, kombu and yuzu from Japan and China, preserved lemons and tahini from Northern Africa and the Middle East, coconut and tamarind from India and South East Asia."

To build complexity and nuance, Brad considers the "length" of flavors in a dish. "Usually," he says, "a diner will taste the fresh herbs in a dish before noticing the spices. By using both, you create a symphony of flavor with each bite."

PUBLIC's crispy fried oysters with shiso, sansho pepper, and a wasabi-yuzu dipping sauce are a good example of Brad's flavor philosophy at work. "With the first bite, you detect the perfumed fresh shiso followed by the richness of the fried oyster," he explains. "As you chew, the acidity from the yuzu in the dipping sauce hits the sides of your tongue, giving a jolt of brightness and cutting through the richness. When you swallow, the heat of the wasabi creeps up the back of your throat and into your nose, followed by the tingly numbness as sansho pepper begins to affects the lips and tongue. For such a 'simple' dish," he continues, "this length and depth of flavor are very complex and memorable – without using stereotypical flavor builders like fat, butter or bacon."

Looking to the future of flavor, Brad – who is an author and television personality as well as an acclaimed chef – sees some definite trends. "First," he notes, "we are heading toward less fat and more flavor across the board. Today, I use a lot of miso to replace fats like butter and cream." Brad is also a fan of unique and house-made vinegars and foresees a growing demand for fresher versions of the dried spices currently available.

Vegetarian Posole Soup

Chef William Reynolds, former Provost, Washburne Culinary Institute, Chicago, Illinois

Yield: 10 cups
10 servings –
1 cup each

This hearty vegetable stew or soup is colorful, delicious and nutrient rich. The recipe is a versatile and excellent option for vegetarians. Substitute red kidney or Great Northern beans for soybeans or black beans for black-eyed peas. The recipe can be made more or less spicy by adjusting the amount of red pepper flakes. Meat can be added for a nonvegetarian version.

Canola or peanut oil	¼ cup
Onions, small dice	2 cups
Garlic, chopped	5 each
Mushrooms, washed, quartered	2 cups
Carrots, peeled, ½ inch dice	3 each
Butternut squash, peeled, ½ inch dice	2 cups
Soybeans, drained and rinsed	1 can (15 ½ ounces)
Black-eyed peas, drained and rinsed	1 can (15 ½ ounces)
Tomatoes, canned with juice	2 cups
Hominy, canned, plus all the can liquid	1 can (15 ½ ounces)
Vegetable stock	1 quart
Cumin, ground	2 tablespoons
Red pepper flakes	2 teaspoons
Cilantro, chopped	½ cup
Salt	1 teaspoon

1. Brown the onions and garlic in the oil. Once brown, add the mushrooms, carrots and butternut squash and saute 2-3 minutes.

2. Add the soybeans, black-eyed peas, tomatoes, hominy and vegetable stock and cook until the vegetables are tender.

3. Add seasonings and simmer 10 minutes. Adjust seasonings as needed.

Per Serving

Calories	220	Cholesterol	0	mg
Fat	9 g	Sodium	400	mg
Saturated Fat	1 g	Carbohydrates	29	mg
Trans Fat	0 g	Dietary Fiber	8	mg
Sugar	8 g	Protein	9	g

What Today's Chef Needs to Know about Flavor

Chef Brad Farmerie offers these flavorful tips.

- Build a great dish by developing richness then cutting it with acidity. Add complex but subtle spices and season with salt, soy or miso as needed.

- Analyze the taste experience of every ingredient and use what you learn to *lengthen* the taste experience.

- Spice is nice; just use a variety. For example, if you put black pepper in every dish, they all taste like black pepper. Why not use fresh or dried chilies to create a similar effect but a broader palette of flavor and nuance.

- Bitter is not a bad thing if it is in balance with other flavors.

Woods Add Flavor in Grilling and Smoking Foods

The best woods for grilling and smoking are hardwoods from certain fruit and nut trees. Grilled foods cook more quickly and thus require a strongly flavored smoking wood in order to pick up the wood flavors. Herbs, such as oregano, sage, thyme, marjoram, rosemary and basil, used both dried and fresh, will permeate meat being smoked with their own particular flavors. Use the woody stems of rosemary and sage as well as the branches and leaves. Place herbs over smoldering wood.

Types of Wood	Characteristics and Typical Use
Alder	This tree originates on the West Coast of the US and generally produces wood that imparts a light, delicate-to-sweet-mild taste. It is the traditional wood used for smoking salmon, particularly in the Pacific Northwest.
Apple	Indigenous to the Northwest, this tree produces wood that imparts a mild and fruity, slightly sweet, taste. Use with sausages, poultry, fresh pork, bacon and ham.
Cherry	Often used with lamb, game birds and venison, cherry wood imparts a taste similar to apple but with a slightly tart finish.
Hickory	The so-called king of woods, hickory trees are prevalent in the South. The wood imparts a sweet-to-strong, hearty taste but is milder than mesquite. Hickory is often used with barbecued steaks, chops and spicy foods and to smoke bacon.
Maple	Maple trees are generally found in the Northeast. Maple wood imparts a sweet and light taste that complements poultry, ham, game and vegetables.
Mesquite	Mesquite flavor can become strong very quickly. Small amounts of mesquite may be added when smoking other woods as the primary heat source. Mesquite is used in Southwestern cooking and with spicy foods.
Oak	Oak, an excellent wood for smoking large pieces of meat for several hours, is also great for steaks, duck and burgers.
Peach	Peach wood chips, which impart a sweet, fruity flavor and leave a nice mellow hint of smoke, are great for poultry or pork.
Pecan	Abundant in the Southwest, pecan wood imparts a medium fruity taste. It will burn cool and offers a richness of character. Pecan is most often used with chicken, duck and game birds.

Other less common woods used for grilling and smoking include guava, almond, walnut, apricot, lemon, orange, bourbon barrel wood chips, wine barrel wood chips and juniper, which is slightly resinous.

Flavor from Processes

Using processes that capture flavor is essential to maximizing the appeal of healthful foods. Easy flavor boosters – lots of fat, sugar and salt – should be avoided in healthful cooking, but chefs can meet the flavor challenge by mastering other techniques and processes.

Infusion and Extraction

Pulling flavor out of ingredients and infusing it into liquids used in food preparation adds flavor to dishes. *Infusion* means steeping a seasoning or food in a hot liquid until the liquid absorbs the item's flavor. Solids are then strained out. Herbed oils and vinegars are common infusions.

Extracts

Extracts, also called essences, are concentrated liquids used to enhance or flavor foods. Plant extracts are obtained by distillation or infusion and include essences of vanilla, almond, orange, lemon, cinnamon and other plants and flowers. Some essences are reductions of a cooking liquid such as mushroom, tarragon, tomato or stock or are made by marinating truffles, garlic, anchovies or other items in wine or vinegar and concentrating that liquid to intensify flavor.

Essential oils are strongly flavored fragrant substances extracted from the flowers, fruit, leaves, seeds or roots of plants. Most essential oils are used to make perfumes and scented and aromatherapy products, but citrus oils, peppermint and almond oils are sometimes used in small amounts to flavor foods.

Extraction and concentration are taken to new levels by some chefs who use specialized techniques and equipment to extract and concentrate all manner of foods and serve them in unique ways. The flavors, aromas, temperatures and textures created through the discipline of molecular gastronomy make it a new art form in cuisine.

Juice

A fruit and vegetable juicer is a valuable piece of equipment in the healthful kitchen. Use a concentrated or reduced juice instead of water to add nutrients and flavor. Adding vegetable juice to poaching liquid, sauce or soup boosts nutrients, flavor and color. Juices can be infused with herbs or spices – for example, apple juice infused with rosemary, zucchini juice with thyme and carrot juice with ginger. Fruit juice will also help sweeten a cooked wholegrain cereal such as oatmeal. Grains such as couscous can be cooked in carrot juice. While juicing concentrates some nutrients and phytochemicals, fiber strained out during juicing is lost.

Stocks and Broths

Stocks are clear, flavorful, unthickened liquids prepared by simmering bones with some adhering meat in water with aromatics until their flavor is extracted. Stock is used as a base for soups, sauces, stews and other preparations. A *broth* is a flavorful, aromatic liquid made by simmering meat or poultry for a long time. Both stocks and broths have an important role in healthy cooking. A good stock is fat free, flavorful, low in added salt, clear and versatile. Many healthful stocks and broths are cooked ahead, concentrated and defatted. Some excellent quality stocks and broths are available but look closely at the sodium content. Cooking grains in stock instead of water adds flavor and nutrients. Stock reduced down to a paste consistency is called a *glace*.

Stocks and Broths

Fundamental Stocks	Other Stocks	Broths
Chicken	Lamb	Shallot
Brown (beef or veal)	Pork	Mushroom
Fish	Game	Lemongrass
Shrimp	Turkey	Onion
Vegetable	Lobster	

Vinegars and Oils

Oils can be infused with garlic, horseradish, citrus zest, shallots, fresh herbs, dried herbs, hot peppers or spices. Infused oils can be used in dishes such as shrimp salad with curry oil or chilled cucumber soup with dill oil. Vinegars can be infused with fresh herbs, dried herbs or fruits and used in salad dressings as well as dressings for vegetables and meat. A small amount of infused oil or vinegar sprinkled over a vegetable can have great flavor impact.

Marination

A **marinade** is an intensely flavored liquid or dry mixture used before cooking to flavor foods and to tenderize tougher cuts of meat. The marinating process may last seconds or days. A liquid marinade is used to soak foods and is typically made of oils, acids and seasonings. Plain yogurt can be used as the base, as in an Indian Tandoori marinade. The acid in a marinade (wine, beer, vinegar or citrus juice) can also "cook" a food by denaturing its proteins, as in fish or seafood ceviche. A dry marinade or **rub** is a mixture of herbs, spices, citrus zests or salt. In some cases, oil or mustard is used to make a paste, which is rubbed over a food. The coated item will absorb the rub's flavors. Adding pineapple to a marinade helps soften meat fibers because pineapples contain an enzyme that tenderizes muscle fiber.

Reduction

Fruit juices, vegetable juices, stocks, broths, wine, spirits and vinegars can be reduced, thus enhancing their flavor through concentration. Aromatics can be added to further develop the flavor. Reductions include:

- Balsamic vinegar
- Cabernet
- Raspberry-Riesling
- Port
- Apple cider
- Pomegranate molasses
- Pure maple syrup
- Agave nectar/syrup

Reduced balsamic vinegar or pomegranate molasses can be drizzled over a salad, meat, fish or a dessert for both flavor and visual effect.

Flavor from Ingredients

Who cannot wait for the first asparagus of spring or the juiciest strawberries from the June farmers' markets? Does tomato salad taste better in the middle of winter or at the height of the season in August? Creating a dish with the best flavor means starting with the best ingredients available. This does not mean flying in exotic items from around the world – although a chef can get almost any ingredient from somewhere year-round. Rather, it means developing menus or special promotions to reflect the seasons and working with local purveyors to get the freshest local products. Freezing or canning can capture seasonal flavor at its peak for use all year, but generally fresh is best.

Many ingredients add flavor during cooking. Plants in the allium family – garlic, leeks, onion, ramps, scallions and shallots – add pungent, spicy flavors and aromas that enhance eating pleasure. Sweet or hot peppers are used in a variety of dishes to add piquancy and depth. They can be raw or cooked, fresh, dried, flaked, powdered, pickled, smoked or in extract form (think hot sauce). Peppers are frequently used raw and chopped in salads or cooked in stir-fries or other mixed dishes. They can be sliced into strips and fried, roasted whole or in pieces, or chopped and incorporated into salsas or other sauces. Favorite hot pepper varieties include chipotle, jalapeno, serrano, habanero and Scotch bonnets. Sweet peppers include ancho, poblano, and green, red, yellow, orange and purple bell peppers.

Prepared condiments can be used in sauces, dressings, soups, stews, stuffings and main items as flavor enhancers. Examples include horseradish, wasabi, ginger, mustards, pickle relishes, soy sauce, olives, capers, salsas (fruit and vegetable), chutneys, catsup, Worcestershire sauce, chimichuri sauce and chili sauce. Light or reduced-sodium soy sauce has good flavor and is easily substituted for regular soy sauce or tamari sauce in a health-concious kitchen.

High-sodium or high-fat ingredients such as cheese, pickles, capers, anchovies and fried onion straws have bold flavors. Sometimes just a small amount can create a big impact. Using a small amount on top, rather than mixed into a dish, creates maximum visual and flavor impact while limiting salt and/or fat.

Herbs and Spices

Herbs and spices create wonderful opportunities for chefs to express their creativity. The flavor lost when fat, salt and sugar are reduced can be replaced with seasonings. Spices and herbs add flavor without calories and many also provide antioxidants and phytochemicals.

Most **herbs**, which are the leaves of aromatic plants, are available fresh, dried and, in some cases, frozen. Some herbs dry more successfully than others. Aroma is a good indicator of quality in both fresh and dried herbs. Some herbs, such as fresh basil, mint and dill, are delicate; others, such as rosemary and thyme, are more assertive. Herbs also can be purchased as pastes or made into pestos. Herbs are generally added toward the end of cooking because their flavor and aroma are more delicate. Many chefs have kitchen gardens that provide fresh herbs for cooking.

Spices are aromatics prepared from the roots, buds, flowers, fruits, bark or seeds of plants. Cinnamon comes from a bark, pepper from a berry, ginger from a root and nutmeg from a fruit. Most spice flavors are intense and powerful. Spices are usually dried and available whole or ground. Whole spices will retain flavor longer than ground spices.

Some spices and seeds used for seasoning can be toasted to make them more aromatic. A few spices, such as cayenne pepper, intensify in flavor during cooking. When changing the yield of recipes, the amount of spices and herbs should be adjusted by taste. A recipe increased from 10 to 50 servings will not need five times the amount of herbs and spices.

case by case

The Blend of Art and Science

At Chicago's renowned Spice House, spices are ground and blended by hand in small batches on the store premises. Owners Tom and Patty Erd and Patty's parents before them have spent a total of five decades finding the best sources and countries of origin for each spice. Patty recommends adding dried herbs to a recipe toward the end of cooking, rather than early on, as is the conventional approach. "In most cases," she explains, "prolonged cooking will diminish dried herbs' essential oils. Compared to spices, herbs have a very low percentage of essential oils."

When it comes to flavor and techniques for creating it, the partnership of art and science in cooking becomes clear. The best way to understand the difference between approaches – dried herbs in early or toward the end of cooking – is to try the techniques yourself and decide which one best achieves the flavor you want to create.

Herb Equivalents

- 1 tablespoon finely cut fresh herbs
- 1 teaspoon crumbled dried herbs
- ¼ to ½ teaspoon ground dried herbs

Cilantro Warning

Be careful with cilantro: It looks tame but can elicit very strong reactions. Some find it refreshing and lemony or lime-like and enjoy it in ethnic cuisines such as Mexican, Indian, Thai and Chinese. Others perceive it as soapy, bitter and foul smelling. If you use cilantro as an ingredient, let it be known so it is not a surprise to those who will reject any food containing it – or simply substitute Mexican oregano instead.

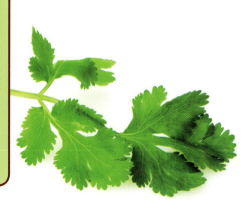

We frequently associate specific grapes with their microclimate and the characteristics of the soil in which they grow. Spices also will acquire different flavor spectrums based on growing conditions. For example, vanilla beans grown in Madagascar display a very pure, clean essence of vanilla. The same plant grown in Mexico has a much spicier bouquet, and vanilla beans grown in Tahiti have an extremely complex floral flavor profile.

Patty Erd, Owner
The Spice House
Chicago, Illinois

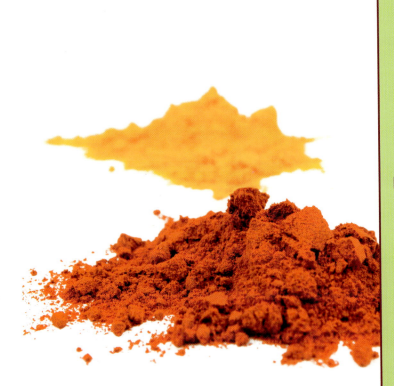

Storing Spices and Herbs

Fresh Herbs

- Refrigerate cut fresh herbs to prevent spoilage. Fresh herbs will keep up to four days in the refrigerator.

- Put fresh herb bouquets in containers, with stems down like cut flowers, and place in the refrigerator. Change the water daily.

- Loosely wrap the herb bouquet in film wrap or perforated plastic bags to extend shelf life. Smaller sprigs and individual leaves should be wrapped in a paper towel or placed in a food-safe plastic bag.

- Wash herbs and slice them into fine strips (chiffonade). Fill an ice cube tray halfway with water. Place a teaspoon or so of the herbs in each square of the tray. Make sure the leaves are down in the water. Place the half-filled tray in the freezer. When the ice cubes are almost frozen, finish filling the tray with water. Place the tray back into the freezer to freeze solid. Once the ice cubes are frozen, remove from the tray and store in zip-closure plastic bags. Use a cube as needed to flavor soup, stock, pasta, sauces or stew.

Dried Herbs and Spices

- Store dried herbs and spices in a cool, dry place in an airtight container. Do not keep containers of herbs near a hot stove. Dried herbs and spices provide flavor because they contain oils that break down faster if they are exposed to air, light and warm temperatures.

- Dried herbs and spices will retain their flavor for about six months. Record the date of delivery on all dried spice and herb containers. Discard a dried spice or herb that has lost aroma or faded in color.

- Avoid buying dried herbs in powdered form. They lose their flavor in a matter of weeks.

Seasoning Tips

The possibilities for using herbs and spices, alone or in combination, are infinite. Creative chefs develop unique balances and flavor contrasts through innovative use of seasonings. Many cookbooks and resources describe flavoring philosophies and provide recipes. The International Association of Culinary Professionals award-winning book *The Flavor Bible: The Essential Guide to Culinary Creativity, Based on the Wisdom of America's Most Imaginative Chefs* is among the best resources a chef can use. [12] Learning to use a wide variety of seasonings requires experience. Here are some seasoning tips.

- Sweet herbs like mint, nutmeg, ginger or anise complement citrus fruits.

- Fresh herbs like savory, chopped basil or cilantro can be added directly to a green salad.

- Salads with strong-flavored ingredients call for peppery dressings. Try some of these additions to a basic dressing:
  - Peppery herbs: red pepper, black pepper, mustard, chives and paprika
  - Strong herbs: oregano, tarragon and dill

- For delicately flavored vegetables such as mashed sweet potatoes, add a sweet spice such as nutmeg to complement the flavor; add a savory spice such as oregano, chives or dill to totally change the flavor.

- Freshly grated cheeses and freshly ground herbs and spices have more flavor, pungency and aroma. When possible, use freshly grated nutmeg, ground pepper and other spices and seeds.

- For strong-flavored vegetables, use peppery spices like basil, black pepper and savory.

- For baked fruits, use spices such as nutmeg, cloves or cinnamon.

- Dry spice blends can be rubbed into cuts of meat the day before cooking as a dry marinade. The flavors are absorbed into the meat before and during cooking.

- The ingredients in seasoning blends may age differently, so taste before seasoning. In lemon-pepper, for example, the pepper fades first, leaving much more lemony flavor.

- Herbs and seeds like caraway, dill, poppy and sesame can be baked into bread or sprinkled on top of breads or vegetables for a nice accent.

- The flavor of ground herbs can be lost quickly. Ground herbs should be added just before the cooking is complete. Adequate time should be allowed for the dried herb to absorb enough moisture to release its flavor.

- Whole spices are best suited to long-cooking recipes. Whole spices should be added as soon as cooking begins for maximum flavor. Whole spices and herbs (fresh and dried) should be removed before the food is served. The use of a **sachet d'epices** makes removal of whole herbs and spices easy.

- Toast whole spices, like fennel, star anise or coriander and mustard or sesame seeds before adding them to a dish for more depth in flavor and to release oils.

- In a fruit recipe, a general rule is to increase the spice by 50% and decrease sugar by 50%. The spice enhances the flavor, reducing the need for sugar.

- Dry mustard as well as horseradish and wasabi powder have no odor. The aroma develops when they are mixed with a cold liquid. Allow 10 to 15 minutes for the full flavor to develop. Mixing with an acid such as vinegar brings out more heat.

- The flavor of spices tends to become more intense in a food over time. If a food such as tomato sauce is cooked the day before and reheated for serving, this timing should be taken into consideration when deciding how much seasoning to use. The longer a food is held after preparation, the more opportunity flavors have to fuse, mellow and develop a full, rich taste.

- For cold foods such as salad dressings and cold salads, add the seasoning at least several hours in advance to allow the flavors to develop.

- In quick-cooking foods such as vegetables, add herbs at the start of cooking.

- In slow-cooking foods such as soups or stews, add herbs in the final 15 to 20 minutes.

- To prepare fresh herbs for use in a bouquet garni, wash in cool water and discard any blemished leaves. If the fresh herbs are to be chopped, the woody stems should be removed and the herb should be chopped to the size appropriate for the food.

- Black sesame seeds, black or red salts, and other colorful seasonings add color and drama to plate presentation.

Traditional Herb and Spice Uses

Meat, Poultry, Fish and Eggs	
Beef	Bay leaf, marjoram, nutmeg, onion, garlic, pepper, sage, thyme
Lamb	Curry powder, garlic, rosemary, mint, thyme, garlic
Pork	Garlic, onion, sage, pepper, oregano, chiles
Veal	Bay leaf, ginger, marjoram, oregano
Chicken	Ginger, marjoram, oregano, paprika, poultry seasoning, rosemary, garlic, sage, tarragon, thyme
Fish	Curry powder, dill, dry mustard, lemon juice, marjoram, paprika, pepper, celery seed
Eggs	Chives, parsley, thyme, paprika, freshly ground pepper, mustard powder, chervil
Vegetables	
Carrots	Cinnamon, cloves, marjoram, mint, nutmeg, parsley, rosemary, sage, allspice, ginger
Corn	Cilantro, cumin, curry powder, onion, paprika, parsley, chile powder
Green beans	Curry powder, dill, lemon juice, marjoram, oregano, tarragon, thyme
Greens	Onion, pepper, nutmeg with spinach
Peas	Ginger, marjoram, onion, parsley, sage, mint
Potatoes	Dill, garlic, mint, onion, paprika, parsley, sage, rosemary
Summer squash	Basil, cloves, curry powder, marjoram, nutmeg, rosemary, sage, thyme
Winter squash	Cinnamon, ginger, nutmeg, onion, allspice, mace
Tomatoes	Basil, bay leaf, chives, cilantro, dill, marjoram, onion, oregano, parsley, pepper, thyme

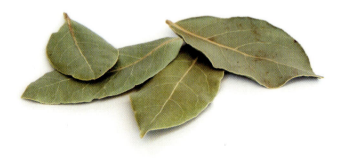

Traditional Herb and Spice Blends

Bouquet garni is a small bundle of fresh herbs such as parsley, thyme, celery leaf, fennel fronds or marjoram, and fresh or dried bay leaf tied with a string or enclosed in cheesecloth to make a sachet. It is used to flavor stocks, braises, stews and other slowly cooked meat dishes. Remove the herb bundle after cooking, before the food is served.

Fines herbes is a time-honored French seasoning composed of fresh minced parsley, tarragon, chervil and chives. It is often used in omelets, on grilled meats and in marinades. The blend is added toward the end of cooking or used fresh in a salad dressing. Try mixing fresh *fines* herbs into bean spread, low-fat mayonnaise, sour cream and cottage cheese or use it as a spread for sandwiches.

Quatre-epices, traditionally used in charcuterie, is a mixture of fresh ground black or white pepper, nutmeg, cloves or cinnamon, and ginger. Use quatre-epices to add a more aromatic nuance to all meats, particularly game, or to add a Caribbean piquance to grilled or stewed meat.

Garam masala, traditionally used in Northern Indian cuisine, literally means "warm spice blend" because it is meant to heat the body. The blend is stirred into curries, pilafs and biryanis toward the end of cooking. Try substituting garam masala for cinnamon and nutmeg in oatmeal cookies. Dry-roast the whole spices in a hot pan over low heat before grinding them. Spices found in garam masala include cardamom, coriander, cumin, black pepper, cloves, cinnamon and nutmeg.

The word *curry* comes from the south Indian word kari, which means sauce. Curry is not a single spice but rather a spice blend with many variations. Spices found in curry may include coriander, cumin, red chili powder, turmeric, ginger, allspice, black pepper, cardamom, cinnamon, cloves, fennel seeds, fenugreek seeds, nutmeg or mace, saffron, asafetida, mustard seeds, nigella seeds, curry leaves, galangal, or sesame seeds. For something different, try adding a little curry powder to a fresh carrot soup. To maximize flavor, dry-roast the whole spices in a hot pan over low heat before grinding them.

Sometimes called *five-spice powder*, five-fragrance powder, five perfumes or five heavenly spices, this traditional Chinese blend of ground star anise, fennel seeds, Szechwan or white pepper, cassia or cinnamon, and cloves is used throughout southern China and Vietnam in stir-fries and in marinades for pork, beef, chicken or duck. It makes a wonderful addition to barbecued ribs or braised leeks.

Although there is no "classic" Latin blend, *chili powder*, composed of ground assorted chile peppers, cumin, Mexican oregano, fresh or ground onion, and garlic, is probably the most common. In Mexico, this powder is added to chili con carne dishes and all sorts of bean and meat chilis. A salt-free blend that adds lots of flavor, chili powder is also used to season fried tortilla chips and other snack chips.

Adobo seasoning, another Latin flavor, is composed of fresh thyme, oregano, cilantro, ground cumin, black pepper and garlic. Ingredients are placed in a blender and mixed with orange juice to make an adobo marinade. The ingredients mixed in their dried form make a spice rub commonly used in South American cooking. Adobo mix is also found on many of the Caribbean islands once occupied by the Spanish.

Ethnic Influences

Countries, regions, cities and even neighborhoods have traditional spice/herb combinations used for seasoning. Spice and herb shops, ethnic markets and catalogs offer single herbs and spices and blends. Some excellent sources for herbs and spices not typically available through food distributors are the Spice House at www.thespicehouse.com; McCormick Spices at www.mccormick.com; and Penzeys Spice at www.penzeys.com.

Selected Spice Mixtures

Mixture	Country of Origin	Traditional Use	Form	Characteristic Spices
Bumbu	Indonesia	Used to flavor rendangs and gulais (spicy dishes served with sauce)	Dry spice mixture combined with coconut milk prior to use	Ginger, turmeric, chiles, cinnamon, cloves, coriander, black peppercorns, tamarind
Ras al Hanout	Morocco	All-purpose flavoring powder	Whole spices ground together	10 to 15 ingredients, usually including allspice, cloves, cumin, cardamom, chiles, ginger, peppercorns, mace, turmeric and caraway seeds
Berbere	Ethiopia	Cure for meats; added to condiments and stews	Ingredients mixed together then simmered prior to use	Chiles, cardamom, cumin, black pepper, fenugreek, allspice, ginger, cloves, coriander, ajowan seed, cinnamon
Harissa	Tunisia, Morocco, Algeria	All-purpose condiment, also used to flavor stews and sauces	Whole spices ground together then mixed with olive oil to moisten	Chiles, caraway, cumin, coriander, garlic
Baharat	Middle East (Lebanon, Syria, Gulf States, Saudi Arabia)	Widely used to flavor all types of dishes, particularly soups and stews	Whole spices ground together	Cloves, nutmeg, cinnamon, coriander, black pepper, paprika, cumin, cardamom, chiles
Curry Powder	Southern India	Used to flavor thin, soupy sauces	Fresh ground spices sauteed in oil at beginning of cooking process	Curry leaves, turmeric, chiles, coriander, black pepper and sometimes cumin, ginger, fenugreek, cinnamon, cloves, nutmeg, fennel seed, cardamom
Garam Masala	Northern India	Usually added at end of cooking to complete seasoning	Spices roasted whole then ground into a powder	Cinnamon, cardamom, cloves, cumin seeds, coriander, black peppercorns, nutmeg, mace
Panch Phoron (Indian Five-spice Mix)	Eastern India and Bengal	All-purpose flavoring for vegetable dishes	Sauteed in hot oil prior to cooking	Whole cumin seeds, fennel seeds, fenugreek, nigella, black mustard seeds
Gaeng Wan (Green Curry Paste)	Thailand	All-purpose flavoring, widely used in soups and sauces	Ingredients ground together in mortar and pestle to form a wet paste	Green chiles, lemongrass, ginger, coriander, cumin, white peppercorns, cilantro, green curry

Mixture	Country of Origin	Traditional Use	Form	Characteristic Spices
Massaman Paste	Thailand	All-purpose flavoring, widely used in soups and sauces	Ingredients ground together in mortar and pestle to form a wet paste	Chiles, coriander, cumin, cinnamon, cloves, star anise, cardamom, white peppercorns
Recado	Yucatan Peninsula of Mexico	Rubbed on food prior to cooking, also used as all-purpose flavoring for sauces and stews	Spices pounded to a paste in combination with vinegar, garlic and herbs	Achiote, cloves, black pepper, chiles, allspice, cinnamon, coriander, cumin, oregano
Chile Powder	Mexico		Stems and seeds removed (if desired); dry toasted until fragrant then ground	Various chiles such as: • Ancho • Pasillo • Guajillo • Chiles de arbol
Chili Powder	Mexico	One of the most common spice blends in Mexican foods	Spices combined	Paprika, cumin, cayenne pepper, oregano, garlic power
Five-Spice Powder	China	Used as flavoring in a wide variety of Chinese dishes; frequently used in marinades	Whole spices ground into a raw powder	Anise, fennel seeds, cloves, cinnamon, peppercorns
Quatre Spices	France	Most often used in patês	Spices combined and then ground into a powder	Pepper, nutmeg, cloves, ginger, sometimes cinnamon
Pickling Spices	Europe	Used to add flavor to pickles and certain liquids	Raw whole spices	Mustard seeds, cloves, coriander seeds, mace, black peppercorns, allspice, ginger, chiles, cinnamon sticks, bay leaves
Cajun Blackening Spices	Louisiana	Used to coat fish prior to cooking	Ground raw spices	Mustard powder, cumin, paprika, cayenne pepper, black pepper, onion, garlic, thyme, oregano
Crab or Shrimp Boil	Chesapeake Bay	Add to water used for boiling crab or shrimp	Ground raw spices	Peppercorns, mustard seeds, coriander, salt, cloves, ginger, ground bay leaves
Mojo	Carribean South America	Marinade	Liquid with sour orange base	Garlic, oil, fresh herbs

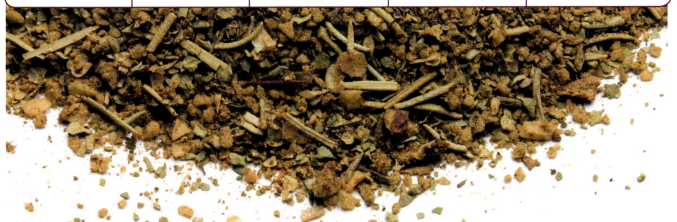

The Issue of Salt

Regular **salt** is sodium chloride (NaCl). Some regular salts have added iodine and anti-caking agents. Sea salts and other natural salts have small amounts of additional minerals that may add color and other subtle flavors. Most sodium in the diet comes from salt added in food processing and preparation. Some comes from high-sodium ingredients like soy sauce. Relatively little comes from adding salt at the table. Successfully reducing the sodium content of foods requires a substantial change to fresher and less processed foods and ingredients. Currently, about three-quarters of the sodium in the American diet comes from processed foods.

As diners try to reduce their sodium consumption, culinary professionals are challenged to reduce salt and sodium-rich ingredients used during cooking. Knowing how much sodium is in a recipe requires calculation. Asian cuisines, such as Thai, Japanese and Chinese, tend to be high in sodium because they use salty fish and soy-based sauces and stocks liberally. Italian cuisine can be high in sodium when salted tomato products and cheese are used. Recipes with particularly high levels of sodium can be adjusted or portion size can be altered.

Salt's most obvious impact is on taste, but it also serves other functions in cooking such as increasing the water-binding capacity of proteins and increasing the juiciness of meat and poultry. Salt also helps stabilize batters and extends shelf life through its antimicrobial effects.

Sodium reduction in the American diet is an emerging concern. After nutrition labeling regulations mandated disclosure of sodium content, many food manufacturers began incrementally reducing the amount of sodium in prepared foods. The average American eats at least twice the amount of sodium recommended for a healthy diet. The *Dietary Guidelines* recommend that everyone gradually reduce sodium intake to 1,500 milligrams per day (1 teaspoon of salt contains about 2,300 milligrams of sodium). [13] This is a major challenge; currently, many menu items exceed the total daily recommendation. In June 2006, the American Medical Association called on the food and restaurant industries to cut salt levels by one-half during the next decade. But some scientists and the Salt Institute argue that individuals who are healthy and not salt-sensitive do not need to limit salt intake. [14]

As awareness of sodium's contribution to health risks increases, there will be more demand for food options with less sodium. Following repeated petitions from the Center for Science in the Public Interest and other advocacy groups, the Food and Drug Administration is considering removing salt from the list of foods it categorizes as "generally recognized as safe" (GRAS). [15]

Types of Salt

White, pink, grey or black – salt comes in many colors and forms and is found all over the world. Each variety has its own special characteristics.

Experiment with unique colors and flavors as garnishes for maximum visual and taste impact. (Remember to reduce the amount of salt in food as it is prepared.)

Type of Salt	Description
Table salt	Table salt is the most common kind of salt. It usually comes from salt mines and is refined with most minerals removed until it is pure sodium chloride. Most table salt is available either plain or iodized. It is mixed with a trace amount of an anti-caking agent such as calcium silicate to prevent clumping. Table salt is often preferred in baking for its fine-grained texture and accuracy of measure. One teaspoon of table salt contains 2,300 milligrams of sodium.
Iodized table salt	American salt manufacturers began iodizing salt in the 1920s after people in some parts of the country were found to be suffering from goiter, an enlargement of the thyroid gland caused by an easily preventable iodine deficiency. People require less than 225 micrograms of iodine a day. Iodized salt can be considered the first "functional food."
Coarse salt	Coarse salt is a larger grained sea salt crystal. It is less moisture sensitive so it resists caking. It is often used for salt crusts on meat or fish.
Kosher salt	Kosher salt is so named because it is used in the preparation of meat according to the requirements of Jewish dietary guidelines. Its craggy crystals make it perfect for curing meat – a step in the koshering process. It contains fewer additives and has a more salty taste than ordinary table salt. Kosher salt generally comes in flakes rather than granules. The flakes dissolve easily and have a less pungent flavor than table salt. Many chefs enjoy using kosher salt because it tends to have a clean, natural flavor and sprinkles more evenly than other salts. This is the salt of choice for creating seasoning mixes. Diamond Crystal kosher salt has half the sodium of regular table salt. Because the crystals are hollow and lighter, 1 teaspoon has only 1,120 milligrams of sodium. Morton kosher salt is not hollow and has the same amount of sodium per teaspoon as table salt.
Rock salt	Rock salt is composed of large, hard, chunky crystals. Rock salt is often used to regulate temperature when making ice cream in an ice cream maker. Sold in large crystals, rock salt has a grayish hue because it is unrefined. Rock salt makes a great bed for serving oysters and clams.
Pickling salt	This salt is commonly used to brine pickles, sauerkraut or turkey.

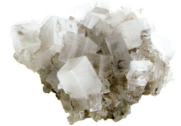

Type of Salt	Description
Sea salt	Sea salt is a broad term that generally refers to unrefined salt derived directly from an ocean or sea. It is harvested by channeling ocean water into large clay trays and allowing the sun and wind to evaporate the water naturally. Manufacturers of sea salt typically do not refine it as much as other kinds of salt, so it contains traces of other minerals including iron, magnesium, calcium, potassium, manganese, zinc and iodine that may impart color or flavor. Sea salt may be coarse or fine.
Smoked sea salt	Smoked sea salts are naturally smoked over wood fires. Smoked sea salts add a unique flavor to a wide range of dishes including roasts, chicken, salads and sandwiches.
Flake sea salt	Flake sea salt is a light crystal reminiscent of snowflakes. Seawater is evaporated using the natural processes of sun and wind, producing salt brine that is fed into an open evaporating pan. The brine is then slowly heated until delicate pyramid-shaped crystals appear.
Celtic salt	Celtic salt refers to naturally moist salts harvested from Atlantic seawater off the coast of Brittany, France. These salts, which are rich in trace minerals, are hand harvested in the traditional Celtic manner, using wooden rakes that allow no metal to touch the salt.
Fleur de sel	Fleur de sel (flower of salt) is an artisan sea salt composed of "young" crystals that form naturally on the surface of salt evaporation ponds. They are hand harvested under specific weather conditions by traditional paludiers (salt farmers). True fleur de sel comes from the Guérande region of France; different areas within Guérande produce salts with their own unique flavors and aroma profiles.
Grey salt	Grey salt is a moist unrefined sea salt usually found in the coastal areas of France. Its light grey, almost light purple, color comes from the clay found in the salt flats. The salt is collected by hand using traditional Celtic methods.
Grinder salt	Grinder salts are typically large dry crystals suitable for a salt mill or grinder. The white salt crystals are easy to grind and the lower moisture content allows the salt to flow through easily.
Hawaiian red alaea clay sea salt	Alaea sea salt is a traditional Hawaiian table salt used to season and preserve. A natural mineral called alaea (volcanic baked red clay) is added to enrich the salt with iron oxide. This mineral gives the salt its distinctive pink color. The clay imparts a subtle flavor that is said to be mellower than regular sea salt. Hawaiian sea salts have a nuance of sweetness that is rarely found in other salts.
Hawaiian black lava sea salt	Black lava Hawaiian sea salt is a unique combination of taste and mineral content. It can add drama and textural contrast when sprinkled over food. This salt is dried in high-tech solar evaporators and retains only 84% sodium chloride, the remainder being naturally occurring mineral elements.
Salt substitutes	Most salt substitutes are partially or entirely made from potassium chloride. They taste somewhat salty.
Light salt	A blend of salt substitute and salt that tries to capture the flavor of salt but with less sodium.

Reducing the Sodium Content of Food

Chefs can reduce sodium by optimizing the size and shape of salt flakes or granules. On a gram-for-gram basis, the sodium level is the same, but the flaky, less dense granules of kosher salt, for example, mean less sodium per teaspoon – and less saltiness. A teaspoon of regular table salt (granular) has 2,300 milligrams of sodium; kosher salt has 1,120 milligrams per teaspoon; and sea salt has about 1,870 milligrams per teaspoon. Tips for reducing sodium include:

- Read labels, become aware of sodium content and choose lower-sodium options as ingredients.

- Purchase ingredients, especially bases, that are labeled "low in sodium," "reduced-sodium" or "lower-sodium." Use reduced-sodium soy sauce. Many Asian sauces are extremely high in sodium.

- Balance the sodium content of a favorite higher-sodium food with food choices naturally low in sodium, such as fresh fruits.

- Decrease salt in recipes whenever possible. In baked goods, leaving out the salt can affect quality and taste, but salt usually can be reduced by half.

- Make salad dressings and sauces with lower-sodium ingredients and with little added salt.

- Rinse canned vegetables, particularly beans, before cooking to reduce sodium content by about 40%.

- Salt provides flavor but no aroma. Use aromatic ingredients and assertive flavors to replace flavors lost when cutting down on salt.

Salt Substitutes

While most chefs will not use salt substitutes, there are situations – for example, cooking for people with severe salt restriction – in which using salt substitutes may be necessary. There are a number of salt substitutes available. The traditional salt substitute is a blend of potassium chloride and sodium chloride. Most people find these blends to have a bitter or metallic as well as salty flavor. Some substitutes use blends of potassium chloride, magnesium sulphate and the amino acid lysine hydrochloride. Other new salt products are blends of natural sea salts (both sodium and potassium chloride). Salt substitutes with potassium may not be a good choice for individuals with type 1 diabetes, kidney or heart problems who may need to limit potassium. Researchers in the United Kingdom are exploring the potential use of seaweed granules to replace salt in processed foods. Seaweed also adds minerals to the diet.

Another approach to salt reduction is to use flavor enhancers such as yeast extracts, yeast-based ingredients or monosodium glutamate (MSG), which activate taste receptors in the mouth and throat to amplify flavor and compensate for less salt as described earlier in this chapter.

Opportunities for Chefs

Providing excellent flavor is a goal of all chefs, including those whose food is especially healthful. Chefs and culinary professionals are uniquely equipped to create healthy recipes that are full of flavor and appeal. Flavor involves the elements of taste, smell, texture, temperature, sight and sound. Herbs, spices, marinades, infusions, juicing and cooking methods can be used to enhance flavors in food. Traditionally, food preparers have relied on salt to add flavor to food. Today, we use other techniques and ingredients to bring out the flavors of foods.

Learning Activities

1. Using a selection of flavored jellybeans, close your eyes and select a bean. Pinch your nostrils closed and chew the jellybean. Can you identify the flavor? Unplug your nose. Can you identify the flavor?

2. Select several recipes (from a cookbook, magazine, website or cooking class). Identify ways to reduce the amount of salt in the recipes and ways to increase the flavor. Prepare recipes and compare the flavor of both versions.

3. Using a common spice (cinnamon, nutmeg, clove, etc.), gather various forms of the spice (ground, whole, toasted, etc.) and compare the smell and flavor of each form.

4. Compare the flavor of three preparations of an onion – raw, sweated and caramelized. Discuss the changes in flavor caused by cooking technique.

5. Conduct a tasting of sea salt, kosher salt, smoked salt and iodized table salt. Identify differences in grind, texture and flavor.

6. View "Reinventing Texture and Flavor," a lecture and demonstration given by Grant Achatz in 2010 at Harvard University School of Engineering, (www.youtube.com/watch?v=dYDe3RASpaO). Discuss in class.

For More Information

- McCormick Spices, www.mccormick.com
- Monell Chemical Senses Center, www.monell.org
- Page K, Dornenburg A. *The Flavor Bible: The Essential Guide to Culinary Creativity, Based on the Wisdom of America's Most Imaginative Chefs*. New York: Little, Brown and Company; 2008.
- Penzeys Spices, www.penzeys.com
- Salt Institute, www.saltinstitute.org
- The Spice House, www.thespicehouse.com
- Taste Science Laboratory, Cornell University, www.tastescience.com
- World of Flavors, Culinary Institute of America, www.worldofflavors.com

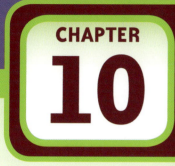

Healthful Cooking Techniques

LEARNING OBJECTIVES

After completing this chapter, you should be able to:

- Describe 15 healthful cooking methods or techniques
- Explain the nutritional advantages and disadvantages of various cooking methods
- Determine which healthful cooking method is best for specific foods
- List the factors that affect nutrient retention in food preparation
- Explain the process for developing and modifying recipes for healthful menus

Putting theory into practice is the purpose of this chapter. Using what you have learned about the essentials of nutrition and nutrition standards, it is time to focus on creating great-tasting, eye-appealing, healthful dishes. This chapter describes the cooking techniques used to create such dishes. When plenty of healthful choices are available on the menu, the service or wait staff should be educated to promote flavor, interesting combinations and the healthful ingredients in these dishes.

Some people perceive healthful cooking as an unpleasant task requiring odd ingredients and unfamiliar techniques. In fact, many traditional cooking techniques from around the world can be used to prepare healthful food, sometimes with just a few modifications. The techniques described in this chapter work well with meat, poultry and fish as well as with vegetables, fruits, legumes and grains, and can help promote overall consumption of foods that are rich in protective nutrients. Proper serving temperature, portion size and attractive presentation also influence the perception of taste, quality and add enjoyment.

Cooking Techniques

There are four fundamental keys to healthful cooking:

1. Start with ingredients at their freshness and flavor peak.
2. Use a minimum amount of the type of fat necessary to provide excellent flavor and texture. Choose healthful fats when possible.
3. Use minimal amounts of added sugar and limit salt and other sodium sources.
4. Cook items at the right temperature and for the right amount of time, using sound cooking techniques.

A Word from the Chef
Fundamentally Speaking

Chef Ron DeSantis, director of culinary excellence at Yale University, is responsible for menu development, food production and culinary professional development at the university. Prior to joining Yale, he was director for CIA Consulting, a group of certified master chefs who offer their clients a wide array of services from menu research and development to facility design to culinary training. Ron began his career at the Culinary Institute of America (CIA) as a chef instructor and advanced to a senior leadership role within the institution.

"Nutrition used to be very clinical," Ron explains, "but it has evolved into what is simply good, fundamental cooking. For the chef, nutrition starts with ingredient selection and continues with menu design and cooking methods. In other words," he continues, "nutrition always has a role in cooking. And if you are executing the fundamentals correctly, good ingredients will result in healthy food."

Ron suggests limiting processed foods but recommends taking a common sense approach to eliminating any ingredient completely. "For example, with a flavor-dense food such as butter," he explains, "it's about cooking with the proper amount to achieve impact. With a properly heated pan, you can use very little fat and have a great finished product. A lot depends on your grasp of culinary basics and technique.

"When you are lazy and don't build flavor," Ron warns, "that's when you end up compromising and cutting corners – for example, adding cream or butter to make it work. Healthy cooking is a commitment," Ron asserts, "and that commitment starts early."

Roasting and Baking

Roasting and *baking* are methods of cooking that cook food in dry heat in a controlled environment, usually an oven. Foods can be roasted or baked at low or high temperatures uncovered, which allows steam to escape. The term roasting typically applies to large pieces of meat, poultry, vegetables and fruits. Cooking on a rotisserie, with food turning mechanically, is also a form of roasting. Baking generally refers to seafood, starches, breads, cakes and pastries. The method of heat transfer in baking is generally the same as in roasting. There are exceptions – for example, pan-roasted salmon. This description has more to do with marketing than any real difference in cooking technique. Pan-roasted salmon just sounds better than baked salmon.

When vegetables and fruits are roasted, the heat caramelizes their natural sugars, making them sweet and soft on the inside but browned and firm on the surface. Roasted fruits and vegetables are a flavorful way to incorporate more produce into menus and create unique flavors, color contrast and attractive plate presentations. Because they have little fat and salt, lots of protective nutrients, and relatively few calories, roasted fruits and vegetables are particularly good options for health-conscious diners and those with dietary restrictions.

When roasting poultry, it is preferable to keep the skin on to retain moisture and add flavor. The skin may be removed before serving or by the diner to reduce calorie and fat content. Most of the fat in poultry skin is unsaturated, so it makes little sense to remove the skin if other fats must be added.

Roasting on a rack allows rendering fats to drip from the food and air to circulate around the food. Generally, no additional fat is needed in preparation, but meat may be seared in a small amount of fat at the start of cooking to develop color and flavor. Tender, more expensive cuts of meat are usually used for roasting. Care should be taken to avoid overcooking roasted meats; use a thermometer to determine the degree of doneness.

Traditionally, fat drippings are used to make a roux for a pan gravy; however, after fat is removed, the pan can be deglazed and browned bits from the bottom of the pan used to make a delicious sauce.

Fruits for Roasting or Baking

Apples	Oranges
Apricots	Peaches
Bananas	Pears
Figs	Pineapple
Grapefruit	Plucots
Mangos	Plums
Nectarines	

Beyond Potatoes and Onions: Great Vegetables for Roasting

Most roasted vegetables benefit from a light brushing of olive oil or a nut oil and the addition of herbs or seasoning before cooking. Go beyond roasted potatoes, sweet potatoes, onions, mushrooms, shallots and garlic with:

Acorn or other winter squashes	Fennel
	Leeks
Asparagus	Mushrooms including Portobellos
Beets	
Bok choy	Parsnips
Broccoli	Scallions
Brussels sprouts	Sweet bell peppers
Carrots	Tomatoes
Cauliflower	Turnips

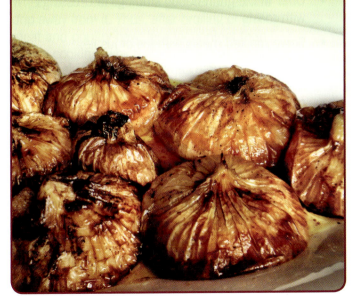

Some limitations of broiling and grilling include:

- Both techniques require relatively tender cuts of meat, fish and poultry that usually are more expensive than less tender cuts.

- Dense vegetables, such as potatoes, other root vegetables and hard squashes sometimes require precooking.

- Grilled foods do not usually hold well in the prolonged heat of a steam table or for extended food service; however, food can be marked by grilling and finished in the oven as needed.

Here are some suggestions for preparing healthful broiled and grilled foods:

- Marinate or season the product prior to grilling.

- Low-fat marinades add flavor. Use herbs, rubs or spices for seasoning.

- Oil the grill to prevent food from sticking. Most of the oil will burn off, so there should be no concern about that added fat.

- Apply sauces with sugar, such as barbecue sauce, toward the end of the cooking process to prevent burning or excessive charring.

Smoke-Roasting or Pan-Smoking

Smoke-roasting or *pan-smoking*, also called *hot-smoking*, is done in a closed container using wood chips and, if desired, aromatics, herbs or tea to make smoke. This technique is best for small, tender, quick-cooking items such as poultry pieces, tender meats, fish, shellfish, game, lean sausages and some vegetables. It adds flavor without adding fat, salt or calories. Foods intended for smoke-roasting are often cured or brined for flavor. This step can easily be skipped to avoid high-sodium content. It is important, however, to season well with other herbs and spices.

Smoke-roasting is an excellent cooking technique for vegetables such as corn on the cob, peppers or tomatoes. It imparts a smoky "meaty" flavor. If left in the smoke too long, however, food may develop a strong, bitter and unpleasant flavor.

Here are some suggestions for preparing healthful smoke-roasted foods:

- Use various woods or aromatics for unique flavors.

- If the food is large or dense, it may be finished in the oven.

- Serve smoke-roasted foods with a lean accompaniment such as coulis, fruit sauce or chutney.

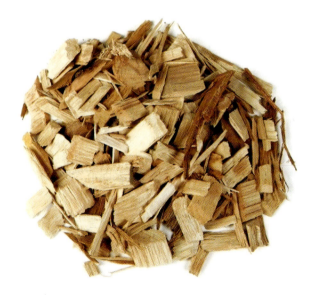

The Grilling Question

Grilling and broiling are excellent cooking techniques and many people love the resulting flavors. Chefs should be aware, however, that dietary advice for the prevention of cancer suggests limiting char-grilled foods.

Substances in the muscle protein of red meat, poultry or seafood react under high heat to form compounds called *heterocyclic amines (HCAs)* that can damage genes, thus triggering development of cancer.

Consumption of HCAs is linked most clearly to cancers of the colon and stomach. One study found that people who eat the most barbecued red meat (beef, pork and lamb) almost double their risk of colon polyps, compared to those who do not eat these foods. The more meat is cooked past ideal temperature, the more HCAs will form. A higher consumption of well-done meat is linked with two to five times more colon cancer and two to three times more breast cancer. Risk of cancers of the stomach, pancreas and prostate may also increase.

To reduce HCA formation when grilling, turn the gas down or wait for charcoal to become low-burning embers. Raise the grilling surface from the heat source to reducing charring and flip meat often.

Also consider cooking meat at lower temperatures, such as roasting or stewing. Pan-frying also should be done at a lower temperature. Research shows that frying meat at a high temperature, which saves only 2 minutes of cooking time, produces three times the HCA content of meat cooked at medium temperatures. In addition, marinating can decrease HCA formation by up to 96%, although studies are still underway to determine which ingredients help the most.

Vegetables and fruits are the best choice for grilling because they don't form HCAs and supply a range of cancer-fighting nutrients. In addition, the phytochemicals in vegetables stimulate enzymes that can convert HCAs to an inactive, stable form that is easily eliminated from the body.

Four factors influence HCA formation:

- **Type of food.** HCAs are found in cooked muscle meats.

- **Temperature.** Temperature is the most important factor in the formation of HCAs.

- **Cooking method.** Frying, broiling and barbecuing produce the largest amounts of HCAs because these cooking methods require very high temperatures. Roasting and baking require lower temperatures, so they result in formation of lower HCA levels. Gravy made from meat drippings, however, does contain substantial amounts of HCAs. Stewing, boiling or poaching are done at or below 212° F; cooking at this low temperature creates negligible amounts of HCAs.

- **Time**. Foods cooked a long time ("well-done" instead of "medium") form slightly higher HCA levels.

To avoid a different class of cancer-causing compounds called *polycyclic aromatic hydrocarbons (PAHs)*, grill leaner meat cuts that will drip less and cause fewer flare-ups and smoke. PAHs form in smoke and are deposited on the outside of meat.

Source: American Institute for Cancer Research, www.aicr.org/site/News2?page=NewsArticle&id=8484&news_iv_ctrl=0&abbr=pr_hf_

Sauteing, Searing, Stir-Frying, Pan-Frying and Deep-Frying

Generally, the term **frying** means cooking foods in hot fat or oil. In all forms of frying, choose as heart-healthy a fat as possible. Fry foods at temperatures that will cause the least amount of fat absorption.

Sauteing

A traditional **saute** is a dry-heat method using some fat and medium-to-high heat. Sauteing is done in a shallow pan, turning or tossing the food to cook the outside surface evenly without overcooking the inside. Sauteing is a technique generally used with delicate foods that cook quickly – scallops, shrimp, tender strips or medallions of meat, poultry, fish fillets, and tender vegetables. In many recipes, onions are sauteed to a light golden color to bring out the natural sweetness and to create and impart flavor to a dish.

Traditionally, sauteed meats are served with a pan sauce with shallots, garlic, pepper, herbs and other seasonings. In the case of seafood, butter is often added and browned and served over the finished product. Omitting this last step will reduce the fat and caloric content of a sauteed dish.

In **dry sauteing**, no added fat is used. High heat is necessary to sear food and there must be enough space in the pan for proper browning without steaming. Nuts, grains and seeds may also be dry sauteed (toasted) to bring out their natural flavors and intensify aromas. Foods, such as onions, receive flavor from caramelizing. For some foods, such as mushrooms, water is released and the natural flavors of the vegetable intensify. Although dry sauteing is an excellent technique for serving health-conscious diners, it does have some disadvantages. Dry sauteing requires tender, often more expensive cuts of meat, poultry or fish. It works best when a food has some internal fat to help with browning.

Dense vegetables, such as carrots and potatoes, usually need to be precooked before sauteing. Generally, sauteed foods are prepared or finished when the order arrives in the kitchen, thus lowering nutrient loss from holding. Sauteed foods do not hold well on the steam table.

Safety of Nonstick Cookware

Nonstick cookware has been used for years to reduce the added fat needed in cooking. The safety of this cookware continues to be examined with no clear answer. At issue is the use of **perfluorocarbon acid** (PFOA). PFOA is used in manufacturing fluoropolymers, which impart fire resistance and oil, stain, grease and water repellency. Fluropolymers are used to make nonstick surfaces on cookware and to waterproof breathable membranes for clothing.

PFOA has been shown to cause cancer, low birth weight and a suppressed immune system in laboratory animals exposed to high doses. Studies have shown the chemical to be present at low levels in the bloodstream of nine out of 10 Americans. And although the effects of PFOA at lower doses in humans are disputed, there does seem to be a link between PFOA and raised levels of cholesterol.

Manufacturers claim that PFOA does not leach into food cooked in nonstick pans made with perflurocarbon acid. Although indicating that the science is still coming in, the Environmental Protection Agency launched a global stewardship program in 2006 that asked companies to reduce the presence of PFOA in products by 95% by no later than 2010 and to work toward eliminating sources of exposure by no later than 2015.

Until science has determined the complete safety of nonstick cookware, follow these guidelines:

- Never leave nonstick pans unattended on an open flame or other heat source.

- While cooking, don't let temperatures get hotter than 450° F. It is best to cook at low-to-medium heat.

- Don't use metal utensils that could scratch the surface of nonstick cookware.

- Wash nonstick cookware by hand using non-abrasive cleaners and sponges (do not use steel wool).

- Do not put nonstick cookware in a dishwasher.

- Don't stack pieces of nonstick cookware on top of each other.

Source: Consumer Reports, www.consumerreports.org/cro/home-garden/kitchen/cookware-bakeware-cutlery/nonstick-pans-6-07/overview/0607_pans_ov_1.htm

Searing, a variation of sauteing, calls for browning foods on all sides in a very hot pan over medium-high to high heat to develop a brown and flavorful crust. A little oil may be used in the pan to prevent sticking. Food is sometimes served seared, such as thinly sliced seared tuna or very rare beef. Often searing is followed by braising or stewing, as in lamb shanks, osso bucco, short ribs and beef stew.

Stir-frying, another variation of sauteing, is traditionally found throughout Asia. Stir-frying is done in a wok or large pan with sloping sides and involves constantly turning food as it cooks. Cut vegetables and boneless meats and shellfish are often stir-fried. Foods are added to the stir-fry in sequence of longest to shortest cooking time so that at service, all ingredients are completely but gently cooked. Take care when seasoning stir-fries. The soy sauce, fish sauce and other Asian condiments included in stir-fry recipes are typically very high in sodium. Reduced-sodium varieties are available and preferable.

Here are some suggestions for preparing healthful sauteed foods:

- In mixed dishes, use more vegetables and less protein. This is a great way to boost the volume of vegetables and moderate the protein portion.

- Use a well-seasoned or nonstick pan so that little or no additional fat is needed.

- Use herbs, spices and aromatics for seasoning.

- Use low-fat liquids to deglaze the pan and make the sauce.

- Use arrowroot or cornstarch to thicken the sauce if appropriate.

- Limit amounts of high-fat ingredients (butter, cream or cheese) to enrich and finish the sauce, or use only if necessary.

- Limit condiments and sauces high in salt or sugar.

- Serve sauteed foods with light, flavorful sauces made from vegetables or fruits.

Pan-Frying and Deep-Frying

Generally, pan-frying, and especially deep-frying, are not healthful techniques because frying in fats and oils usually creates a product that has a considerable amount of added fat. Eating fried foods frequently is likely to increase calories and weight. On healthful menus, fried foods are limited, portions of fried-foods are modest and while fried foods can be requested as side dishes, they should not be routinely served as accompaniments to main course items. In fact many food service kitchens (especially in schools and healthcare facilities) no longer include fryers.

To **pan-fry** means to cook in a moderate amount of fat, typically a vegetable oil. To **deep-fry** means to cook a food submerged in hot fat. While frying may not seem to be compatible with healthful cooking, it can be used prudently. Modest amounts of fried foods can be used to add visual appeal, crunchy texture and unique flavors – for example, crispy fried leeks used as a garnish on a poached fish or a fried sage leaf on top of butternut squash soup. When fried foods are incorporated in healthful cooking, they should be front and center – used for visual and flavor impact in the first bites.

Limiting the fat in fried foods depends on cooking technique. Less fat is absorbed if no batter or breading is used. After a food has been fried, it should be removed from the oil and drained on an absorbent surface or rack. Most foods are fried at 350° F to 375° F. The fat should be hot enough to sizzle when food is added but not hot enough to smoke. Frying at too low a temperature usually causes excessive greasiness and contributes to excessive fat absorption in fried foods. When foods are pan-fried or deep-fried, care should be taken to choose oils that are mono- or polyunsaturated and trans-fat free.

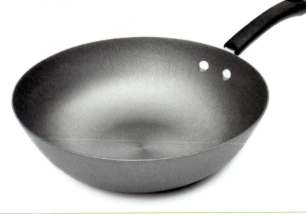

Microwave Cooking

Microwave ovens can cook some foods, but their main use is to reheat quickly. Foods like soups, stews, many sauces and grain dishes can be prepared in advance, divided into small batches and reheated before serving. Sometimes microwaving can also be used to precook root vegetables before finishing by grilling. Microwaving reduces the need to keep large batches of food hot through service, which can result in nutrient loss, reduced food quality and waste.

Poaching, Simmering, Boiling, Sous Vide and Blanching

Poaching, simmering, boiling and blanching are methods of gently cooking food in a liquid. Poached, simmered and boiled food can take flavor from the liquid used. Flavorful liquids include stock, broth, wine, vegetable or fruit juices or spiced teas often with aromatics added.

To **poach** means to cook in a small amount of liquid that is hot but not bubbling, about 140° F to 180° F. Often, the poached food (especially fruit) is cooled in the liquid to absorb its flavors. If the poaching liquid is flavorful, it is sometimes reduced to make a sauce that can be thickened with arrowroot or cornstarch. Poaching is a good technique for tender, delicate fish fillets, chicken breasts, eggs, some meats and fruits. Some classic recipes even poach filet mignon.

To **simmer** means to cook in a liquid that is bubbling gently, at a temperature no higher than 185° F to 205° F. Simmering may also be used to reduce the volume of a liquid, such as when making a tomato sauce thicker or reducing a wine or fruit sauce. Because simmering is done at a higher heat than poaching, it has a tenderizing and rehydrating effect. It is a good technique for cooking dense vegetables, grains, legumes, poultry and meat.

To **boil** means to cook in a rapidly bubbling liquid, often water or stock, at about 212° F. Boiling is typically used for certain vegetables and starches. Boiling toughens the proteins in meats, fish, poultry and eggs and breaks up delicate foods.

Sous vide (the French term for "under vacuum") or reduced-oxygen packaging (ROP) is a method of cooking in vacuum-sealed plastic pouches at precise temperatures. The result is a final product with superior texture and concentrated flavors. Sous vide is being used to serve food to large numbers of people at hotels and casinos, on airplanes and cruise ships and in the military. It is also a favorite of many top-tier chefs, who say the technique can be used to create unique, individual dishes for their discriminating clientele. It is an effective way to consistently turn out the same quality dish day after day and saves a great deal of time.

The sous vide plastic-film packaging prevents the loss of moisture and flavors. Consequently, flavors are concentrated and fewer spices and less salt is required, lowering the overall sodium content of sous vide foods. Seasoning can be a little tricky when cooking sous vide. While many herbs and spices act as expected, others are amplified and can easily overpower a dish. Additionally, aromatics (such as carrots, onions, celery, bell peppers, etc.) will not soften or flavor the dish as they do in conventional cooking because the temperature is too low to soften the starches and cell walls.

Sous vide is a very healthful method of cooking. Little or no fat is needed in the preparation and nutrients are preserved. Essential minerals are typically leached into cooking water, reducing the mineral content of foods processed by traditional means. The pouch eliminates mineral loss, preserving the mineral content of fresh foods. All the flavor and most of the nutrients are retained.

The drawback is that the sous vide process cannot produce a browning of surfaces or crispy texture. In addition, cooking produces no food aroma. Food safety, however, is probably the biggest concern with sous vide cooking. The hermetically sealed plastic bags form oxygen barriers that slow the growth of **aerobic bacteria**, delaying spoilage. While this certainly can be a benefit, the downside is that anaerobic bacteria may thrive under the right conditions. Unfortunately, the most deadly food-borne illness is **botulism**, caused by *Clostridium botulinum*, an anaerobic bacteria. Because of this, foods must be of the highest quality and handled within strictly maintained temperature ranges according to Hazard

Analysis Critical Control Point (HACCP) procedures. The Food and Drug Administration's 2009 Food Code sets out strict procedures, including chilling the bagged products to 34° F and storing them for no more than 30 days to eliminate the possibility of listeria or botulism poisoning. [1]

Blanching is a two-step process. First, the food is completely submerged in boiling water for a short time. Then it is removed and plunged into ice water. The quick chill stops the cooking process and sets the color, especially bright oranges and greens. Since vegetables with green, orange, deep yellow and red pigments are particularly rich in vitamins, minerals and phytochemicals, every effort should be made to serve as many of them as possible to maximize the healthfulness of menu offerings.

Crudités platters with blanched rather than raw carrots, broccoli, green beans, asparagus, cauliflower, sugar snap peas, etc., are more attractive, colorful and taste better. Blanching also increases the bioavailability of some vitamins.

Blanching can also be used to:

- Speed the peeling process (for tomatoes, peaches, etc.)
- Soften herbs
- Remove excessive saltiness
- Reduce strong flavors from meats and game
- Precook vegetables prior to stir-frying

The amount of nutrients lost during poaching, simmering, boiling and blanching depends on the heat stability of the nutrients present and the length of cooking time. Some vitamins, but not all, are destroyed by heat, especially when there is a long cooking time. In some cases, nutrients from vegetables leach into the cooking liquid. If the liquid is used in a soup or reduced sauce, those nutrients are consumed. Often, however, the cooking liquid is discarded. Every effort should be made to save the cooking liquid for use in soups and sauces. For many vegetables, cooking softens the fibers and makes the nutrients more available. Cooked carrots,

for example, are more nutrient rich than raw carrots. In doing nutrient calculations, it is important to enter the values of vegetables in the state they are eaten, rather than how they are listed on the ingredient list. The same vegetable, raw or cooked, has different nutrient levels.

Here are some suggestions for preparing healthful poached, simmered, boiled and blanched foods:

- Use flavorful cooking liquids, such as juices, wines and stocks.
- Trim surplus fat from food before cooking.
- Use cooking liquid for sauces or retain for use in soup when possible.
- Cook food only as long as necessary.
- Maintain proper cooking temperatures.

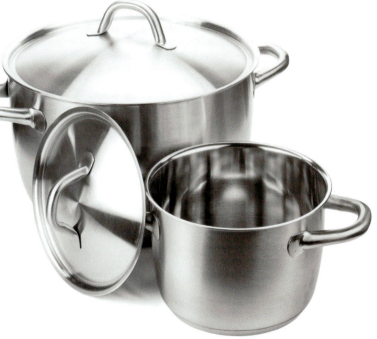

Poached Chicken Breast with Root Vegetables

Yield: 10 servings

Orange zest and ginger create a flavorful poaching liquid and enhance this appetizing dish. Lightly searing the chicken breast before poaching adds to both flavor and appearance. This main course is beautiful in its simplicity and perfect for most guests with special dietary needs or restrictions.

Broth:

Chicken broth, defatted, high-quality	1 ½	quarts
Red onion, chopped	¾	cup
Garlic, minced	2	cloves
Orange, peel of	1	each
Ginger, fresh, peeled, chopped	1	tablespoon
Bay leaf	1	each

Chicken:

Chicken breasts, fat trimmed, with wing bone and skin	10	5 ounces each
Salt	½	teaspoon
Black pepper, freshly ground	½	teaspoon
Olive oil	2	tablespoons

Vegetables

Carrots, baby	30	each
Fingerling potatoes	20	each
Pearl onions, peeled, fresh or frozen	2	cups
Asparagus, top half only	40	baby
	20	medium
Orange zest, julienne	2	tablespoons

Garnish:

Garlic cloves, peeled, roasted	20	each
Chives, cut or parsley, chopped	1	tablespoon

1. In a large pot, combine broth ingredients and bring to a boil. Reduce heat and simmer 15 minutes. Adjust seasonings as needed.

2. Season chicken with salt and pepper. Heat fry pan with olive oil and sear chicken breast on both sides until lightly browned but not cooked through.

3. Add chicken pieces to seasoned broth. Add the carrots, potatoes and pearl onions. Cover and simmer 20 minutes until chicken and vegetables are cooked.

4. Add orange zest and asparagus tips. Cook 5 minutes more. Remove bay leaf.

5. To serve, put 1 chicken breast in each flat bowl, top each with potatoes, carrots, pearl onions and asparagus. Add ½ cup broth to each bowl. Top with 2 roasted garlic cloves and cut herbs.

Per Piece

Calories	310	Cholesterol	75	mg
Fat	8 g	Sodium	250	mg
Saturated Fat	2 g	Carbohydrates	28	mg
Trans Fat	0 g	Dietary Fiber	3	mg
Sugar	4 g	Protein	30	g

Adapted from Chicken Breast in Herb Broth with Root Vegetables and Roasted Garlic. Gielisse V, Kimbrough M, Gielisee K. *In Good Taste: A Contemporary Approach to Cooking.* Upper Saddle River, NJ: Prentice Hall; 1999.

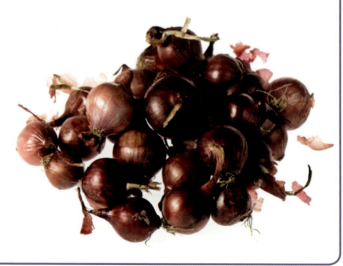

Steaming

Steaming cooks foods by surrounding them with a vapor bath. Many kitchens have pressure steamers that create steam under pressure to cook foods quickly while preserving nutrient value. Pressure steamers are typically used for vegetables, especially in large volume.

Steaming is a very quick cooking method that retains a maximum of nutrients. Although used mostly for vegetables, steaming can also be used for seafood and shellfish, chicken breasts, doughs, some grains and other foods. Steaming helps food retain its shape, color, flavor and texture better than boiling, simmering or even poaching. Foods must be carefully placed within the steamer so they cook evenly. Sometimes foods for steaming are encased in a wrap such as seaweed, cornhusks, banana leaves, leek strips or cabbage leaves. Steamed foods can easily be overcooked.

In *pan-steaming*, foods are placed in a closed vessel, above – but not touching – the liquid. The heat must be high enough for the liquid to boil and create steam to cook the food. Ingredients placed in the liquid can infuse delicious flavors and aromas into steamed food. Mussels and clams are often steamed with aromatics, such as lemon zest, and the pan liquids are served as the sauce. The flavored liquid used to pan-steam vegetables may be reduced to make a sauce or glaze. Chinese cooking techniques include steaming many foods over water or stock, including filled buns, pot stickers and seafood in stacked bamboo baskets.

En papillote is a variation of steaming in which the main item, often fish and accompanying ingredients such as vegetables and herbs, are encased in parchment paper and cooked in a hot oven. The natural juices of the fish and vegetables create their own sauce. When the packet is opened for the diner, aromatic steam is released.

Braising and Stewing

Braising is a method of cooking that involves both dry and moist heat. It is an ideal way to prepare less tender cuts of meat and sturdy root vegetables. Braised meat is generally seasoned and seared in a large roasting pan and then covered and simmered slowly in the oven in liquid with mirepoix and aromatics. *Stewing* is similar to braising but the main item is cut into bite-sized pieces. Legumes, poultry and non-root vegetables can also be braised or stewed.

The amount of liquid used should cover the product by one-third to two-thirds, depending upon how much sauce is desired. The long cooking process tenderizes the meat and produces a concentrated flavorful liquid. The addition of tomato products adds flavor and tenderizes meat. Vegetables are added partway through the process to avoid overcooking them. The liquid is strained and seasoned and the meat and vegetables are returned to the liquid to cool. Braises and stews are best prepared a day ahead and refrigerated so the cooking liquid can be absorbed into the product and the fat can rise to the top to be easily removed before reheating the dish to serve.

The long cooking times of braised and stewed dishes allow the development of wonderful flavors. Because the liquid is consumed as part of the dish, nutrients that are not destroyed by heat are retained and consumed.

When wine or an alcohol-containing liquid is added to food during cooking, some of the alcohol is "burned off." In fact, in a long, slow braise, such as Beef Bourguignon, most of the alcohol has been released in the steam after two hours of cooking. Although long cooking times and very high heats cause alcohol loss, the alcohol flavor remains in the food. Virtually all the added alcohol remains, however, when food is uncooked or cooked only briefly.

Because some individuals choose not to consume alcohol for various reasons, any food with alcohol as an ingredient should be described in a way that mentions the source of the alcohol. Recipes with alcohol-containing ingredients need to be calculated carefully, and the calories must be adjusted for the amount of retained alcohol. Refer to Chapter 6 for information regarding the amount of alcohol retained during the cooking process.

Here are some suggestions for preparing healthful braised and stewed foods:

- Use lean meats or poultry.
- Trim excess fat before stewing.
- Where suitable, marinate food to tenderize and add flavor.
- Use little or no fat for searing.
- Skim the sauce to remove extra fat.

Sauces

Sauces have always added interest, flavor and moistness to menu items, but it is no longer mandatory that sauces be roux- and cream-based, calorie- and fat-laden mixtures. Sauces have evolved into flavorful, colorful and nutritious additions to many meals. Traditional grand or leading sauces – béchamel, veloute, brown, tomato, and hollandaise – are making room for lower-fat and calorie-reduced coulis, salsas, infusions and natural reductions.

A flavorful poultry, meat, fish or vegetable stock can be the foundation of many good sauces and adds few calories and little fat. Ideally, stocks should be made on-site and without added salt. If this is not possible, look for good quality, reduced-sodium stocks. Salt, if needed, can be added when preparing the sauce.

A *reduction* is often used with sauteed items. The saute pan is deglazed with a liquid – often stock, juice or wine – to capture the flavorful bits left on the bottom of the pan. Other flavoring agents are added and the sauce is reduced by simmering to the desired consistency. Sometimes a thickening agent, such as arrowroot or cornstarch, is used. Garnishes, such as bruinoise of vegetables or juniper berries, can be added. Reductions can add flavor and moisture with minimal calories or added fat. Because of the intensified flavor of a reduction, little added salt is necessary.

In addition to adding color and flavor to any dish, salsa adds healthful fruits or vegetables. The traditional *salsa* is a Mexican, tomato-based mixture used for dipping chips. Today's chefs, however, are creating salsas using a wide variety of fruits and vegetables. Examples include mango and red pepper salsa, watermelon and red onion salsa, pineapple and green pepper salsa and strawberry and mint salsa.

Coulis are fruit- or vegetable-based purees. Like salsas, they add color and flavor to a dish as well as fruit and vegetables. Typically, coulis have little added fat and are generally low in calories. Examples of popular coulis are carrot, fresh pea, roasted red pepper coulis, raspberry or mango coulis and applesauce (although it is not strained as other coulis sometimes are).

Rich cream-based and roux-thickened sauces can be modified to be more healthful. Start with a full-flavored stock. For cream, substitute lower-fat dairy products such as evaporated skim milk, which has better body and a more cream-like flavor than skim milk. Buttermilk, which ironically has no fat and no butter, is another substitute suitable if its acidic flavor is appropriate. Yogurt and reduced-fat cream cheese also work well in some sauce recipes. For thickening, try starches such as arrowroot or cornstarch.

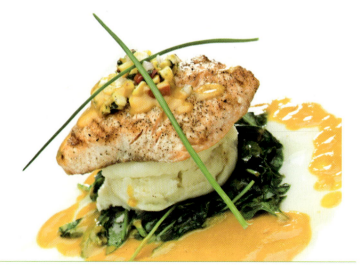

Nutrient Retention

Nutrients – especially vitamins, minerals and phytochemicals – are found in a wide variety of food products, from meat, fish, poultry and dairy to fruits, vegetables and whole grains. The nutrient content of food can vary and is affected by how the food is handled and processed. Factors such as degree of maturity at harvest, length of transportation time, storage time and exposure to the elements – heat, oxygen (air), light, extremes in pH (acidity or alkalinity) and moisture – affect nutrient content before a food is eaten.

The range of nutrient loss will vary among different produce. One study showed that vitamin C loss in cut fruits stored for six days can range from 5% (for cut watermelon) to 25% (for cut cantaloupe). Carotenoid loss ranged from none in kiwifruit to 25% loss in pineapples. This same research concluded that cut and whole fruits deteriorate nutritionally at about the same rate in refrigerated temperatures. [2]

What Is Fresh?

Keep in mind that "fresh" is not always truly fresh. Fresh-picked produce and the same produce after a week or more of storage and distribution can have differing amounts of nutrients. Buying local produce from known sources will help ensure freshness. The nutrient value of frozen produce will usually be comparable to (or better than) fresh produce. Generally, produce is frozen within hours of being picked, and freezing slows down nutrient loss. Drying fruits and vegetables will decrease vitamins A and C and folate. Drying fruits will also concentrate calories and sugar. Fruits dried on iron racks will absorb some iron, which is why raisins are higher in iron than grapes and dried plums (prunes) are higher in iron than fresh plums.

Often, the same procedures used to maintain food quality will also protect nutrients. For example, refrigerating most produce will maintain quality and preserve vitamins; likewise, cooking vegetables properly will maintain both quality and nutrients. Vitamins and, to a certain extent, minerals will leach into the water when cut vegetables and fruits are washed or cooked. Removing the peel will expose even more of the vegetable's flesh (and will remove fiber as well). In cases such as peeled tomatoes, asparagus and potatoes, however, maintaining sophisticated culinary standards often overrides maximizing nutrient retention.

To minimize nutrient loss, wash food just before cutting. Minerals are quite stable and are unaffected by high temperatures. To preserve vitamins, however, avoid high heat and use the shortest appropriate cooking times. Steam vegetables instead of boiling them. Reserve nutrient-rich cooking liquids for use in preparing soups and stocks, to braise or poach meats, poultry and fish, and to cook starches. [3]

Cooking Methods

To cook most vegetables, steam them over rapidly boiling water for a short time until just done. Remove and serve or, if not served immediately, stop the cooking process by plunging the vegetables into ice water and then draining them quickly and thoroughly. Cover and refrigerate until ready to serve. If steaming is not practical, blanch vegetables for a short period in rapidly boiling water. Follow the same ice-water process for maximum nutrient retention. Avoid adding acid during cooking or holding as acid will destroy the color of vegetables. An often-used trick for maintaining the color of vegetables is to add baking soda (alkaline) to the cooking water; however, this addition will change the texture of the vegetable and rob it of nutrients. When possible, cook vegetables from the raw state and serve them immediately.

Using the microwave to reheat starches and soups is an ideal way to decrease cooking time and retain quality and nutrients. To maximize the nutrient value of soups, avoid holding them in a steam table. Some restaurants prepare the soup; cool it immediately; portion it into cups or bowls; reheat portions in the microwave and garnish immediately before serving. A more common practice is to cook and chill soup and then reheat in batches on the stovetop.

Starches, such as rice, pasta and potato, held on a steam table will overcook and dry out, thus increasing nutrient loss. When precooking any starch, make sure that it is cooled and stored properly and reheated in a microwave or oven.

Proper storage is crucial to maintaining the quality of a food product and its nutritional value. Know your inventory needs. Overstocking anything may lead to serving poor quality products with deteriorated nutrient content. It is important to follow "the first in, first out" (FIFO) procedure in order to rotate stocks, fresh produce, fish, meats, poultry and dairy products. Allocate time and staff to make sure this procedure is followed to maintain quality while reducing spoilage and holding down food costs.

Cooking Vegetables to Retain Nutrients

1. **Cook vegetables in the smallest amount of liquid possible.**

   Vegetables have some vitamins that dissolve in water and are lost when the cooking liquid is discarded. Water-soluble vitamins include C and the B vitamins riboflavin, thiamin and niacin. Liquids in which vegetables are cooked can be added to soups and stocks to boost flavor and nutrient content. Commercial steamers are excellent for cooking large quantities of vegetables while retaining maximum nutrients.

2. **Cook vegetables for the shortest amount of time to desired tenderness.**

   Vegetables contain vitamins that are destroyed by heat. Prolonged cooking can reduce vitamin and phtyochemical levels. Use a commercial steamer or a microwave oven, if possible.

3. **For vegetables with skin, scrub well and cook with the skin on whenever possible. If the skin must be removed, peel the vegetable as thinly as possible.**

   Vegetables such as potatoes, carrots, parsnips and turnips have a valuable layer of nutrients right under the skin. Peeling will remove these nutrients as well as fiber. Fiber is also removed when a tomato or stalk of asparagus is peeled.

4. **When cutting vegetables, use a sharp blade and cut pieces as large as possible to suit the recipe. Pieces should be uniform to allow for even cooking. Large pieces help preserve the nutrient content of the vegetable. This guideline contradicts the "green advice" that smaller cuts reduce cooking time. In practice, choose the cut that makes the most sense for the dish you are preparing.**

   A sharp cutting blade will make a clean cut without bruising the vegetable. Bruising causes a rapid loss of vitamin C in green, leafy vegetables such as cabbage.

5. **Cook vegetables just before service.**

   Holding vegetables after cooking causes some nutrient loss and diminishes quality. Vegetables may be precooked, chilled and reheated at service. Batch cooking, preparing vegetables in small quantities as needed, is recommended for maximum nutrition and quality.

Effects of Processing on Nutrients in Foods

Nutrient	Food Source	Effect of Processing
Fat	Vegetable oils, butter, lard	• Oxidation and spoilage accelerated by light
Protein	Meat, fish, poultry	• Structure altered by heat and acids
Vitamin C	Citrus fruit, tomatoes, strawberries, peppers, broccoli and greens	• The least stable of all vitamins • Decreases during storage, drying, heating, oxidation, chopping
Thiamin (B_1)	Pork, organ meats, whole grains, enriched grains and cereals	• Sensitive to light in alkaline and neutral condition • Moderately heat stable under neutral conditions • Sensitive to heat under alkaline conditions
Riboflavin (B_2)	Milk, liver, eggs, cereal/grains, dark leafy greens	• Sensitive to light in alkaline and neutral conditions • Moderately heat stable under neutral conditions • Sensitive to heat under alkaline conditions
Vitamin B_6	Whole grains, vegetables, meat and fish	• Heat stable • Pyridoxal (a form of vitamin B_6) changes when heated
Niacin	Lean meats, whole grains, eggs and legumes	• Stable to heat and light • Leaches into cooking water
Folate	Beef liver, pinto beans, asparagus, lentils, avocado, enriched cereal, leafy green vegetables	• Decreases with storage or prolonged heating • Lost in cooking water
Vitamin B_{12}	Beef, pork, cheese, tuna, fish	• Destroyed by light and high acidity
Vitamin A	Dark leafy greens, yellow vegetables, cantaloupe, milk and eggs	• Easily destroyed by heat • Easily oxidized (exposure to air)
Vitamin D	Fortified milk	• Destroyed when exposed to heat and light
Vitamin E	Vegetable oils, whole grains, cereals, leafy vegetables, nuts and beans	• Oxidizes readily
Vitamin K	Leafy vegetables, vegetable oils, wheat bran	• Destroyed by acids and light
Minerals	Many foods	• Generally stable but leaches into water or other cooking liquid

Source: Adapted from: Morris A, Barnett A, Burrows O. Effect of processing on nutrient content of foods. Cajanus: The Caribbean Food & Nutrition Institute Quarterly. 2004. 37(3). www.paho.org/English/CFNI/cfni-caj37No304-art-3.pdf

Healthful Recipe Development

Understanding the *Dietary Guidelines for Americans*, applying what you know about nutrition, selecting appropriate cooking methods and adding a generous portion of your own creativity will result in recipes that delight and meet the nutritional needs of your customers.

When creating healthful recipes, think about the ingredients and components, flavoring agents and seasonings, garnishes and accompaniments, and cooking methods.

- **Ingredients:** Start with healthful ingredients – lean meats, fish and seafood, whole grains, and plenty of fruits and vegetables. Can you use a whole grain as a crust on the protein item? How about using fruit for the base of a sauce?

- **Flavoring agents and seasonings:** Look for ingredients that add lots of flavor but little fat or sodium. If you are creating an ethnic-inspired dish, look to the flavoring agents commonly found in that region.

- **Garnishes:** Almost as important as the center-of-the plate item, garnishes should complement the dish and blend with the flavors. Remember to ask yourself, "Does it make sense?" An orange slice adds color to a dish, but does it make sense with the food? Thoughtful garnishes add flavor and nutrients, such as vitamins, minerals and phytochemicals.

- **Accompaniments:** Look beyond "vegetable-of-the-day." Vegetable and starch accompaniments should complement the dish and are an opportunity to add healthful ingredients. Sauces should be low in fat and full of flavor. Explore ways to use legumes, fruits and vegetables (whole and juices) in sauce preparation.

- **Cooking methods:** Selecting the appropriate cooking method is as important as choosing the right ingredients. For example, deep-frying or pan-frying tilapia can undo the best healthful intentions. Select cooking methods that add flavor while minimizing added fat and calories. Identify challenging areas and consider alternatives. For example, with fried fish the challenge might be added fat from frying. In this case, consider baking the fish using a panko crumb crust to create the crunchy texture. An understanding of how ingredients function is important when thinking about substitutions: Is the sugar part of the structure of a dessert, or is it just adding sweetness?

Modifying favorite recipes to create more healthful alternatives can be a challenge when you know customers will inevitably compare the two versions. "This low-fat crème brulée is almost as good as … " is not a compliment. If a particular favorite food does not lend itself to modification, and a substitute with a good nutritional profile is not a reasonable option, serve a smaller size portion of "the real thing." Balance an indulgence with several healthful choices at the same meal. Make as many of the foods you serve as healthful as you can, but keep in mind that even the most nutritious food will not be enjoyed unless it tastes delicious.

casebycase

Fresh, Fast and Healthy

Panera Bread Company operates more than 1,350 company-owned and franchise-operated bakery-cafes in 40 states and in Ontario, Canada, under the monikers Panera Bread® Saint Louis Bread Co.® and Paradise Bakery & Café®. Panera knows bread. In fact, the company mission is "a loaf in every arm."

"My vision is 'the magic of the bakery,' which is the magic of who we are as a company," explains head baker Tom Gumpel, who was a member of the grand prize-winning American team at the 1999 World Cup of Baking in Paris and is now Panera's vice president of bakery development. "We are deeply rooted as a bakery; it's one of the ways Panera is special. So we're going to put pressure on ourselves and our partners to raise the bar on our baked goods."

Panera restaurants bake more bread each day than any bakery-cafe concept in the country. Every day, at every location, trained bakers craft and bake each loaf from scratch, using the best ingredients to ensure the highest quality breads. Panera's comprehensive menu makes it easy for guests to make healthful choices such as whole-grain sandwich bread; an apple accompaniment instead of chips; and half-sized soups, salads and sandwiches to control portion size. In addition, Panera's chicken is antibiotics-free.

Panera has garnered many awards, including recognition as the country's healthiest chain restaurant, awarded by *Health* magazine in 2009. *Health*'s panel of judges looked at criteria such as use of healthy fats and preparations, healthy sodium counts in entrees, and the use of organic produce. In 2010, the Zagat Fast-Food Survey named Panera Bread the most popular large restaurant chain in the United States. Panera topped the list of 90 restaurants in its category (chains with less than 5,000 locations). Panera also nabbed the number two spot in the healthy options category.

In early 2010, acting ahead of federally mandated restaurant menu labeling, Panera Bread Company posted calorie information on menu boards in all company-owned units. Franchise-operated locations followed suit by the end of 2010. This move made Panera Bread the first national concept to voluntarily post calorie information on menu boards across the country. "People were trying different products they wouldn't have tried otherwise," says Scott Davis, Panera's chief concept officer. "There are a lot of great ways for people to eat healthy – more than they realize."

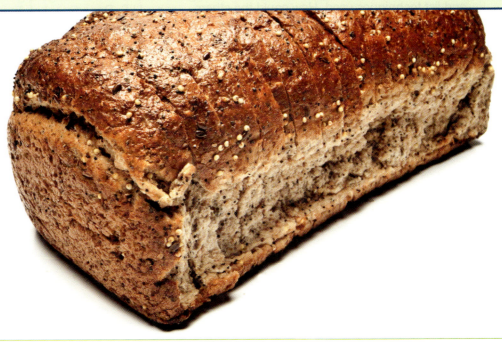

Bottom line: What's the point of preparing healthful, great-tasting food, if no one is going to eat it? Because "healthy" can mean different things to different people, it's important to understand how to promote healthful menu items. In the past, these foods met with customer resistance because they didn't look as appealing or taste as good as "regular" menu items. Many customers are still stuck in this old mindset. Consequently, while they say they want healthful food options, they order everything else. Appealing, high-quality, healthful food can change this behavior pattern. Patrons who know your food is both delicious and nutritious are likely to become regulars.

The menu is the most common tool for communicating nutrition to your guests and customers. Newsletters, websites, blogs, social media and media stories also shape messages to your guests. Increasingly, chefs are using their status and influence to communicate nutrition and health messages. Service staff are also important tellers of your nutrition story and should be properly trained to communicate your message.

Healthy: What's in a Word?

In everyday conversation, most people use the terms "healthy" and "healthful" to describe certain foods and menus. The U.S. Food and Drug Administration (FDA), however, takes these terms very seriously. FDA considers them "implied claims" and sets guidelines for their use on food labels. These guidelines also apply to restaurant menus.

The term "*healthy*" and related terms ("health," "healthful," "healthfully," "healthfulness," "healthier," "healthiest," "healthily" and "healthiness") may be used if the food meets the following requirements:

- An individual food or main dish must contain no more than 3 grams of fat per standard serving. For seafood, meat and game, the guideline is less than 5 grams of total fat and less than 2 grams of saturated fat per 100-gram portion. Note that 100-gram portions are smaller than what most restaurants serve, so the amount of fat and saturated fat must be calibrated to the portion served.

- An individual food must have less than 480 milligrams of sodium per standard serving size (referred to as *RACC* or *reference amount customarily consumed* per eating occasion, the amount used on food labels) or 50 milligrams if the RACC is 30 grams or less. Meals or main dishes may have up to 600 milligrams per serving.

- Seafood, meat, game and main dishes or meals must have 90 milligrams or less of cholesterol.

- An individual food must contain at least 10% of the Daily Value per standard reference serving size of one or more beneficial nutrients – vitamins A or C, calcium, iron, protein or fiber. Main dish products must have at least 10% of the Daily Value of two nutrients; meals must contain at least 10% of the Daily Value for three beneficial nutrients.

- All raw fruits and vegetables and frozen or canned single-ingredient fruits and vegetables are considered "healthy."

- Enriched cereal or grain products that conform to standards of identity are considered "healthy."

Source: U.S. Food and Drug Administration. Guidance for Industry: A Food Labeling Guide, www.fda.gov/Food/GuidanceComplianceRegulatoryInformation/GuidanceDocuments/FoodLabelingNutrition/FoodLabelingGuide/ucm064916.htm

Nutrition on the Menu

There are several schools of thought – and even some controversy – concerning the best way to identify healthful items on menus. One approach uses symbols or icons to designate items as healthier alternatives. Clear and concise, symbols eliminate guesswork and help guests make their selections without a lot of server assistance.

Designing a separate menu or menu section is another approach. The obvious benefit for the guest is that healthier alternatives are easy to identify. Research is needed to determine if people are more likely to order healthier items if they are integrated in the main menu or presented separately.

A third approach – offering but not highlighting healthful alternatives – is based on the concept that special labeling sends a negative message and may lead guests to wonder, "If these items are healthy, does that mean the rest of the menu is unhealthy?" A more positive approach is to let menu items speak for themselves and rely on a combination of guests' knowledge and personal interest in healthful selections and servers' ability to promote the items appropriately.

A fourth approach is to position a restaurant as a provider of healthful foods, serving only foods that are under certain calorie levels, using only heart-healthy fats and focussing on nutrient-rich ingredients. While some consider this a limited market, chains and restaurants such as Seasons 52, Rouge Tomate and others have loyal clientele.

Yet another approach is to offer **small plates** or reduced portions of entrees, salads or desserts. Pricing can be a problem with this approach. A guest may expect a 4-ounce portion of a protein entree to be priced at half the price of an 8-ounce portion when typically, the half portion is priced at about 75% of the larger portion. Overhead, dishwashing, service, utensils and labor are cost factors independent of the difference in portion size. For many patrons, a better choice might be sharing one entree, ordering two appetizers and no entree, ordering a salad or soup and an appetizer as an entree, or splitting desserts. Many people think that sharing limits portions and calories. This approach works only if less total food is ordered. Two people sharing two entrees or two desserts does not cut calories; it just redistributes them.

Menu Labeling and the Healthcare Reform Act

The Patient Protection and Affordable Care Act, commonly known as the **Healthcare Reform Act**, was signed into law in March 2010. One section of the bill – Section 4205 – requires restaurants with 20 or more locations nationally to add calorie counts to menus, menu boards and drive-thru menu boards for standard menu items. It also requires those restaurants to make additional nutrition data available to guests upon request. [1] This mandate provides a single, consistent national standard for nutrition disclosure in restaurants that helps consumers make choices that are best for themselves and their families. The federal standard provides uniform nutrition-labeling requirements that multi-state restaurants can implement nationwide. Before the law, restaurant operators had to comply with a patchwork of state and local menu-labeling regulations. The differing requirements made it difficult for restaurants to comply and consumers to understand.

Restaurants and similar retail food establishments that are covered under the new federal rules are no longer subject to state or local menu labeling laws, except to the extent they are identical to the federal requirements. Smaller chain and individual retail food establishments are not subject to the new federal law; however, they may still be subject to all state and local nutrition-labeling laws and associated regulations. If these restaurants and similar retail food establishments voluntarily register with the Food and Drug Administration (FDA), they will no longer be subject to state or local nutrition-labeling requirements.

The law also requires those restaurants to make available additional written nutrition data about standard menu items upon request. The term **standard** is used to designate items that generally appear on the menu and are usually available. Daily specials or menu items being introduced are not required to have full information.

The nutrition-disclosure requirements also apply to restaurants that are part of a chain that operates 20 or more locations under the same trade name, regardless of the ownership type of the locations, which offer "substantially the same menu items" for sale. The law also applies to retail food establishments that are similar to foodservice operations. It doesn't define those establishments. Based on the way the FDA has interpreted other parts of the Food, Drug and Cosmetic Act, it likely means that the new restaurant labeling requirements apply to any establishment owned by a company with 20 or more locations under the same trade name where food is served for immediate consumption. For example, this category could include foodservice facilities in hospitals or schools, food at convenience stores served for immediate consumption, and food served from mobile carts. The law also applies to vending machines owned by companies that operate 20 or more machines.

Covered restaurants are required to provide the following information for standard menu items:

- Number of calories per standard menu item. The calorie count per serving must appear next to the menu item name. This count is based on actual serving size of a single portion, not on a predetermined amount or RACC (reference amount customarily consumed). FDA will provide more details on how restaurants must display this information.

- A prominent, clear and conspicuous statement about the availability of additional nutrition information. Additional information includes values for:

  - Calories
  - Calories from total fat
  - Saturated fat
  - Cholesterol
  - Sodium
  - Carbohydrates
  - Sugars
  - Dietary fiber
  - Protein

- A succinct statement concerning suggested daily caloric intake posted prominently on the menu to help guests understand calories in the context of a daily diet. FDA will specify the language for this statement in its regulations.

Congress recognizes that there is variation in preparing restaurant meals. A main course salad, for example, might not have the same amount of vegetables, croutons or exactly the same amount of dressing each time it's prepared. As a result, the new law doesn't require an exact count for prescribed nutrient levels. It does, however, require that restaurants show they have a reasonable basis for the nutrition data they present. Restaurants must demonstrate that they have used reasonable means to derive their information, such as nutrient databases, cookbooks, laboratory analysis and other reasonable means described in FDA regulations and related guidance.

The law directs the FDA to look at all the factors that could cause variations in restaurant nutrition content. Some factors the FDA must consider in determining restaurant compliance include:

- Reasonable variation in serving size and formulation of menu items
- Standardization of recipes and preparation methods
- Inadvertent human error
- Employee training
- Ingredient variations

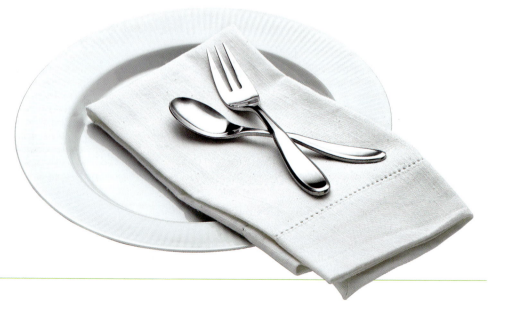

Benefits and Obstacles of Menu Labeling

According to a *2010 Mintel Healthy Dining Trends* survey, 44% of consumers support government intervention in menu transparency (menu labeling laws). Further, almost half of respondents agree that nutritional information should be posted on menus along with recommended Daily Values for key nutrients. [2]

Some of the benefits of menu labeling include:

- Increased consumer education. Theoretically, consumers will use calorie counts to make informed food choices.

- Reformulation of products. As foodservice operators look at menu balance from a nutrition viewpoint, they may choose to create a broader spectrum of food choices. Questions to ask include:

  - What menu items will I keep?
  - What items will I remove?
  - What items will I change?
  - How will I change these items?
  - What items will I add?
  - What commonly used ingredients will I substitute for currently used products?

- Right-sized portions. As calorie amounts are revealed, portion distortion will become more obvious, which may lead to a reduction in portion size, lowered food costs and more healthful options.

Some of the potential obstacles of menu labeling include:

- Restaurants and cafeterias that do not use standardized recipes may unintentionally provide inaccurate information.

- Cooks will require more training to ensure they consistently measure ingredients and use standardized recipes.

- Labeling may limit flexibility in changing the menu.

- Providing nutrition information might be costly.

- Providing nutrition information might lead to reduced demand for profitable menu items.

- Customers may not return to a restaurant that has many menu items that they perceive as having too many calories.

- Training employees to respond to questions about menu labeling will take time and may be difficult.

Does Calorie Knowledge Lead to Calorie Control?

In a June 2009 synthesis of existing menu research titled *Menu Labeling: Does Providing Nutrition Information at Point of Purchase Affect Consumer Behavior?* The Robert Wood Johnson Foundation reported:

- Eating out frequently, particularly at quick-service or fast-food restaurants, is related to greater weight gain and obesity.

- Frequently eating in restaurants is related to higher intakes of fat, sodium and soft drinks, and lower intakes of nutrient-dense foods such as vegetables.

- Most consumers underestimate the number of calories and fat in away-from-home foods and tend to make greater errors when menu items are high in calories.

- Most consumers would like to see nutrition information at places where they go out to eat; however, only limited research has explored how well this information is understood by consumers and which consumers may be most likely to use menu labels in making decisions about what to purchase.

- Consumers may be influenced not to select an item when they read on the menu label that it contains more calories and fat than they had thought.

- Requiring restaurants to provide point-of-purchase nutrition information could help reduce obesity by promoting the introduction of healthier menu options.

Source: The Robert Wood Johnson Foundation, *Menu Labeling: Does Providing Nutrition Information at the Point of Purchase Affect Consumer Behavior?* June 2009, www.rwjf.org/pr/product.jsp?id=45048

Menu Descriptions

What compels a diner to order a particular menu item? Personal food preferences, health concerns, economics, peer pressure and taste generally dictate what people order at a restaurant. How a menu item is described gives diners the information they need to make a selection. Menu descriptions can also provide clues about the healthfulness of an item.

- **What is it?** Healthful key ingredients – for example, scallops, salmon, greens, whole grains, legumes or organic fruit – are a guest's first indication that the menu item may be among the restaurant's healthier choices.

- **How is it prepared?** Poaching, steaming, grilling, roasting and infusing are generally low-fat, high-flavor cooking methods. Indicating preparation method can suggest the healthfulness of the dish. Fried foods, on the other hand, are not considered healthful unless the fried item is used in small amounts as a garnish, such as fried sage atop a pasta with sundried or chopped fresh tomatoes and herbs. Adjectives like "crispy" or "crunchy" generally suggest a food is fried. "Creamy" suggests use of cream or a high-fat product.

- **What are the food's special qualities?** Foods that are free range, organic, grass fed and/or locally grown indicate that ingredients have been carefully selected for nutrition and taste and are "green" – that is, grown in ways that are good for the environment. More and more restaurants are featuring the source names of the farm, ranch, cheesemaker or grower.

- **What are the ingredients?** Words like "creamed," "buttered," "larded" and "glazed" are indications that a menu item may be higher in fat or sugar. "Fruit coulis," "vegetable puree," "beans" and "whole grains" are telling patrons that the menu item is probably healthier.

- **What is the serving size?** Words like "abundant," "bountiful," "generous," "big," "giant" and "heaping" suggest super-sized portions. "Small," "4-ounces" and "garnished with" indicate modest portion sizes. Inviting customers to share an appetizer, salad, pasta, side dish or dessert encourages sales and moderate eating. The trend to small plates, half-portions and bite-sized desserts helps patrons enjoy a wide variety of foods without excess.

Sharing Your Story

Newsletters, websites, blogs, social media and media articles are viable avenues to share your story and promote your foodservice operation. These are excellent places to expand your nutrition message and garner customer support. Some ideas for sharing your story include:

- Post pictures of your restaurant garden and share how you are using more vegetables on the menu.

- Include short biographies or photos of the farmers or growers and producers you patronize on your website.

- Have you recently improved your health? Maybe you have lost weight? Share your success with your guests and let them know that you can help them, too.

- Share your healthful recipes in your newsletter or website to highlight your expertise.

- Showcase your most healthful recipes when teaching classes, hosting events, contributing products to charity events or doing demonstrations.

Garnering Recognition for Healthful Foods

- Give cooking demonstrations or classes for the community. Choose items that feature healthful ingredients and cooking techniques.

- Market the restaurant through cooking competitions, food tastings and media interviews that promote healthy dining.

- Offer getaway weekends with cooking demonstrations, nutrition seminars, exercise workshops and other lifestyle enhancers.

- Tie into hotels or fitness centers with a juice and smoothie bar, healthy snack items, body-fat testing and a menu for the hotel/fitness center restaurant.

- Become the restaurant of choice or caterer of events sponsored by health-related organizations (American Heart Association, American Diabetes Association, etc.) or organizations of health professionals such as district dietetic associations.

- Work with hotels that host conferences to provide special food and/or nutrition seminars for programs or lifestyle-enhancement seminars such as healthful entertaining, how to survive business lunches, staying fit on the road and eating to increase productivity.

- Be sure your establishment is included in listings of healthful restaurants in your community.

- When being quoted or when providing recipes to the media, use your most healthful recipes.

Community and Professional Involvement

Building a reputation for doing the right thing can be the best marketing plan. Many chefs and foodservice professionals are realizing they have a responsibility to use their influence to foster change. Celebrity chefs are leading campaigns to improve school meals, lose weight, increase produce consumption and be more physically active. How can you become part of this movement? Consider:

- Working in the kitchens of a local school district

- Supporting and promoting local farmers and growers

- Supporting community food pantries and hunger organizations

- Donating left-over food to homeless shelters and hunger organizations or volunteering to provide or cook meals

- Teaching a series of cooking classes at the local Boys and Girls Club

- Inviting students to dine in your restaurant

- Teaching parents or guardians how to prepare easy and healthful meals

- Conducting demonstrations at your local farmers' market

- Pushing your local, state and federal legislators to support more healthful food choices at schools and community feeding sites

Cause-related marketing allows you to help non-profit organizations within your community and reap the rewards from the publicity surrounding charitable events.

- Establish a connection with a community-service organization to galvanize positive public perception about your business. Find charitable organizations through your customers, employees or vendors. Pick a cause that employees are excited about so they will continue to participate in your community-service project. Spark employee activism by exchanging an afternoon or evening off for donating a certain number of hours to charity events.

- Be sure the charity or event acknowledges your restaurant to let the community learn of your efforts.

- Maximize publicity by printing T-shirts with your restaurant's logo for employees to wear while they perform volunteer service.

- Distribute bumper stickers urging the public to support your chosen organization. The stickers should include your establishment's name and logo.

- Post a bulletin board in your restaurant where customers can see photos of your staff's volunteer activities. Display flyers urging patrons to sign up as well.

- Include your charitable activities in your restaurant's newsletter and website.

- Have staff wear buttons promoting your charitable organization or event so customers will inquire about it.

- Work with a publicist to increase business. Highlight that your operation has added menu items to meet the needs of health-conscious diners in your publicity and public relations efforts.

casebycase

Marketing Healthful Menus: Five Ways to Use Social Media

With the rise of social media, it's easier than ever to promote your establishment – even with a limited marketing budget, according to food blogger and public relations executive Janet Helm, MS, RD, who is the chief food and nutrition strategist for Weber Shandwick, one of the world's leading global public relations firms.

"Social media is all about storytelling and visuals, which makes it an ideal platform for food," Helm explains. "It's about building a community, starting conversations and providing content that people want to share. All of that can translate to customers for you."

When you have a good story to tell about a healthful menu, that's even better. "Food and health are two of the major topics that people search for online," Helm says. "So you have a tremendous amount to gain if you build your social profile and elevate your online presence." Here are five steps to get you started:

1. **Create a Facebook page**. Set up a business page and let people "like" you. Share photos of your healthful menu items, promote specials and converse with diners. Consider offering a discount to fans or people who check in using Facebook Places, or other location-based social tools such as Foursquare.

2. **Connect on Twitter**. Many of the country's top chefs have developed large followings on Twitter. Set up your own profile and begin connecting with people. It's a great way to create a personality for your establishment and to network. You can use Twitter to post pictures and to enter conversations about food and nutrition that give you a chance to talk about your healthful offerings. Get yourself in the minds (and phones) of your followers!

3. **Post pictures on Flickr.** Flickr is a media-sharing site and is one of the best places to post pictures. Take photos of your healthful menu items and use captions to describe each dish. Under a Creative Commons license (http://creativecommons.org), you can allow others to use your pictures with attribution, which means more exposure for your establishment.

4. **Get to know social networking food sites**. Foodies flock to sites such as Yelp, Urbanspoon and Foodspotting or forums on Serious Eats, Chow and other food sites. Make sure your information is up to date and that you are listening to what's being said about your establishment

5. **Combine your online activities with offline publicity**. Offer to do a cooking segment for a local TV station and use it as an opportunity to showcase new healthful menu items and to provide recipes for viewers to make at home. Bring food to radio DJs and ask them to talk about special items and promotions. Be a resource to the food editor of your local newspaper.

Non-Commercial Foodservice

Many innovations that are focused on quality foods are happening in the healthcare arena. Culinary teams led by certified and/or culinary-trained chefs are partnering with registered dietitians to create nourishing quality meals. The traditional trayline is being replaced by the room service model in which patients are able to have more control over what and when they can eat a meal. Patients can order what they feel like eating when they are ready to eat rather than at set mealtimes. As hospitals and other healthcare operations try to differentiate themselves from the competition, they often look to value-added services. The food served is certainly an area for differentiation, and good food is always appreciated. The days of strict diets have been replaced with a more liberal approach to the menu in hospitals and in healthcare and senior-living facilities.

Students and people of all ages in residential facilities appreciate the strides foodservice directors are making to serve food that is both healthful and delicious. Many food establishments are adding salad bars, baked potato bars, soup and sandwich lines, vegetarian and stir-fry entrees, homemade whole-grain breads, low-fat entrees and dairy products, light salad dressings, and grilled and petite meat portions. Many facilities are planting gardens or featuring produce from local sources. Display cooking – moving the final stages of preparation to the front of the house – has become popular in colleges and hospitals.

New food options can be promoted in newsletters to students, parents or residents, on websites, on bulletin boards and posters, on table tents in the cafeteria, and in presentations to classes or group meetings. Let the dietary department of your local hospital and dietitians who do counseling in your community know that your operation is serving more heart-healthy or moderate-calorie options so that they may suggest your restaurant. Of course, it helps to instruct the cooking and serving staff, residents and teachers on nutrition benefits and reasons for change first. Caring about customers' health and well-being, as well as your own and your staff's, can increase sales and create the dividend of better health for all.

A Word from the Chef
Chefs Move to Schools

Schools also have a role in meeting the nutrition needs of children as many children have one, and sometimes two meals, a day at school. The national school meal program serves healthful breakfasts, lunches, after-school snacks and summer meals to hungry children around the country. More than 31 million children eat school lunch and more than 11 million enjoy healthy breakfasts each day. The Healthy, Hunger-Free Kids Act of 2010 brought major improvements to these programs with greater emphasis on fruits, vegetables, whole grains and lower-sodium menu items.

To help accomplish the new goals of the national school meal program the Chefs Move to Schools, an integral part of First Lady Michelle Obama's Let's Move! initiative, was founded in May 2010 with the goal of solving the childhood obesity epidemic within a generation. It has matched thousands of chefs and schools around the country to create partnerships in their communities with the mission of collaboratively educating kids about food and healthy eating.

First Lady Michelle Obama is fully behind the movement and shares that "We are going to need everyone's time and talent to solve the childhood obesity epidemic and our Nation's chefs have tremendous power as leaders on this issue because of their deep knowledge of food and nutrition and their standing in the community."

Chefs and schools have a unique opportunity to work together to teach kids about food in a fun, appealing way. The Chefs Move to Schools program seeks to utilize the creativity and culinary expertise of chefs to help schools ensure that America's youngest generation grows up healthy.

Chefs Move to Schools focuses on the interests and expertise of each chef volunteer and the needs of each school. There are many ways the partnership can work to positively impact the eating habits of children both in the classroom and the cafeteria.

To become a part of this important initiative go to www.chefsmovetoschools.org.

Turkey Meatloaf

Chef Ann Cooper, Director of Foodservice,
Boulder Valley School District, Boulder, Colorado

Yield: 51 ounces
Serves: 12 slices, 4 ounces each

This delicious, mild-flavored meatloaf can be adapted for many audiences. It can be used in schools, long-term care or family-style restaurants.

Onion, small dice	4	ounces
Garlic, minced	1	teaspoon
Carrots, shredded	2	ounces
Canola oil	1	tablespoon
Turkey, ground	3	pounds
Parsley, chopped	1	tablespoon
Japanese (Panko) bread crumbs	½	cup
Eggs	3	
Kosher salt	1	teaspoon
Black pepper, freshly ground	¼	teaspoon
Ketchup	3	tablespoons

1. Preheat oven to 350° F. Prepare a 9 inch x 5 inch loaf pan with non-stick spray.

2. Saute onions, garlic, and carrots in oil until soft. Remove from heat and allow to cool slightly before transferring to a separate bowl.

3. Combine the sauteed ingredients with the turkey, parsley, bread crumbs, eggs, salt and pepper and mix well.

4. Pack meat into prepared loaf pan, coat top with ketchup, and bake until cooked through to an internal temperature of 165° F.

Per Piece

Calories	220	Cholesterol	120	mg
Fat	10 g	Sodium	340	mg
Saturated Fat	2.5 g	Carbohydrates	10	mg
Trans Fat	0 g	Dietary Fiber	1	mg
Sugar	2 g	Protein	25	g

Recipe reprinted with permission from *Lunch Lessons* by Ann Cooper and Lisa M. Holmes (Harper Collins, 2006).

Butternut Squash Soup with Fried Sage Leaves

Chef Ann Cooper, Director of Foodservice,
Boulder Valley School District, Boulder, Colorado

Serves: 12, 1 cup servings

Butternut squash is a mainstay during the late summer and early fall. It can be prepared countless ways, but this soup is one of our favorites because it combines the sweetness of the squash with the perfume of the sage and the spiciness of cloves and herbs.

Olive oil, extra virgin	¼	cup
Sage leaves, whole	16	
Butternut squash peeled, seeded, roughly chopped	1	large (2 ½ pounds)
Beet, peeled and roughly chopped	1	medium
Onion, peeled and roughly chopped	1	large
Carrots, peeled and chopped	1	each
Celery, peeled and chopped	2	stalks
Parsley, minced	¼	cup
Garlic, minced	4	cloves
Thyme, fresh, minced	1	teaspoon
Cloves, ground	⅛	teaspoon
Vegetable broth	7	cups
Salt	1	teaspoon
Black pepper, freshly ground	⅛	teaspoon

1. In an 8 quart stock pot heat the oil and fry sage leaves until crisp—about 45 seconds. Remove them from the oil and reserve.

2. In the same pot, saute the squash, beet, onion, carrots and celery for 15 minutes.

3. Stir in the parsley, garlic, thyme and cloves. Cook for 5 more minutes.

4. Add the vegetable stock, cover and simmer 5 minutes until all of the vegetables are tender.

5. Crush 4 sage leaves into soup. Season with salt and pepper.

6. Puree with an immersion blender.

7. When serving, top each bowl with one whole fried sage leaf.

Per Piece

Calories	100	Cholesterol	0	mg
Fat	5 g	Sodium	260	mg
Saturated Fat	0.5 g	Carbohydrates	14	mg
Trans Fat	0 g	Dietary Fiber	3	mg
Sugar	5 g	Protein	2	g

Staff Development

Inadequate staff training is a primary reason for the failure of a healthful dining program. To keep momentum high, both kitchen and service staff must buy into the program's philosophy wholeheartedly.

Training for the back-of-the-house staff should include:

- Basic nutrition information explaining any changes. When staff members understand why changes are being made, they are better able to execute them.

- Portion control and ingredient-measuring techniques for standardized recipes.

- Across-the-board reductions in salt, fat and sugar in cooking.

- Switching to reduced-sodium sauces and heart-healthy oils.

- Proper cooking techniques and the need for conscientious application every time a dish is prepared.

- Translating customers' special requests into specific menu items (such as broiling fish instead of sauteing, frying or cooking *a la minute*).

- Importance of careful ingredient and technique control, especially while preparing foods for patrons with food allergies, intolerances or on special diets.

Training for the front-of-the-house staff should emphasize basic nutrition information as well as information about cooking techniques and ingredients. With this background, wait staff can respond to guests' individual needs and communicate special requests to the kitchen staff. There should be a designated individual who can answer questions on nutrient values and ingredients.

Some diners have allergies, intolerances or medical conditions that can be triggered by food choices. The patron who asks if there is cream in the soup or if a menu item has nuts requires a correct response. Sometimes, busy servers do not bother to check, especially if the food item is new to the menu. An incorrect response can lead to a medical emergency.

An effective training program should teach servers their many responsibilities, including how to sell menu items.

- Start by hiring job applicants who have the potential to be effective servers and sales people. Look for candidates who are friendly, personable, good at listening and persuasive. You should be able to ascertain many of these qualities during a job interview.

- As part of training, ensure that servers know about each menu item, including ingredients and preparation method. Provide opportunities for new staff members to taste each menu item. Employees who are informed about menu items will be able to give more knowledgeable answers to customer questions and thus boost sales.

- Consider having new employees learn the ropes by shadowing or trailing experienced servers. Start the shadowing experience on the right foot by selecting your best employees to serve as trainers. Compensate and recognize trainers with higher wages or some other incentive, such as gift certificates.

- Before new servers hit the floor, have them do a test run by serving experienced staffers or managers. Provide feedback on their performance, including their selling skills.

- Remember that training is a continuous process. Use pre-shift meetings to remind employees about selling techniques, to notify them about menu items you particularly want to sell and to provide food tastings.

Having a registered dietitian with culinary experience available to an operation provides credibility and reliability for any healthful dining initiative. A dietitian can be a source of information for staff, management and marketing and also can help to generate local support by encouraging his/her clients and colleagues to enjoy healthy meals at your restaurant. Registered dietitians can also work with chefs to develop more healthful menu items and provide nutrient calculations for the menu and additional information as required by law.

Making a Nutrition Claim

Any restaurant (defined by the government as a place that serves food ready for consumption, including typical sit-down and carryout venues, as well as institutional foodservice, delicatessens and catering operations) that uses nutrient content claims or health claims on its menu must comply with Nutrition Labeling and Education Act (NLEA) regulations. [3] These regulations also apply to menus that use symbols – such as a heart, an apple or a checkmark – to signify healthful items.

Many of the nutrient and health claims used in food labeling (see Chapter 2) also apply to menus. A *nutrient claim* makes a statement about a specific nutrient or food component of a menu item or meal. It typically includes words such as "reduced," "free" or "low." Claims such as "low in fat," "sugar-free" or "cholesterol-free" are common on menus. For example, when an airline provides a special "low-sodium," "reduced-sodium," or "low-fat," meal, it is making a nutrient content claim. Not only must the meal meet the definition(s) for the claim(s), the airline must provide information on the nutrients that underlie the claim(s) – "low-fat," for example, means the meal contains only 10 grams of fat. This information must be provided by "reasonable means" such as a card identifying the meal as a special request or in a binder available from the flight attendants.

A *health claim* links the food or meal with health status or disease prevention and usually mentions a specific disease. Health claims are relatively uncommon on printed menus, but there are government-mandated rules for terminology. For example, a dish that is low in fat, saturated fat and cholesterol might carry a claim about how diets low in saturated fat and cholesterol may reduce the risk of heart disease. Health claims may appear on the menu in simple terms, such as "heart healthy."

The government strictly regulates health claims and has approved only 12 for which there is sufficient scientific support. These claims are also used on food labels (see Chapter 2). Some customers may be familiar with them. Foodservice operators are not permitted to make up their own health claims or alter the approved healthy claim statements in any way. For example, an operator cannot claim that a pomegranate blueberry smoothie is high in antioxidants and thus may help prevent cancer. There is no approved health claim for that relationship even if it is believed to be true.

When a nutrient or health claim is used, regulations require there be a reasonable basis for believing the food is qualified to make the claim. Although regulations allow foodservice operators some flexibility in establishing that reasonable basis, they must be prepared to show, on demand, that the menu claims are consistent with the definitions established under the NLEA. Foodservice operators may determine nutrient levels using computer databases, nutrient analyses, cookbooks or some other reasonable source that can provide assurance that the food or meal meets claim requirements.

The Food and Drug Administration (FDA) does not subject restaurant foods to chemical analysis to determine whether nutrient levels are properly declared. Rather, FDA will assess whether the restaurant's basis for a claim or other nutrition information is or is not reasonable. For example, if a restaurant claims a meal is "low-fat," FDA may look at the recipe, nutrient calculations and any other information used by the restaurant in determining whether the meal meets the definition of "low-fat" – that is, containing no more than 3 grams of fat per 100 grams of food.

Claim It. Prove It.

If a menu uses any of the following words or symbols representing these words, documentation is required.

Free	High/Excellent Source of/ Rich in
Low	
Reduced	Lean/Extra-Lean
Light/Lite	Fresh
Provides/Contains/ Good Source of	Natural
	Healthy

The FDA offers operators a number of ways to present nutrient data information to patrons. Information is required only for nutrients for which a claim is made. For example, if the menu makes a claim about the cholesterol content of an item, the operator must provide information on the amount of cholesterol but does not have to provide information about the item's calorie, fat or vitamin content. Of course, it would be helpful to guests if all nutrition information were provided.

The nutrient information does not have to be in a special format, such as the Nutrition Facts label found on food products; it simply must be available – for example, in a brochure, on a poster or in a notebook. A statement from a server, such as "a low-fat meal contains less than 10 grams of fat," is the equivalent of full nutrition labeling. As a backup, a restaurant should also have nutrition information in writing to ensure that whatever servers communicate is accurate. It makes sense that restaurants know what they are serving from a nutrition perspective, even if they are not required to share this information with customers or guests or choose not to do so.

Where Does 'Fresh' Fit?

Although the word "fresh" is not a nutrient claim, federal regulations include a definition of what constitutes a "fresh" food item. Many foodservice establishments use the term *fresh* without knowing its legal definition – a food that is raw, has never been frozen or heated, contains no preservatives other than approved waxes or coatings, and may be washed with mild acid to clean. (Irradiation at low levels is allowed.) The term "fresh" also can be used to describe a product such as fresh milk or freshly baked bread.

In its *2012 Restaurant Industry Forecast*, the National Restaurant Association reported keen interest in fresh produce among restaurant operators. And according to research presented at the Produce Marketing Association's 2009 Foodservice Conference & Exposition, opportunities abound for using fresh produce on restaurant menus. [4] The research showed that restaurant operators see fresh produce as a way to differentiate themselves from the competition. Forty-one percent said they expect to serve more fresh produce in the next two years; 56% said they expect to serve about the same amount.

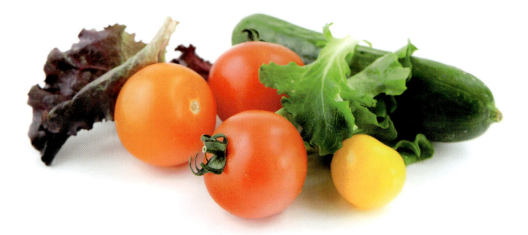

Calculating Nutrient Data

Providing nutrient data for recipes is a common practice today as restaurants, cookbook authors, culinary demonstrators and food media respond to consumer demand for information on the healthfulness of food. On the surface, gathering these data may seem like a simple process. For example, a recipe for fruit salad containing a specified amount of select fruits per portion involves calculating the nutrient contribution of the edible portion of each fruit, totaling the nutrient values and dividing by the number of servings. This nutrient calculation is fairly straightforward. Few are so easy. Accurate nutrient calculations require more than simply inputting numbers from a database based on an ingredient list. Recipe calculation also calls for understanding how ingredients will react and the nutritional implications of various cooking techniques.

Even though nutrient calculations involve specific measurements and deliver precise-looking data, the numbers are approximate at best. Many factors – including seasonal variations, soil conditions, animal diet, storage conditions, cooking methods and variety of product used – affect the nutrient content of ingredients and the final product. Many restaurants hire registered dietitians with culinary nutrition expertise and experience to calculate nutrient data accurately.

Sometimes, to meet a nutritional goal, the amount of fat, salt or sugar used in a recipe must be adjusted or a pan size must be changed to yield more cuts and thus smaller portions. Sometimes a cooking method must be revised. With any change, a recipe must be retested and recalculated.

Analysis versus Calculation

True *nutrient analysis* refers to an assay of select nutrients done by laboratory analysis using incinerated ash or chemical extraction to determine the actual content of various components. Newer techniques are used for the extraction of bioactive chemicals. Each analytical laboratory has specific procedures for sample management and collection as well as procedures for quality assurance and control. The procedures usually include collecting samples from different batches and obtaining values of the blended samples.

True nutrient analysis is typically used when precise data are essential; when the analysis will be entered into databases to be widely used; when nutrition claims will be made; when there are gaps in nutrient data; or when it is impossible to obtain data by calculation. While the advantage of this method is accuracy, the disadvantages are expense, collecting the appropriate number and type of samples, and the time needed to perform laboratory analyses. Although a nutrient analysis will report exactly what is in the sample(s) provided, because of seasonal variations and variations in cooking techniques from sample to sample, even with excellent quality control, the resulting data are still, at best, estimates, although they are far more accurate than calculated values.

Most foodservice operators will use computerized databases for estimating the nutrient content of foods. This procedure is commonly called *nutrient calculation*. Some practitioners refer to the process as nutritional analysis by calculation or nutrient analysis by database. Many nutrient databases are available. Nutrient calculation software offers the advantages of ease, speed and reduced cost, but is less accurate than true nutrient analysis. Certain additional skills, including culinary expertise, are necessary to ensure optimal results. Operators should keep files of all nutrient calculations - the source of the data, the person calculating, and the date of the calculation. When recipes are modified they need to be recalculated.

Only a few studies have compared the calculated and analytic nutrient values for foods. Differences between calculated and actual analytic results may reflect the effects of different types of cooking equipment, surface area of food contact exposure, length and temperature of cooking, and the volume of the product.

Nutrient Databases

Interpreting base nutrient data supplied by the U.S. Department of Agriculture (USDA) National Nutrient Database for Standard Reference, original research, nutrient calculation software, or commodity boards and manufacturers presents a number of challenges. USDA's extensive database is available at www.nal. usda.gov/fnic/foodcomp/search/ and is free to all. Many of the existing data, however, were determined when analytical methods were less precise. Years ago, for example, there was no analysis for trans fat, bioactive substances, phytochemicals, specific types of fiber and other substances of concern today. Consequently, there are gaps in most databases.

Despite the many claims that organic, heirloom or artisanally grown products provide higher or different values of certain nutrients than do conventional varieties, most nutrient databases do not reflect differences that may exist. Much research on the antioxidant and phytochemical content of organic foods is underway. Nutrient data for ethnic and imported ingredients are becoming available as these foods grow in popularity and become subject to nutritional labeling. Information on nutrient composition, however, may be limited to only the specific nutrients required on the label.

Accurate nutrient calculations require far more skill than selecting the right data based on the recipe ingredient list. For many ingredients, there are numerous item numbers from which to choose, reflecting differences in form or variety. Choosing the correct item number is essential to accuracy.

One common error made when calculating nutrient data is ignoring a blank space in a database or substituting a zero for a blank. A blank space means that reliable data has not been collected. A zero indicates that the food item contains none of that nutrient or substance. It may be necessary to contact the manufacturer, grower or commodity board; check labels of currently available products or other databases; or use experience and professional judgment to estimate the missing value from a comparable product. While databases are useful tools, dietetics professionals often must dig deeper for complete and accurate information for nutrient calculation.

Standardization

The first step in calculating nutrient data is standardizing the recipe. It is important to be specific both with ingredients and amounts. For example, the ingredient "chicken" should specify with or without skin and bones, white or dark meat, and cooking method. If a recipe calls for 1 cup of fresh spinach, the calculator must know or decide if it is raw whole-leaf spinach with or without stems, baby spinach or mature leaves. When using a database and determining which item to select that most closely resembles a certain ingredient, calculators must look for key terms in the definition of the item. They also may weigh the ingredient and compare it to the weight or volume of a similar ingredient in the database. Experienced nutrient calculators maintain files detailing the weights of many foods in various forms so that they know, for example, how many grams of a vegetable in various cuts equal a cup or other measure of volume. A very common error is to confuse weights and measures. One cup of a food by measure can weigh as little as 2 ounces or as much as 10 ounces by weight. Recipes often mix weights and measures.

Seasonings, especially high-sodium ingredients such as salt, should be listed by amount, not "to taste" or "as needed." Saying "salt to taste" gives the calculator no information to determine sodium content. (Omission of seasoning in a calculation creates a false impression; however, it is acceptable to note that salt may be omitted to reduce the sodium content of the recipe.)

The calculator may want to prepare the recipe or observe its being prepared to clarify exact ingredients and amounts. Chefs may add oil and seasonings to food (and to flat grills) during cooking and then make final flavoring and seasoning adjustments. As a result, they often have no idea how much oil or salt they actually use. In this case, it may be necessary to put generous premeasured weighed amounts of oil and salt on the mis-en-place tray, watch the chef prepare the food, and then measure the amount of oil and salt left after the dish is prepared. For calculation purposes, the difference between "before" and "after" is the amount actually used in the recipe. In addition to the amount of salt used, it is also important to clarify the type of salt. Kosher salt may have less sodium per teaspoon than regular table salt.

Cooking Method

It is important to remember that items in an ingredient list may not be the same in the finished product, and it is the finished product that must be calculated. A thorough understanding of food preparation and cooking methods is often necessary, especially when not all ingredients in a recipe will be consumed. For example, when a chicken breast is marinated prior to grilling and the unabsorbed marinade is discarded, only the absorbed marinade is calculated. A larger surface area will absorb more marinade (chicken tenders versus chicken breast), as will a product that is more porous (mushrooms versus red peppers). If the food is cooked on a grill, some marinade will burn off. In addition, sodium in the marinade will extract liquid from the product being marinated.

A nutrient calculation for stock made with beef bones and mirepoix (a combination of carrots, celery and onion) that is later discarded must account for nutrients that have been infused into the stock (with less sodium). In this situation, the calculation can substitute a laboratory-analyzed value of the most similar product, perhaps a canned stock. Special consideration is also needed in calculating the nutrients in pureed and strained fruits and vegetables. For example, strained sauces must be adjusted for fiber and other nutrient losses. A registered dietitian with culinary expertise might estimate a percentage of loss or estimate remaining fiber based on values of other strained sauces. Examples such as these illustrate that a high level of culinary expertise is necessary to make adjustments for food preparation and cooking methods when calculating the nutrient content of a recipe.

Sub-Recipes

Determining the per portion nutrient contribution of sub-recipes is usually a more complex task than calculating the value of one recipe with several components that are plated and served together as one dish. This step in the nutrient calculation process can also require culinary expertise beyond what packaged software offers.

Some recipes have several sub-recipes. For example, many fine restaurants serve a main item on a bed of something, surrounded by a small amount of one or more sauces and topped with an edible garnish. The dish as served may use varying amounts of each sub-recipe. Consequently, a sauce sub-recipe may make 16 servings of 1 tablespoon each, while the bed of vegetables or salad sub-recipe makes enough for 8 servings. In this case, it is necessary to determine the single-serving portions of each sub-recipe and then total the values for 1 serving of the main dish fully plated. A photo of the plated food can be used to confirm the amount of sauce served per portion and is always provided with the standardized recipe. (Mary Abbott Hess used this process when calculating recipes for Charlie Trotter's *One & Only Palmilla Spa Cuisine*.)

Yield

Yield is used to calculate per portion nutrient content. A very large volume of ingredients that yields only 4 or 6 servings or a low volume of ingredients that is meant to serve many will raise a red flag to an experienced calculator. This situation often requires that the full recipe be prepared, the yield weighed and measured, and the number of portions reevaluated. Yields may be determined by:

- Preparing the recipe, then measuring volumes and determining the number of servings

- Using the yield given by the standardized recipe

- Adding the volumes of the served ingredients in prepared form (if there are multiple ingredient components)

- Measuring container size (e.g., 1 gallon) that holds finished product

Yield is best determined by an actual weight or measure of the finished product. Results can be inaccurate when weights and/or volumes of raw ingredients are used to determine yield. Combinations of ingredients and cooking methods significantly alter yield volume. For example, when reducing a sauce or baking a cake, moisture is lost, thus reducing final yield weight and increasing nutrients per portion.

If the recipe calls for a specific weight of raw meat to be added and cooked, and data exist for the nutrient content of cooked meat, one must apply a yield factor to the amount of raw meat needed in order to determine the amount of cooked meat that will result, and then calculate the nutrient content of that amount. Understanding cooking method is also necessary for determining nutrient values. For example, a sauteed entree is usually served in a sauce made from the drippings remaining in the pan. Sometimes rendered fat will be poured off before the pan is deglazed, and a sauce will be prepared by reducing added liquid (stock, wine or juice) and seasonings. The amount of fat removed must be subtracted from the calculation. The reduced liquid will lower volume but not calories. Some of the calories from alcohol, however, such as a wine or brandy used to deglaze a pan, may burn off during cooking, depending on cooking time and total volume of liquid. These losses must be estimated and subtracted.

Basic Rules for the Yield Factor Method

- Use the form and portion of the food as served.

- Select raw if not heated or cooked.

- Select cooked if cooked before serving, using the database food code for the cooked ingredient.

- Convert or adjust the amount of the raw ingredient in the recipe by using a yield factor.

Where to Get Help

Foodservice operators, especially those who are required to provide calorie and nutrient information for the first time, may need assistance to generate accurate, defensible data. Many operators will want to work with a registered dietitian (RD) with culinary expertise. Your local or state dietetic association, the Food & Culinary Professionals Dietetic Practice Group (www.foodculinaryporf.org) or The Academy of Nutrition and Dietetics (www.eatright.org) can help find someone to assist you in determining the nutritional composition of existing menu offerings and perhaps modifying offerings to enhance the healthfulness of the total menu. Onsite help, perhaps with observation to clarify techniques and standardize recipes, may be warranted.

There are also services that employ individuals experienced in calculating nutrient values. This approach works only if recipes are standardized and requires substantial communication to clarify techniques, volumes and yield for proper calculation. For difficult-to-calculate items or when accuracy is essential, the best option is nutritional analysis not calculated values.

Presenting Nutrient Data

Given the ease and power of computerized nutrient calculation, resulting data are often carried out to several decimal points. The specificity of these numbers creates a false sense of accuracy and confidence in the numbers. All nutrient calculations are estimates; numbers calculated for recipes should be rounded according to the Food and Drug Administration's (FDA) rounding rules for product labels. In addition, nutrient calculation information should always include a statement that the values are an estimate based on calculations from whatever databases were used along with the professional judgment of the person who performed the calculation.

The following table summarizes FDA's rounding rules.

Guidance for Industry: Food Labeling

Nutrient	Increment Rounding	Insignificant Amount
Calories **Calories from fat** **Calories from saturated fat**	< 5 calories - list as 0 ≤ 50 calories - round to nearest 5-calorie increment > 50 calories - round to nearest 10-calorie increment	< 5 calories
Total fat **Saturated fat** **Trans fat** **Polyunsaturated fat** **Monounsaturated fat**	< .5 grams - list as 0 < 5 grams - round to nearest .5-gram increment ≥ 5 grams - round to nearest 1-gram increment	< .5 gram
Cholesterol	< 2 milligrams - list as 0 2-5 milligrams - report as "less than 5 milligrams" > 5 milligrams - round to nearest 5-milligram increment	< 2 milligrams
Sodium **Potassium**	< 5 milligrams - list as 0 5-140 milligrams - round to nearest 5-milligram increment > 140 milligrams - round to nearest 10-milligram increment	< 5 milligrams
Total carbohydrate **Dietary fiber**	< .5 grams - list as 0 0 < 1 gram - report as "contains less than 1 gram" or "less than 1 gram" ≥ 1gram - round to nearest 1-gram increment	< 1 gram
Soluble and insoluble fiber sugars **Sugar alcohol** **Other carbohydrate**	< .5 gram - list as 0 < 1gram - report as "contains less than 1 gram" or "less than 1 gram" ≥ 1gram - round to nearest 1-gram increment	< .5 gram

Nutrient	Increment Rounding	Insignificant Amount
Protein	< .5 gram - list as 0 < 1 gram - report as "contains less than 1 gram" or "less than 1 gram" or report as 1gram if .5 gram to < 1 gram ≥ 1gram - round to nearest 1-gram increment	< 1 gram
Nutrients other than vitamins and minerals that have RDIs as a % DV	Round to nearest 1% DV increment	< 1% DV

Vitamins and minerals (% DV)	< 2% of RDI may be listed as:
	  a) 0
	  b) 2% DV if actual amount is 1% or more
	  c) an asterisk that refers to statement "Contains less than 2% of the Daily Value of this (these) nutrient(s)"
	  d) for Vit A, C, calcium, iron: statement "Not a significant source of _____ (listing the vitamins and minerals omitted)"
	≤ 10% of RDI - round to nearest 2% DV increment
	> 10% - 50% of RDI - round to nearest 5% DV increment
	> 50% of RDI - round to nearest 10% DV increment
		< 2% RDI

Beta-Carotene (% DV)	≤ 10% of RDI for vitamin A - round to nearest 2% DV increment > 10%-50% of RDI for vitamin A - round to nearest 5% DV increment > 50% of RDI for vitamin A - round to nearest 10% DV increment	

Note: *To list nutrient values to the nearest 1-gram increment, for amounts falling exactly halfway between two whole numbers or higher (e.g., 2.5 grams to 2.99 grams), round up (e.g., 3 grams). For amounts less than halfway between two whole numbers (e.g, 2.01 grams to 2.49 grams), round down (e.g., 2 grams).*

When rounding % DV for nutrients other than vitamins and minerals, when the % DV values fall exactly halfway between two whole numbers or higher (e.g., 2.5 to 2.99), the values round up (e.g., 3 %). For values less than halfway between two whole numbers (e.g., 2.01 to 2.49), the values round down (e.g., 2%).

Adapted from: www.fda.gov/Food/GuidanceComplianceRegulatoryInformation/GuidanceDocuments/FoodLabelingNutrition/FoodLabelingGuide/ucm064932.htm

Round and Round and Round

The nutrient calculation report indicates that a recipe contains 277.62 calories, 464.49 milligrams of sodium, 39.221 grams of protein and 5.811 grams of fat per serving. The specificity of these numbers suggests a high degree of accuracy. To avoid the impression of unwarranted accuracy and to make nutrition labeling easier for customers to read and understand, foodservice operators should follow FDA's rounding rules. The above values should be listed as 280 calories, 460 milligrams of sodium, 39 grams of protein and 6 grams of fat.

Opportunities for Chefs

Nutrition is big business. Providing healthful choices to your guests can increase your bottom line and guest loyalty. How you communicate your nutrition message to guests can influence how healthful items are purchased, promoted and positioned. Additionally, federal regulations and laws mandate that the foodservice industry provide nutrition information. Calculating nutrient data is a challenging task for foodservice operators. Consulting a registered dietitian with culinary expertise can help ensure accuracy of nutrient data.

Learning Activities

1. Using a nutrient calculation program, calculate the nutrient content of three recipes.
2. Identify a health-related cause and develop an action plan for supporting it and getting visibility for your establishment's participation.
3. Investigate the nutrient content of three chain restaurant concepts. (This information is commonly available on the company website.) What percentage of items have more than 500 calories per portion? Which items would you identify as healthful?

For More Information

- National Nutrient Database for Standard Reference. Available at http://ndb.nal.usda.gov/. Accessed August 4, 2012.

- National Restaurant Association. Q&A: New Federal Nutrition-Disclosure Rules for Certain Restaurants, April 7, 2010. Available at http://restaurant.org/pdfs/advocacy/menulabeling_faq.pdf. Accessed August 4, 2012.

- Peregrin T, Next on the Menu: Labeling Law Could Mean Career Opportunities for RDs. *J Am Diet Assoc.* 2010:110(8):1144-1147.

- Powers C, Hess MA, Kimbrough M. How accurate are your nutrient calculations? Why culinary expertise makes a difference. *J Am Diet Assoc.* 2008;108(9):1418-22.

- Stein, K. A National Approach to Restaurant Menu Labeling: The Patient Protection and Affordable Health Care Act, Section 4205. *J Academy of Nutrition and Dietetics.* 2011; 111(5):S19-S27.

- Taylor CL, Wilkening VL. How the nutrition food label was developed. Part 1: The nutrition facts panel. *J Am Diet Assoc.* 2008;108(3):437-442.

- Taylor CL, Wilkening VL. How the nutrition food label was developed. Part 2: The purpose and promise of nutritional claims. *J Am Diet Assoc.* 2008;108(4):618-23.

- U. S. Food and Drug Administration. Claims That Can Be Made for Conventional Foods and Dietary Supplements. September 2003. Available at www.fda.gov/Food/LabelingNutrition/LabelClaims/ucm111447.htm. Accessed August 4, 2012.

- U.S. Food and Drug Administration. Food Labeling Guide. Available at www.fda.gov/Food/GuidanceComplianceRegulatoryInformation/GuidanceDocuments/FoodLabelingNutrition/FoodLabelingGuide/default.htm. Accessed August 4, 2012.

Free Nutrient Calculation Software

- USDA MyPlate SuperTracker, www.choosemyplate.gov/SuperTracker/default.aspx

- USDA National Nutrient Database for Standard Reference, www.nal.usda.gov/fnic/foodcomp/search

- FoodCount.com

- Nutrition Analysis Tool (NAT), Food Science and Human Nutrition Department, University of Illinois, http://nat.illinois.edu

- CondéNet, www.nutritiondata.com

- Papaya Head, www.papayahead.com

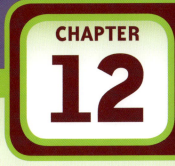

Food For Healthy Living

LEARNING OBJECTIVES

After completing this chapter, you should be able to:

- Plan menus that are appropriate and nutrient rich for children and adolescents
- Identify issues specific to menu planning for aging adults
- Explain meal planning for athletes
- Discuss nutritional menu planning for weight management
- Plan healthful menus for vegetarians and vegans
- Describe dietary practices, restrictions and rationale for eating behaviors of people of the world's major religions
- Describe basic requirements for kosher meal preparation
- List foods permitted and foods to be avoided for halal meals

Everybody eats – but not everybody has the same needs and expectations when it comes to the foods they choose. Age, lifestyle, weight concerns and religion/culture affect how people incorporate food into their daily lives. In this chapter, experts from around the country – our Essentials Experts – have contributed their knowledge and practical advice about serving children, aging adults, athletes, vegetarians, dieters and patrons with strong religious/cultural food traditions. A boost in flavor here and a portion adjustment there may be all it takes to appeal to some guests. Others, however, have more complicated requirements and strict rules dictating what they can and cannot eat. Knowing the special needs of patrons is step one. Learning to meet those needs is what sets the successful chef apart from others.

Meeting the Needs of Children

ESSENTIALS EXPERT

Catharine Powers, MS, RD, LD, co-author of this book, has worked with school nutrition programs around the country and was project manager for the National Food Service Management Institute's award winning Cooks for Kids *video program and* Culinary Techniques for Healthy School Meals *training program.*

Whether served at home, in a restaurant or at school, children's food should be healthful and their meals well balanced. Too many children don't get enough of the nutritious foods growing minds and bodies need. Some eat only a few foods over and over again. Others eat too many highly processed, high-fat and/or high-sugar foods. While it is primarily the responsibility of parents and caregivers to provide a healthful diet to children, schools also have a role as most children have one and sometimes two meals a day at school. Chefs can play an important role by providing food options that are interesting, nourishing and expand children's food experiences.

Nearly one in three American children is overweight or obese and thus at risk for a lifetime of obesity and serious diseases associated with obesity. And even overfed children can be undernourished. Most American children do not regularly eat enough of the foods that promote optimal health and growth. Ninety-six percent of children ages 2 to 12 fall short of the recommended 2 to 5 cups/day of fruits and vegetables. [1] Only 15% of teens in grades 9 through 12 consume at least 3 servings of vegetables per day. [2] Overall, only 2% of school-aged children consume the recommended daily number of servings from all major food groups. [3]

The *Dietary Guidelines for Americans 2010* identified shortfall nutrients for children as vitamins A, C, D, E, and calcium, magnesium, phosphorus, potassium and dietary fiber. Increasing intakes of vegetables (notably dark-green and orange vegetables), legumes, fruits (particularly whole fruits), whole grains, fluid milk and milk products, meat and beans, and oils will help address these shortfall nutrients. A growing body of evidence links low intakes of essential nutrients, particularly vitamins D, C and E and omega-3 fatty acids, to increased rates of respiratory problems such as coughing and asthma, weak bones, and impaired immunity. [4]

Researchers also have found that the majority of children, especially dark-skinned children, do not get enough vitamin D to build healthy bones. Dark-skinned children are vulnerable because the melanin that makes skin dark blocks ultraviolet rays that the body uses to make vitamin D. Consequently, additional sources of vitamin D, particularly fortified milk, are important for these children and their families as well. [5]

Key Nutrition Points

- Children need to eat every 4 to 6 hours. Make sure both snacks and meals are nutrient-rich.

- At least half of the grain products children eat should be whole grains. Serve whole-grain cereals and breads often and encourage use of whole grains whenever possible. Limit refined grains such as white breads and white rice.

- Children ages 2 to 8 years should drink 2 cups/day of fat-free or low-fat milk or equivalent milk products such as cheese or yogurt. Children age 9 and older should drink 3 cups/day of fat-free or low-fat milk or equivalent dairy products. Use cheese and yogurt in cooking, mixed dishes and salads, and smoothies.

- Total fat intake should be between 30% and 35% of calories for children ages 2 to 3 and between 25% and 35% of calories for children and adolescents ages 4 to 18. Most fats should come from polyunsaturated and monounsaturated fatty acids found in fish, nuts and vegetable oils. Just as for adults, food for children should limit saturated fat and eliminate trans fats.

- Many children don't consume enough dietary fiber. Adding whole fruits, dried fruits, vegetables, legumes, nuts and whole-grain products to the diet increases fiber intake.

- Avoid excessive calories from added sugars. While an occasional soft drink is okay, these beverages are not healthful and may train the brain to seek more sweets. Sweetened foods that provide few nutrients reduce diet quality and contribute to weight gain.

- Lack of iron can affect behavior, mood and attention span. Serve iron-rich foods such as lean meat, enriched cereals and legumes. Ground meats (in meat sauces, chili, meat balls and burgers) are easier for young children to chew. A source of vitamin C, such as red or green peppers or citrus fruit, increases the amount of iron absorbed from enriched grains, eggs and vegetables.

Best Choices

- Use primarily whole foods such as fruits, vegetables, legumes, lean meats, poultry and fish, whole grains, and low-fat milk and dairy products.

- Serve roasted, grilled or poached foods such as baked apples, grilled shrimp and scallops, and roasted potato strips.

- Serve fruits whole or cut to provide more nutrients and fiber. Place apple and orange wedges, a small bunch of grapes, a few cherries, or berries on plates to add color, texture and boost fruit intake.

- When serving juices, choose 100% juice rather than sweetened fruit drinks. Add 2 ounces of juice to 6 ounces water or sparkling water for a refreshing, healthful and lower calorie option.

- Serve vegetables – carrot or jicama sticks, zucchini or summer squash coins, blanched green beans or sugar snap peas, bell peppers, or edamame – as healthful crunchy meal enhancers.

- Provide dips and sauces that are appealing to kids. Allow them to select from several sauces with their meal to encourage eating more fruits and vegetables. Include complementary sauces with menu items.

  - Savory: mild salsa, sweet and sour, barbecue, cheese, hummus, Asian dipping sauces, chutney, fruited vinaigrette, tzatziki (Greek cucumber sauce), ranch dip and peanut butter

  - Sweet: small amounts of caramel, chocolate, fruit purees, chutney

- Include nutrient-dense beverages with each meal, such as low-fat milk or 100% fruit juice. If sweetened beverages are served, make them lightly sweetened.

- Provide healthful side dishes as an option. Include seasonal fruits, vegetables, whole grains and legumes to add variety, color and new taste experiences to meals. Be specific in menu descriptions.

- Serve whole-grain breads, buns, crackers, tortillas, wraps and pitas when possible.

- Make low-fat milk or equivalent dairy products available at meals and with snacks. If white milk or plain yogurt is not popular, try flavored milk or fruited yogurt.

- Use brown rice and other whole grains. Use whole-wheat breadcrumbs for breaded items.

- Serve graham crackers and oatmeal raisin or other cookies with some healthful ingredients.

Foods to Limit

Generally, the foods to limit for children are the same as for adults making healthful choices. Limit portion size by serving kid-sized portions in a small cup, bowl or container.

- Fried foods

- Foods containing trans or saturated fats

- Refined grains, white rice

- Breads, cereals, crackers, pasta and pretzels made from refined flour

- Soft drinks, slushies and other highly sweetened beverages (liquid candy)

- Milkshakes and similar beverages

- Foods with added sugar

- Foods high in sodium

- Processed foods containing artificial colors, flavors and additives

casebycase

Kids Are Customers, Too!

Kids LiveWell, a collaborative initiative between the National Restaurant Association and Healthy Dining Finder, works with restaurants nationwide to develop and promote a selection of healthful menu choices that emphasize lean proteins, fruits, vegetables, whole grains and low-fat dairy products. Launched in July 2011, this first-of-its-kind program grew to include 100 restaurant brands and more than 25,000 locations in just one year – and continues to build momentum. Participants range from Burger King and Arby's to Bonefish Grill and Outback Steakhouse.

Restaurants pay a nominal fee to join the program and commit to offering healthful menu choices for children, with a particular focus on increasing consumption of fruit and vegetables, lean protein, whole grains and low-fat dairy, and limiting unhealthy fats, sugars and sodium. Menu items must meet certain nutrition criteria based on leading health organizations' scientific recommendations, including the *Dietary Guidelines*. Healthy Dining's team of registered dietitians works with participating restaurants to identify and validate menu choices that meet the Kids LiveWell criteria:

- At least one full children's meal (an entrée, side and beverage) that is 600 calories or less; contains 2 or more servings of fruit, vegetables, whole grains, lean protein and/or low-fat dairy; and limits sodium, fats and sugar.

  - ≤ 35% of calories from total fat
  - ≤ 10% of calories from saturated fat
  - < 0.5 grams trans fat (artificial trans fat only)
  - ≤ 35% of calories from total sugars (added and naturally occurring)
  - ≤ 770 mg of sodium

- Offer at least one other individual item that has 200 calories or less, with limits on fats, sugars and sodium, and contains a serving of fruit, vegetables, whole grains, lean protein or low-fat dairy

  - ≤ 35% of calories from total fat
  - ≤ 10% of calories from saturated fat
  - < 0.5 grams trans fat (artificial trans fat only)
  - ≤ 35% of calories from total sugars (added and naturally occurring)
  - ≤ 250 mg of sodium

For a more details on the Kids LiveWell program, visit www.restaurant.org/foodhealthyliving/kidslivewell

Tips for Chefs

Children have more taste buds than adults. As a result, they often dislike very strong-flavored and highly salted foods. This increased sensitivity to flavor along with a biological preference for sweet foods is part of the reason children often have strong food likes and dislikes, repeatedly requesting favorite foods and rejecting others. Children often enjoy brightly colored, mild-flavored foods such as corn. Crisp and chewy foods develop a child's chewing skills.

While parents play the primary role in providing healthful foods for their children, chefs can help by making the foods children should have more available and accessible. Eating away from home also provides opportunities for children to try foods not usually served at home. All segments of the food-service industry need to move beyond the narrowly focused traditional children's menu of breaded chicken tenders, macaroni and cheese, burgers and pizzas. Children need a greater variety of food than what is provided at popular foodservice outlets.

- Offer a variety of food that appeals to different age groups and preferences.

- Serve small bites and hand-held food items.

- Use child-sized utensils and unbreakable plates.

- Minimize choking hazards for young children by avoiding foods that are round and about the size of a nickel such as grapes and cherry tomatoes. Remove pits from fruits and be sure fish is boneless.

- Be aware of common allergens. Peanut butter is popular, but peanuts are a common allergen. (See information on allergens in Chapter 13.)

- Serve foods and use flavors children know. Sweet flavors are most appealing to children. Some children also enjoy salsas and dips with a little heat and spiciness.

- Serve appropriate portions. Make half-size muffins, pancakes, meatballs, etc.

- Use healthful cooking techniques like grilling, baking and steaming, while minimizing fried items. For example, serve grilled chicken or chicken skewers rather than fried chicken fingers.

- Introduce new options in familiar ways – jicama or sugar snap peas with a dip, grilled cheese on whole-wheat bread, mashed butternut squash or an interesting-shaped pasta tossed with roasted vegetables.

- Serve colorful, nutrient-rich foods that add eye appeal – for example, broccoli, red peppers, red and yellow grape tomatoes, and cantaloupe.

- Put produce on every plate, making fruits and vegetables the side dish of choice.

- Add variety to children's menus by offering half portions of foods from the regular menu.

- For sandwiches, offer low-fat deli meat and sliced lean turkey, chicken or pork or reduced-fat cold cuts. Add extra vegetables, such as tomatoes, roasted red peppers or sliced cucumbers.

- Put healthful appetizers from the regular menu on the children's menu to provide interesting options beyond traditional kid-friendly offerings. Many children enjoy a shrimp cocktail or small crab cake as a healthful entree.

A Word from the Chef
Get on the Bandwagon Now

Chef Marvin Woods is an Emmy Award-nominated television host, restaurateur and best-selling author known for his commitment to health-conscious cooking as well as his innovative approach to Low Country cuisine and its North African, South American, Caribbean roots. Marvin believes that food can be prepared healthfully, cost-effectively and conveniently without sacrificing flavor. "Each year, I get better at it," he says. "Through travel and research, I discover and learn about using new ingredients, like seaweeds instead of table salt and agave for sweetening instead of refined sugar. And I have adopted new techniques, like dehydrating ingredients and raw food preparation. Five years ago, I wasn't doing any of these things," Marvin notes. "Now healthy cooking is a part of me. It's a lifestyle.

"We are bombarded daily by the media, corporations, dietitians and doctors about healthful food and healthy lifestyles," Marvin continues. "Some people listen, but most don't because it is usually portrayed negatively and they are sick of hearing about it. We need to get away from defining food as 'healthful.' That word turns people off. Just prepare a recipe from scratch with a minimum amount of good oil and less sodium than you would get in a processed food and you are on your way to good food that is better for you."

Since 2006, Marvin has traveled the country educating and motivating children and parents with his own program, "Droppin' Knowledge with Chef Marvin Woods," which focuses on reducing childhood obesity and other child and adult health issues. He also has been involved with First Lady Michelle Obama's Let's Move campaign for children and families.

Marvin is currently redefining the concept of healthy food and challenging what is now considered American cuisine. His next restaurant, Covet, will embody what he believes to be his culinary evolution. "This is just the beginning," Marvin predicts. "In the next five years, all menus are going to look a lot different. Chefs need to get on the bandwagon now."

For More Information

- Action for Healthy Kids, www.actionforhealthykids.org
- American Institute of Wine & Food, Days of Taste, www.aiwf.org/site/days-of-taste.html
- American Culinary Federation, Chef and the Child Foundation, www.acfchefs.org
- Healthy Kids Choice, Inc., www.healthykidschoice.org
- Let's Move, www.letsmove.gov
- National Food Service Management Institute, www.NFSMI.org
- Nutrition Explorations, Kids' Nutrition at its Best, National Dairy Council. www.nutritionexplorations.org
- School Nutrition Association, www.schoolnutrition.org
- U.S. Department of Agriculture, Food and Nutrition Services, Child Nutrition Programs, School Meals, www.fns.usda.gov/cnd
- U.S. Department of Agriculture, Food and Nutrition Services, Team Nutrition, www.teamnutrition.usda.gov/Default.htm

Meeting the Needs of Aging Adults

ESSENTIALS EXPERTS

Becky Dorner, RD, LD, is one of the nation's leading experts on nutrition, long-term healthcare and healthcare communities. She has more than 25 years' experience as a speaker, consultant and author. Becky Dorner & Associates, Inc., publishes and presents continuing education programs and information on nutrition care for older adults. Her other company, Nutrition Consulting Services, Inc., which employs registered dietitians and dietetic technicians, registered, has provided services to healthcare facilities in Ohio since 1983.

Joseph M. Carlin, MS, MA, RD, LND, FADA, has spent almost 40 years of his professional career as a public health nutritionist with the Administration for Community Living specializing in nutritional gerontology. In addition, he is a recognized food historian, cooking school instructor and award-winning photographer.

Chefs feed aging adults everywhere, not only in restaurants and in healthcare communities such as skilled nursing facilities, assisted living facilities, and retirement and senior communities, but also on cruise ships and in resorts and fast-food outlets. Chefs also play a critical role in providing the 250 million meals served yearly at senior centers and to Meals on Wheels recipients in their homes. As the population ages, these opportunities will increase. In 2010, there were 40.2 million Americans age 65 or older and 6.1 million over age 85. By 2030, there will be twice as many older Americans (more than 72 million) as there were in 2000, and at least 70% of people over age 65 will require long-term healthcare services at some point in their lives. [6]

Many older people are environmentally savvy and put a high priority on farm fresh and locally grown foods from sustainable sources. Today's seniors are more highly educated and share many of the same values about food as those half their age. They are well read, keep up with the literature on what is good to eat and make critical purchasing decisions based on how food will improve their health, wellbeing and longevity. The Canyon Ranch philosophy of food is an excellent model for healthy eating for most older Americans.

Joseph Carlin, MS, MA, RD, LND, FADA
Administration for Community Living

Key Nutrition Points

- The nutrition concerns of aging adults are often driven by the onset of chronic diseases and the inability to participate in the normal activities of daily living.

- More than 80% of people age 65 or older have one or more chronic conditions that are affected by nutrition and/or food choices. As they age, Americans are likely to be concerned about sodium, cholesterol, fiber, trans fats and concentrated sweets.

- Diabetes is common in older adults (about 25% of all nursing home residents have diabetes) and requires some dietary modifications.

- Older adults need more nutrient-dense foods to meet nutritional requirements in fewer calories. In each decade after reaching adulthood, the body requires fewer calories to maintain a healthy weight. Some people with chronic diseases and conditions, however, may require additional calories, protein or other nutrients. For example, those who have pressure ulcers (commonly known as bed sores) may need up to 50% more calories and protein than those who do not.

- Many older adults are on therapeutic diets, but liberal diets are recommended for those who live in long-term care facilities. Promoting enjoyment of food and enhancing quality of life are important goals. Overly restrictive diets may reduce food intake and cause unintended weight loss, which can have devastating health effects. Some long-term facilities now offer a glass of wine or beer with the dinner meal.

For More Information

- Becky Dorner & Associates, free information and resources, publications, menus and recipes, and continuing education programs, www.beckydorner.com

- Centers for Medicare & Medicaid Services (CMS), www.cms.gov

- State health departments for regulations on nursing homes and assisted living facilities (including food safety, sanitation and nutrition)

- Carlin, JM. Older Americans. *Dietitian's Pocket Guide to Nutrition.* Herbold N, Edelstein S, eds. Sudbury, MA: Jones and Bartlett Publishers; 2010.

- Dorner B. *Policy & Procedure Manual: Food and Nutrition Guidelines for Health Care.* Akron, OH: Becky Dorner & Associates, Inc; 2013.

- Dorner, B. *Diet Manual: A Comprehensive Nutrition Care Guide.* Akron, OH: Becky Dorner & Associates, Inc; 2011.

- Hume S. Never too old to rock n' roll: Baby boomers still wield enormous influence on food-service's future. *Restaurants & Institutions.* December 2007;117(18):16-17.

- Position of the Academy of Nutrition and Dietetics: Food and Nutrition for Older Adults: Promoting Health and Wellness. http://www.eatright.org/About/Content.aspx?id=8374.

- Position of the Academy of Nutrition and Dietetics: Individualized Nutrition Approaches for Older Adults in Health Care Communities. http://www.eatright.org/About/Content.aspx?id=837&terms=position+paper+older+adult

Meeting the Needs of Athletes

ESSENTIALS EXPERTS

Jacqueline R. Berning, PhD, RD, CSSD, is associate professor and chair of the Biology Department at the University of Colorado at Colorado Springs. Jacqueline is board certified as a specialist in sports dietetics. She is sports dietitian for the Cleveland Indians and Colorado Rockies.

Nancy Clark, MS, RD, CSSD, counsels both competitive athletes and casual exercisers. Her successful private practice is located in Newton, Massachusetts. Nancy is an internationally known sports nutritionist and is board certified as a specialist in sports dietetics. She focuses on nutrition for exercise, wellness and the management of eating disorders. Her clients have run the gamut from Olympians and members of the Boston Red Sox, Bruins and Celtics, to high school and college athletes, to "ordinary mortals," fitness exercisers and weekend warriors. She is the author of Nancy Clark's Sports Nutrition Guidebook. *Her nutrition advice and photo have even been on the back of the Wheaties box!*

Whether feeding the casual exerciser or the professional athlete, there are some important points to keep in mind. Depending on the intensity and frequency as well as the type of activity, an athlete may require 3,000 to 6,000 calories per day. The optimal number of calories also depends on age, body composition and environmental conditions. High-calorie, healthful foods are best for football and ice hockey players and for active high school boys who need to maintain or increase their weight and muscle mass. In contrast, gymnasts, figure skaters, lightweight rowers and dancers must remain slim, so they seek healthful, low-calorie but high-satiety foods.

For people who exercise intensely for 90 minutes or more per day, refueling during exercise can be beneficial. Marathon runners, elite athletes and recreational sports participants who practice and train on a regular basis should pay extra attention to replenishing fluid and nutrient losses to maintain optimal blood sugar levels and maximize performance.

Key Nutrition Points

- All types of athletes should start every day with breakfast.

- Athletes need to eat evenly sized meals across the day for sustained energy.

- Hydration is critical. Athletes must drink plenty of beverages daily. It is recommended that athletes drink .6 ounces of fluid per pound of body weight per day. For example, a 150-pound person should drink 90 ounces of fluids (.6 x 150) daily. While weight-conscious athletes will want calorie-free beverages, athletes trying to maintain or gain weight will want juice, flavored low-fat milk, smoothies and shakes.

- Serve a lean protein source at each meal.

- Serve foods rich in fiber. Athletes need approximately 25 to 35 grams of fiber per day.

- Pre-game (pre-competition) meals should consist of foods that offer easily digested carbohydrates and lean proteins, such as pasta with tomato sauce and grilled chicken. Athletes should eat about 3 or 4 hours before competition to allow time for food to clear the stomach before the event. During the hour before the event, some athletes might want another light meal, for example yogurt with fruit; oatmeal or granola with low-fat milk; a banana and peanut butter; or a smoothie made with low-fat yogurt, fruit and wheat germ. Avoid high-fat protein foods such as cheeseburgers or fried chicken. Offer plenty of beverages.

- Carbohydrates from food (used to maintain blood sugar or stored as glycogen in the muscles) and fat are the primary fuel sources for exercise. For most athletes, 55% to 65% of calories should come from carbohydrates. Thirty percent or less of calories should come from fat. Protein needs are 1.2 to 1.7 grams of protein per kilogram of body weight, depending on the type of athletic activity.

- The goal of a post-competition or post-workout meal is to replenish nutrients lost during exercise. Replacing lost fluid is an essential part of recovering. Good choices include water, juices, and high-water-content fruit such as watermelon, grapes and oranges. Replenishing muscle glycogen stores is accomplished by eating carbohydrate-rich foods within an hour after the workout has ended. Athletes should aim for 1 gram of carbohydrate for every 2 pounds of body weight per hour, taken at 30-minute intervals over 4 to 5 hours. Replacing the sodium, potassium and electrolytes lost through sweating is easy enough to do with food. Supplements are generally not recommended. Recovery foods high in essential electrolytes include potatoes, yogurt, orange juice, bananas and soup.

- The goal of recovery nutrition is to convert the body from a **catabolic state** (breakdown of muscle cells) to an **anabolic state** (building up of muscle cells). Immediately after exercise, the window is open for rapid nutrient delivery to muscle cells. Recovery is a three-step process – a meal or snack immediately after training, a meal approximately 1 hour later, and then frequent snacking on wholesome foods. Meals for recovery should contain carbohydrates (45 to 75 grams) and lean protein (15 to 25 grams). Ideas for a snack immediately after exercise include chocolate milk, fruit smoothie made with a yogurt base, trail mix or sandwiches. The recovery process is not complete until the athlete eats a meal within 30 minutes after training.

Weight Management

ESSENTIALS EXPERTS

Cheryl Forberg, RD, is a James Beard award-winning chef, a New York Times *bestselling author and the nutritionist for NBC's "The Biggest Loser," where her role is to help overweight contestants transform their bodies, health and ultimately, their lives. As a culinary expert and registered dietitian, she has shared cooking and nutrition tips with the contestants for eight seasons.*

Marilyn Majchrzak, MS, RD, is the corporate menu development manager at Canyon Ranch in Tucson, Arizona. She has been at Canyon Ranch since 1990 and is responsible for coordinating menu development with the chefs for all Canyon Ranch properties and projects.

Over the last 20 years, the problems of overweight and obesity in the United States have grown to epidemic proportions. Two-thirds of Americans are overweight or obese. The latest data from the National Center for Health Statistics show that 35% of U.S. adults age 20 and older – more than 60 million people – are obese. [9] Most Americans are either trying to lose weight (55%) or maintain their weight (22%) while 3% are trying to gain weight. [10] James O. Hill, MD, PhD, director of the Center for Human Nutrition at the University of Colorado Health Sciences Center and founder of the National Weight Control Registry, has found that the average American adult gains weight gradually – 1 to 2 pounds each year. This gain reflects eating about 100 calories more each day than needed to maintain weight. That means that all most adults need to do to prevent gaining weight is eat 100 fewer calories each day or exercise enough to burn 100 calories. [11] The solution might be as simple as lightening up a favorite coffee drink with nonfat milk, reducing the fat used in sauce preparation, trimming fat from meat, baking crispy foods instead of frying, or skipping soft drinks and switching to sparkling or plain water or low-fat milk. Another useful strategy is to simply reduce portion sizes.

The World Health Organization considers obesity to be one of the top 10 causes of preventable death worldwide. [12] Overweight or obese individuals are at a higher risk for coronary heart disease, stroke, type 2 diabetes, certain types of cancers, hypertension (high blood pressure), sleep apnea and respiratory problems, osteoarthritis, and other health problems.

When it comes to weight loss, there's no lack of diets promising fast results. But fad diets, which often eliminate foods or food groups that provide essential nutrients, can be unhealthy and tend to fail in the long run. Weight loss programs that promote fasting and special cookies or soups may result in quick weight loss, but they cannot be sustained. The key to achieving and maintaining a healthy weight isn't about short-term dietary changes. It's about a lifestyle that includes healthy eating and regular physical activity to achieve a healthy weight and then maintain energy balance. Ensuring that the number of calories consumed is about equal to the number of calories the body uses for maintenance and activity will maintain that healthy weight.

Because genetics, amount of muscle mass, age and other factors influence a person's metabolic rate, different people need different levels of calories to lose, gain or maintain weight. Many Americans are fairly sedentary and do not exercise regularly, so their calorie needs are quite low. If they are not mindful of what they eat, they will gain weight. If they continue their same eating and exercise patterns as their metabolic rate decreases, they will gain weight.

Healthy weight management is about small steps that add up. Little changes in eating and activity level have a more positive impact on health than drastic changes, if for no other reason than it is easier to stick with smaller changes over time. Extreme diets, diets requiring purchasing "special" foods or products, and fast and intensive exercise regimens may work well at first, but their effectiveness rarely lasts.

The American public has long been obsessed with weight-loss programs and diet books. Plans come and go, but the truth is that any program or combination of plans that results in fewer calories consumed than needed to maintain weight will result in weight loss. Lack of exercise in conjunction with a low-calorie diet will cause the loss of both fat and muscle. People claim success on diets high in carbs, low in carbs, high in fat, low in fat, liquid diets, raw diets, home-delivered foods, frozen entrees and on and on. Most diets ultimately fail, however, because the dieter returns to his or her former eating habits and the lost weight returns, often plus more. The only weight-loss diets that seem to work in the long run are those that focus on portion size, include all food groups, reduce empty-calorie foods, increase nutrient-rich foods and incorporate healthy eating habits that can be sustained. WeightWatchers® is an example of such a program. It includes lifestyle changes that increase its success for long-term weight control.

Increasing physical activity and addressing behavioral and psychological issues that lead to emotional overeating are also important to long-term weight loss and maintaining desirable weight. People who lose weight and keep if off successfully usually exercise daily and are physically active.

Body Mass Index

Body mass index (BMI) is a useful measure of overweight and obesity and is calculated from height and weight. It is an estimate of body fat and a good gauge of risk for diseases that can occur with more body fat. The higher your BMI, the higher the risk for certain diseases such as heart disease, high blood pressure, type 2 diabetes, breathing problems, and certain cancers. (See Appendix E for a BMI table.)

BMI Categories	BMI
Underweight	Below 18.5
Normal	18.5–24.9
Overweight	25.0–29.9
Obesity	30.0 and Above

Do the Math

Managing a healthy weight can be a challenge, and the causes of obesity are complex, but the body's energy balance is straightforward. Maintaining weight is a matter of balancing calories consumed (from food and beverages) with calories expended (through exercise and maintaining body functions). Consuming more calories than the body needs results in weight gain in the form of stored energy or body fat. Consuming fewer calories than the body needs results in weight loss because the body will take energy from stored fat.

A pound of body fat is about 3,500 calories of stored energy. In other words, eating 3,500 more calories than the body needs results in the body's storing a pound of fat. Losing a pound of body fat entails eating 3,500 calories less than the body needs. Most successful weight loss is achieved at a rate of 1 to 2 pounds per week. Losing 1 pound of fat per week means eating 500 calories less than the body needs each day (3,500 calories divided by 7 days = 500 calories per day). An adult who needs 2,500 calories per day to maintain his or her weight would eat 2,000 calories per day (2,500 calories - 500 calories = 2,000 calories) and lose about a pound a week.

It is generally recommended that daily calorie intake not dip below 1,500 to 1,800 calories. When people consume too few calories, it is a challenge to get the vitamins, minerals, fiber and protein the body needs each day. And it is difficult to sustain a low-calorie diet when hunger sets in because of severe dietary restriction. The body will adapt to fewer calories and try to maintain itself to protect from starvation. The result can be that even calories are needed to maintain weight.

Canyon Ranch Nutrition Basics

For the past 30 years, nutrition has been an exciting and integral part of the food and culinary program at the legendary Canyon Ranch. "We don't believe in dieting or in 'watching what we eat,' " explains Marilyn Majchrzak, MS, RD, corporate menu development manager at Canyon Ranch in Tucson, Arizona. "It's all about adopting a healthy weight philosophy – a lifelong strategy that involves understanding your own personal needs for food and being physically active enough so that weight management becomes achievable, sustainable and permanent," she says. "We believe in balance, moderation and savoring all the pleasures of eating well. We believe in food that nourishes the body and soul."

Canyon Ranch's corporate chef Scott Uehlein, who trained at the Culinary Institute of America, concurs. "Healthful cooking is real world cooking," he says. "Extreme diets are unsustainable – for chefs and customers. We stick to our basic philosophy: balance."

Canyon Ranch chefs work with a staff of nutritionists to ensure that every meal that comes out of the kitchen meets an exacting set of nutritional standards. "We start with fresh, clean and wholesome foods," says Marilyn. "At Canyon Ranch, fresh means foods that are local and regional, seasonal, and from sustainable sources. We define clean foods as free from pesticides and herbicide residues, hormones and antibiotics, unnecessary additives and preservatives, contaminants, and food-borne pathogens. Wholesomeness," she continues, "captures that old-fashioned sense of goodness. All really fresh food that's been cleanly grown and handled is wholesome. Eating it is an excellent way to support your health, manage your weight and live healthier longer."

"Guests at our resorts can 'self-monitor' their food intake," Scott explains. "At all our destination resorts, we have a comprehensive list of all the ingredients in everything we serve. People with special dietary needs can see exactly what they are eating."

Key Nutrition Points

Here are some key nutrition points from Canyon Ranch's Marilyn Majchrzak.

- Downsize protein portions and upsize nutrient-dense carbohydrates like vegetables, fruits and whole grains.

- Use a wide variety of plant ingredients. Vegetables, fruits, whole grains, beans, nuts and seeds, and herbs and spices are not only delicious and satisfying but also have the most power to prevent disease.

- Emphasize fiber from a wide variety of plant foods. The good news about fiber's health benefits appears to be never-ending.

- Use minimal added sugar and no artificial sweeteners. Canyon Ranch recipes call for a variety of natural sweeteners in moderate quantities, including cane sugar, honey and molasses.

- Provide meals and snacks that include protein, carbohydrate and small amounts of healthy fat. This combination satisfies both nutritional needs and appetite. Canyon Ranch chefs strive to balance each meal, including vegetarian options, with some protein-rich food. Protein offerings include beans plus soy foods, fish, eggs, low-fat dairy products, and the leanest cuts of poultry and red meat.

- Use healthy fats in moderation. Canyon Ranch chefs use special care in selecting fats and oils that are beneficial to health. Preferred choices are extra virgin olive oil and expeller-pressed canola oil, both rich in flavor and antioxidants. Also emphasize omega-3 fatty acids (found mainly in fish and flax seeds) and fats from other plant sources, including avocado and nuts. Minimize saturated fats and never use trans fats. Use cooking techniques such as braising, sauteing, grilling, broiling, baking and stir-frying. Use fat sparingly.

- Season foods with an array of herbs and spices. Keep a careful eye on sodium, however, because most Americans regularly consume more salt than recommended. The goal is to allow the natural flavors of the food to shine. Canyon Ranch chefs prefer sea salt, which is a little lower in sodium and higher in other minerals than table salt.

Best Choices

- Serve plenty of real food that is fresh – lots of fresh fruits and vegetables, whole grains, lean proteins such as pork loin, chicken and turkey, occasional lean red meat, fish, lean dairy products, vegetable proteins such as beans and legumes, and good fats – avocado, flax, nuts, seeds and olive oil.

- If fresh produce is not available or affordable, frozen fruits and vegetables are good substitutes. Nearly any fruit and vegetable is better than no fruit and vegetable.

- Serve all food in moderate and appropriate portions.

- Prepare food with minimal fat and limit added sugar and salt.

Foods to Limit

- Refined grains like white rice, all-purpose flour and pasta

- Foods or ingredients high in sugar including granulated sugar, soft drinks, etc.

- High-fat cheeses, dairy products and sauces

- Foods with trans and/or saturated fats

- Fried foods unless used sparingly as a garnish

- Sugar and highly sweetened foods and sauces

- Salt and high-sodium sauces, prepared foods and condiments

- Highly processed foods

- High-fat meats and processed meats

- Processed fat-free products

- Large portions

- Beverages containing alcohol (one per day)

Help or Harm? Low-Calorie Sweeteners and Beverages

Diet beverages are widely available, and the general assumption has been that they are better than high-sugar beverages for people who want to lose weight. While drinking a reasonable amount of diet soda, such as a can or two a day, isn't likely to cause harm, diet beverages are not a health drink. A few studies have suggested that low-calorie sweeteners may cause cravings for more sugar and/or lead to weight gain, but these studies have not changed the overall scientific consensus that low-calorie sweeteners can aid in weight management if the diet beverage replaces a sugared beverage that would ordinarily be consumed. While diet beverages do not have calories, they also do not have vitamins, minerals and phytochemicals that are in other beverage options.

A review of studies conducted over the past two decades has shown that low-calorie sweeteners can help with weight loss and/or maintenance if they are part of a healthy diet and exercise regimen. Certainly diet beverages and other sugar-free products that use low-calorie sweeteners are useful for people who have diabetes or other medical reasons to reduce sugar intake.

Concerns about the potentially negative effect of carbonated beverages on bone health and concerns about artificial colors and flavors persist. Numerous other beverages choices are healthier, provide necessary liquids along with nutrients and are better for your guests, especially for children.

The quality of calories is just as important, if not more so, than the quantity.

Cheryl Forberg, RD
Nutrition advisor to television's
"The Biggest Loser"

Tips for Chefs

- Many guests will have personal beliefs about dieting and what they want to fit into their diet regimen. Offer a variety of healthful choices that are low to moderate in calories.

- Offer skim milk, low-fat or fat-free salad dressing, sugar substitutes, diet soft drinks, unsweetened teas and other foods as options that dieters may expect – and delight them with plenty of other healthful options.

- If guests are on fad diets, low-carb, raw or other regimens for weight control, offerings should include some options suitable for them.

- Look critically at the menu: Are there broth-based and vegetable soups without cream? Are there interesting salads that do not contain bacon, cheese, croutons or other high-fat ingredients? Are portions appropriate and not excessive? Are there a few desserts that are moderate in sugar and fat? Are half or smaller portions available? Are there whole-grain breads, rolls or crackers? Are there healthful olive oil dips or spreads for breads? Are raw, steamed, grilled or roasted vegetables available and abundant? Are there interesting options that feature legumes, seafood, poultry and lean meats? Do vegetarians have a reasonable selection? Is fresh fruit available as an appetizer, salad or dessert option? Are healthful cooking techniques used throughout the menu?

For More Information

- *Chemical Cuisine,* a guide to food additives when packaged foods are a more convenient choice, www.cspinet.org

- Consumer Union, food label information and current food product and eco-labeling advice, www.consumersunion.org/food.html

- *Eat Wild,* guide to grass-fed and organic meat, poultry and dairy products including a list of suppliers of pasture-raised products, www.eatwild.com

- *Eating Well* and *Cooking Light* magazines provide reliable current information on food and nutrition for home cooks and culinary professionals.

- Field to Plate, seasonal produce, www.fieldtoplate.com/guide.php

- Forberg C. *Flavor First: Cut Calories and Boost Flavor with 75 Delicious, All-Natural Recipes.* New York: Rodale; 2012.

- Forberg C. *The Biggest Loser Simple Swaps: 100 Easy Changes to Start Living a Healthier Lifestyle.* New York: Rodale; 2009.

- Institute for Agriculture and Trade Policy, guides to healthy choices, www.iatp.org

- Local Harvest, sourcing local foods and community supported agriculture, www.localharvest.org

- Mullen MC, Shield J. *ADA Pocket Guide to Pediatric Weight Management.* Chicago, IL: American Dietetic Association; 2009.

- Rolls B, Hermann M. *The Ultimate Volumetrics Diet: Smart, Simple, Science-Based Strategies for Losing Weight and Keeping It Off.* New York: HarperCollins Publishers; 2012.

- Rolls B. *The Volumetrics Eating Plan: Techniques and Recipes for Feeling Full on Fewer Calories.* New York: Harper Paperbacks; 2007.

- Uehlien S. *Canyon Ranch: Nourish Indulgently Healthy Cuisine.* New York: Viking Studio; 2009.

- Wansink, B. *Mindless Eating: Why We Eat More Than We Think.* New York: Bantam; 2007.

Cold Watermelon Ginger Soup with Mango

Chef Scott Uehlein, Corporate Executive Chef,
Canyon Ranch, Tuscon, Arizona

Serves: 10 servings, ¾ cup each

Watermelon,
cubed, 2 quarts . . . . about 4 pounds
Ginger, minced, fresh. . . . . 2 tablespoons
Green chili, chopped . . . . ¼ cup
Lime juice, fresh . . . . ¾ cup
Evaporated cane juice . . . . ⅓ tablespoons
Sea salt . . . . ½ teaspoon

Garnish
Mango, diced, fresh . . . . ¾ cup
Cumin, whole seed. . . . . 1 teaspoon

1. Place all ingredients except for garnish in a blender container and puree until smooth. Strain through a sieve.

2. Place ¾ cup soup in a bowl and top with 1 tablespoon diced mango and a pinch of whole cumin seed.

Per Serving

Calories	60	Cholesterol	0	mg
Fat	0 g	Sodium	200	mg
Saturated Fat	0 g	Carbohydrates	16	mg
Trans Fat	0 g	Dietary Fiber	1	mg
Sugar	12 g	Protein	1	g

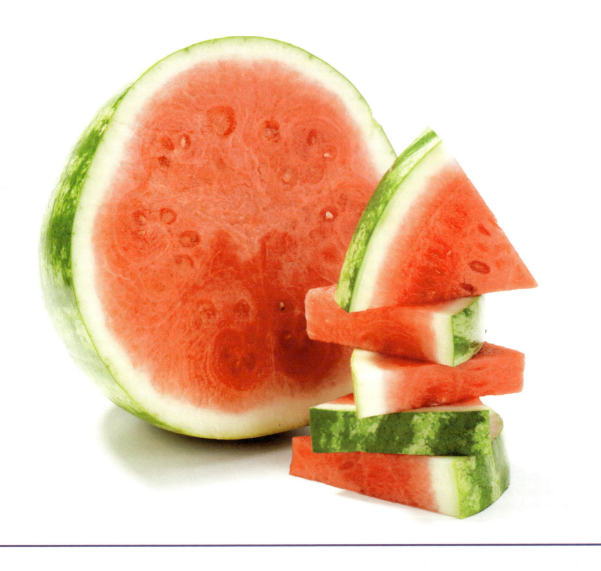

Seared Beef Tenderloin with Tomato Confit, Kale and Sage Polenta

Chef Scott Uehlein, Corporate Executive Chef,
Canyon Ranch, Tuscon, Arizona

Yield: 2 ½ cups
Serves: 10, 1 filet with ¼ cup Tomato Confit,
¹/₃ cup Sauteed Kale and
¹/₃ cup Sage Polenta

Tomato Confit   Yield: **2 ½ cups**

Roma tomato concasse	2 ½	cups
Olive oil, extra virgin	2	tablespoons
Sea salt	1	teaspoon
Black pepper, freshly ground	½	teaspoon
Garlic cloves	2	minced
Fresh thyme, chopped	2	tablespoons

Beef Tenderloin

Beef tenderloin filets	10	4-ounce
	(2 ½	pounds)
Sea salt	½	teaspoon
Black pepper, freshly ground	½	teaspoon

Sauteed Kale   Yield: **3 ½ cups**

Shallots, sliced	¼	cup
Kale, fresh, stems removed	2	bunches
	(2	pounds)
Olive oil, extra virgin	1	tablespoon
Sea salt	1	teaspoon
Black pepper, freshly ground	½	teaspoon
Water	½	cup
Cider vinegar	⅓	cup

1. Preheat oven to 300° F.
2. Toss all ingredients for Tomato Confit together on a baking sheet. Roast for 20 to 30 minutes or until vegetables are cooked through and slightly caramelized.
3. Preheat grill or broiler.
4. Lightly season beef tenderloin filets with salt and pepper. Grill tenderloin filets for 3 to 5 minutes on each side or to desired doneness.
5. In a large saute pan over medium heat, saute shallots in olive oil. Add kale leaves, salt and pepper. Add water to steam and soften vegetables. Finish with vinegar.
6. Serve each beef tenderloin topped with ¼ cup Tomato Confit. Serve with ⅓ cup Sauteed Kale and ⅓ cup Sage Polenta.

Sage Polenta   Yield: **3 ¾ cups**
Serves: 10- **⅓ cup each**

Onion, finely minced	½	cup
Unsalted butter	2	tablespoons
Soft corn, cut from the cob	½	cup
2% milk	3 ¾	cups
Polenta	¾	cup
Sea salt	½	teaspoon
Black pepper, freshly ground		Pinch
Evaporated cane juice	1	tablespoon
Parmesan cheese, grated	⅓	cup
Sage, fresh, chopped	1	tablespoon
Chives, fresh, chopped	2	tablespoons

1. In a large saucepan, saute onion in butter over medium heat until translucent. Add corn and saute briefly, about 30 seconds.
2. Add milk and bring to a boil. Using a wire whip, lightly whisk in polenta, salt, pepper and evaporated cane juice. Cook until thickened, about 3 minutes.
3. Add cheese, sage and chives and stir until cheese is melted.

Per Serving

Calories	320	Cholesterol	90	mg
Fat	14 g	Sodium	460	mg
Saturated Fat	4 g	Carbohydrates	13	mg
Trans Fat	0 g	Dietary Fiber	3	mg
Sugar	2 g	Protein	36	g

Meeting the Needs of Vegetarians

ESSENTIALS EXPERT

Jill Nussinow, MS, RD, aka *The Veggie Queen™*, *is an expert in vegetarian, vegan and pressure cooking. In the past 25 years, she has taught thousands of people about the joys and delights of eating fresh, in-season plant foods. She is a speaker, writer and consultant on plant-food related topics.*

According to The Academy of Nutrition and Dietetics and most health authorities, well-planned vegetarian diets are healthful and nutritionally adequate. People choose to become vegetarians for many reasons – including health, environmental, animal welfare, religion and ethics. Family or friends influence some people to become vegetarians.

Vegetarians are becoming more and more common as restaurant guests, in schools and on college campuses. In a Vegetarian Resource Group 2009 poll conducted by Harris Interactive®, 3% of the U.S. population was identified as vegetarian and about 1% of the population as vegan. [13] In a Vegetarian Resource Group 2008 poll conducted by Zogby International, more than 55% of those polled said they sometimes, often or always ordered a dish without meat, fish or fowl. [14] All foodservice operators need to be creative in meeting these guests' preferences.

Generally, there are six different types of vegetarians:

- *Strict vegetarian* or *vegan*: Excludes all animal products including meat, poultry, fish, eggs, milk, cheese and other dairy products as well as ingredients from animal sources such as gelatin.

- *Lacto-vegetarian*: Excludes meat, poultry, fish and eggs but includes dairy products.

- *Lacto-ovo vegetarian*: Excludes meat, poultry and fish but includes eggs and dairy products. Most vegetarians in the United States fall into this category.

- *Raw vegan*: Includes raw vegetables and fruits, nuts and nut pastes, grain and legume sprouts, seeds, plant oils, sea vegetables, herbs and fresh juices. Excludes all food of animal origin, and all food cooked above 118° F.

- *Flexitarian*: A mostly vegetarian diet with an occasional meat consumption – "semi" or sometimes vegetarian.

- *Pescetarian*: A mostly vegetarian diet that includes fish and shellfish but excludes mammals and birds.

Eating more raw foods is certainly healthful and an easy way to incorporate more whole foods. Eating raw often takes as much work if not more, as eating cooked food, especially if you are relying on sprouting, dehydrating and fermenting, all of which take advance planning. Consequently, few people have the patience or desire to do it regularly. For example, you cannot decide to serve house-made sprouts on the spur of the moment; it takes several days to grow them.

Chefs can often rely on vendors to supply prepared ingredients, but they are typically more expensive. Preparing sprouts or fermented foods is relatively inexpensive and can add a certain modern panache to a restaurant dish, hence the interest in "microgreens," which are truly sprouts (grown in soil). Dehydrated foods are great for when there is abundance. In my opinion, there's nothing quite like eating kale chips as a special treat. But again, advanced planning is needed.

Jill Nussinow, MS, RD
The Veggie Queen™

Tips for Chefs

- Chefs can show off their creativity with vegetarian and vegan appetizers, salads, soups, entrees and desserts. Generally, there should be a vegetarian option in each menu category plus at least one vegan entree.

- Feature combination dishes that provide a variety of plant proteins to boost overall availability of protein – such as sandwiches on whole-grain bread and pita with hummus or portobello mushrooms and red peppers; red or brown rice with black beans; eggplant and sundried tomatoes on whole-grain pizza crust; bean and cheese burritos on whole-wheat tortillas; and beans in vegetable soups and in salads.

- Because meats, poultry, fish, etc. are not options for them, many vegetarians frequently serve pasta dishes at home. Chefs, however, should provide a variety of creative vegetarian options in addition to traditional pasta entrees.

- Canned beans typically have a lot of salt added to preserve texture. If liquid from the can is used, reduce the amount of salt in the recipe. If beans are drained, rinse them to reduce sodium.

- Roasted and grilled seasonal vegetables and fruit dishes, interesting salads, legumes and legume-vegetable combinations, hearty vegetable soups, ethnic foods without meat or dairy products, grain-vegetable combinations, flat breads or pizzas with vegetable toppings, and risottos and other grain-based dishes offer vegetarians options that may be popular with other guests as well.

- A combination of side dishes and garnishes from other menu items can make an interesting daily vegetarian offering.

For More Information

- Berkoff N. *Vegan in Volume: Vegan Quantity Recipes for Every Occasion.* Baltimore, MD: Vegetarian Resource Group; 2000.

- Davis B, Melina V. *Becoming Vegan: The Complete to Guide to Adopting a Healthy Plant-Based Diet.* Summertown, TN: Book Publishing Company; 2000.

- Dragonwagon C. *The Passionate Vegetarian.* New York: Workman Publishing Company; 2002.

- Dragonwagon, C, *Bean By Bean: A Cookbook: More than 175 Recipes for Fresh Beans, Dried Beans, Cool Beans, Hot Beans, Savory Beans, Even Sweet Beans!,* 2012, Workman Publishing Company, New York.

- Madison D. *Vegetarian Cooking for Everyone.* New York: Broadway Books; 2007.

- Melina V, Davis B, Berry R. *Becoming Raw: The Essential Guide to Raw Vegan Diets.* Summertown, TN: Book Publishing Company; 2010.

- Melina V, Davis B. *The New Becoming Vegetarian: The Essential Guide to a Healthy Vegetarian Diet.* 2nd ed. Summertown, TN: Healthy Living Publications (Book Publishing Company); 2003.

- Natkin, M, *Herivoracious: A Flavor Revolution with 150 Vibrant and Original Vegetarian Recipes.* Boston, MA: The Harvard Common Press; 2012.

- Nussinow, J, *The New Fast Food: The Veggie Queen Pressure Cooks Whole Food Meals in Less than 30 Minutes.* Santa Rosa, CA: Vegetarian Connection Press; 2012.

- Nussinow J. *The Veggie Queen: Vegetables Get the Royal Treatment.* Santa Rosa, CA: Vegetarian Connection Press; 2005.

- Polenz K. *Vegetarian Cooking at Home with The Culinary Institute of America.* New York: John Wiley & Sons, Inc.; 2012.

- Sando, S. and Barrington, *V. Heirloom Beans.* San Francisco: Chronicle Books; 2008.

- Vegetarian Resource Group, www.vrg.org

- *Vegetarian Times* magazine, www.vegetariantimes.com

Black Bean Quinoa Burger

Jill Nussinow, MS, RD, The Veggie Queen™
Santa Rosa, California

Serves: 10

This recipe will likely work with any cooked grain or bean with slight adjustments in amounts. It is good served with a fruit or vegetable salsa. Use canned, drained and rinsed black beans. If prepared in advance, finish in a saute pan or on a griddle.

Quinoa, cooked	¾	cup
Black beans, cooked	1	cup
Onion, chopped	¾	cup
Garlic cloves	3	
Fresh herbs such as parsley, basil or cilantro	¼	cup
Nutritional yeast	2	tablespoons
Salt, only if using fresh cooked, not canned, beans	½	teaspoon
Hemp seeds (optional)	2	tablespoons

1. Preheat the oven to 350° F

2. Put the quinoa, beans and onion in the food processor. Pulse a few times until slightly mixed. Add the garlic, herbs, yeast and salt, if using. Pulse again, adding 1-2 tablespoons bean liquid if it needs it. Stir in hemp seeds. Form into patties.

3. Bake on oiled baking sheet for 10 minutes. Turn over and bake another 10 minutes.

Per Serving

Calories	80	Cholesterol	0	mg
Fat	1	g	Sodium	280	mg
Saturated Fat	0	g	Carbohydrates	14	mg
Trans Fat	0	g	Dietary Fiber	3	mg
Sugar	1	g	Protein	5	g

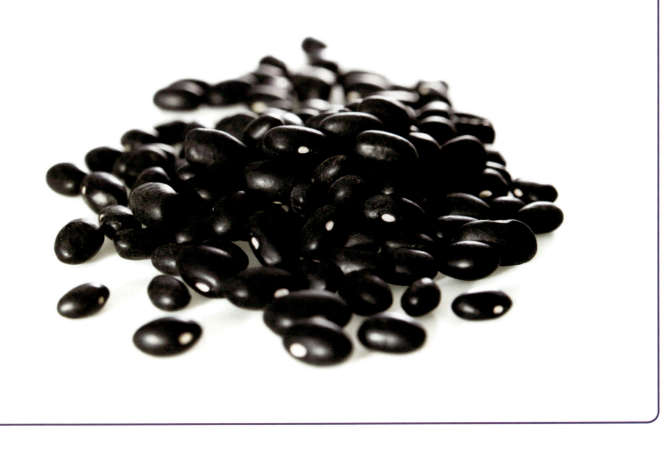

Kosher

ESSENTIALS EXPERT

Tina Wasserman is the author of Entrée to Judaism, A Culinary Exploration of the Jewish Diaspora and the food authority for the URJ Reform Jewish movement for a decade. She is a highly respected food educator, lecturer and Jewish culinary historian. For more than 40 years, her hands-on approach to all facets of food has had broad appeal to students throughout the United States and Europe.

"The word 'kashrut,' " Tina Wasserman explains, "refers to the body of Jewish law dealing with what foods we can and cannot eat and how those foods must be prepared and eaten. Kashrut comes from the Hebrew root *kaf-shin-reish*, meaning fit, proper or correct. The more commonly known word **kosher**, also comes from this root and describes food that meets these standards."

According to the 2000 National Jewish Population Survey, 21% of American Jews report that they keep kosher in the home. [15] This number includes the vast majority of the Orthodox community as well as many Conservative, Reform and Reconstructionist Jews. Some keep kosher at home but will eat "kosher style" while dining out. This means that they will eat foods that are allowed by law but are not certified kosher (chicken or hamburger, for example), and they won't eat dairy products and meat products together on the same plate. Others will avoid breaking the laws of kashrut when dining out by eating a vegetarian dish or fish (not seafood that is un-kosher) and dairy products. People who are strictly kosher will not eat in any facility that isn't supervised by a rabbi.

According to a 2009 Mintel report, however, only 15% of all the people who buy kosher foods do so for religious reasons. In fact, most people buy kosher food for its quality, safety and healthfulness. [16] The Kosher and Halal Food Initiative, a research project at Cornell University, found that 40% of foods sold at grocery stores is kosher or halal. [17]

Many vegetarians (not vegans) pick kosher foods because a **pareve** label means no meat or dairy products are included as ingredients. Rules for the humane treatment of animals make kosher and halal attractive to individuals concerned about animal welfare. Kosher meat and other kosher foods must be inspected and certified by authorized rabbis who follow strict rules for sanitation.

Keep in mind, however, that a kosher label does not mean a food is the most healthful choice. For example, the washing and salting of kosher poultry reduces the possibility of salmonella but increases sodium content. Many highly processed packaged cookies and snacks carry a kosher insignia.

Key Nutrition Points

- Shellfish, fish without scales, and pork are not allowed.

- Kosher cuts of meat come only from the front of the animal above the sciatic nerve. Sirloin, tenderloin, rump roast, etc. are non-kosher cuts.

- If certified-kosher meat or poultry is used, always reduce the amount of salt in the recipe. The raw meat has been salted and rinsed to conform to Jewish dietary laws, and some salt remains.

- Do not include milk-based foods in recipes or meals containing meat. Dairy foods and meat foods may not be served at the same meal. For example, fried chicken is acceptable and so is macaroni and cheese, but serving them together at the same meal is not appropriate; chicken cannot be soaked in buttermilk before breading.

- Do not include chicken or beef base in a sauce that will contain butter or milk products.

- Different plates and eating and cooking utensils must be used for meat and dairy foods.

- Dairy products, fish products and egg products may be served together according to most kosher authorities. Fish, eggs, fruits, vegetables and grains are neutral and can be served with either milk or meat products.

- Just about any ethnic cuisine can conform to keeping kosher.

- Thousands of products bear symbols indicating they are certified kosher. Look for a U within an O to represent the Union of Orthodox Rabbis or a K in a triangle to represent the Conservative Jewish Movement's stamp of approval. Other symbols exist, but these two are the most prevalent. Some very observant Orthodox Jews require the seal of specific certifying groups in addition to the circle U or K designation.

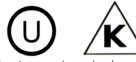

- Foods that are kosher and marked pareve have no milk or meat ingredients and can be used with either meat or dairy/milk meals. Mayonnaise (certified kosher) may be used for all food preparations if listed as pareve. Some non-dairy creamers contain thickeners made from gelatin (or animal products) and may be used only with meat meals if certified kosher. Cream or milk may be used only with milk/dairy meals.

- Adherence to Jewish dietary laws varies among people of the Jewish faith. Many do not adhere to any of the dietary laws and eat everything; some will not eat pork and/or shellfish; while others will eat only in kosher restaurants or homes and will eat only foods prepared and packaged in kosher kitchens. Kosher kitchens have strictly separated equipment, dishes and tools used to prepare dairy and meat products. Authorized rabbis must inspect these kitchens regularly.

Best Choices

- Fish and kosher chicken are the easiest to prepare given normal kitchen routine and recipes. Many favorites such as hamburgers are acceptable as well; however, cooking equipment must be used exclusively for kosher food.

- Vegetarian dishes using cheese and tofu as the protein base do not have to be adjusted.

- Soy creamers and coconut milk are kosher substitutes for the cream in cream-style sauces.

- All oils are kosher.

- Vegetable oils may be used in all types of dishes.

- Serve plenty of fruits, vegetables and grains. All can be served with meat or dairy meals.

- Grilled, marinated meats (such as lamb chops or shish kabobs) and recipes that use small cubes of meat are popular because many tender cuts of meat are not kosher. These cooking techniques tenderize tougher cuts.

- Sauteed, grilled, roasted or oven-fried chicken is popular as are fried cutlets (schnitzel).

- Prepare pizza with (kosher) meat but no cheese or pasta with cheese but no meat. Either type of pizza may have vegetables. Kosher non-dairy, soy-based cheese substitutes are available.

- Use pareve margarine (no milk solids) and soy-based creamer instead of butter or cream in any meal containing meat and in making a béchamel or other sauces served with meat. Pareve non-dairy whipped topping, cream or coffee lightener may be used as well but note that non-dairy creamers are often sweetened and may need testing when used in place of cream in cooking.

Foods to Limit

Foods prohibited in the diets of those who keep kosher include all pork products, all shellfish and mollusks, fish without fins and scales (shark, sturgeon, catfish, octopus, squid, swordfish), cuts of meat from the hindquarters of animals (loin, sirloin, strip and porterhouse steaks, filet mignon, round, flank, etc.) and meat from animals that do not have cloven hooves and chew their cud (most game meats). Eating hare (rabbit), camel, birds of prey, reptiles, eel and insects is also forbidden. All meat that is non-kosher, that has not been slaughtered, salted, inspected and blessed by specially authorized rabbis, is not eaten. Most people who keep kosher eat foods that bear kosher symbols that ensure that food is appropriate. Some individuals who keep kosher will buy produce only from certain purveyors or restaurants (even kosher ones) because vegetables such as broccoli may have insects that would make these usually neutral foods un-kosher.

In addition to selecting only kosher foods, the chef must be particularly careful to avoid serving any meat or meat-derived ingredient with a dairy meal or any dairy-based ingredient with a meat meal.

Tips for Chefs

- A kosher kitchen has separate sets of utensils, dishes, etc. for meat/poultry and dairy/milk meals. Another set of dishes and utensils are used only for Passover. Kosher-certified cleaning products are required, but most detergents are certified. Disposables are often used to ensure that there has been no prior contact with either meat or milk meals.

- Unless a kitchen is strictly kosher and supervised by rabbis, chefs can serve only "kosher-style" food. In many situations, including catering, food-service operators purchase prepared kosher foods in sealed containers to serve to kosher guests or customers.

- Read ingredient lists carefully. Look for kosher symbols on packaged foods. Remember that although there are kosher meats and kosher dairy products, they cannot be served together.

- Use vegetable broth when cooking foods for dairy meals.

- All foods in the same meal must be entirely meat or dairy. For example, if the entree or salad contains meat, the dessert or salad dressing at that meal cannot contain any dairy products. Neutral foods can be served with either.

- For those who keep kosher, several hours must elapse between meat and milk meals; the time varies based on personal religious practices.

- Dried mushrooms or sun-dried tomatoes will add a salty or umami taste and may be used in place of small amounts of bacon or smoked meats in some recipes.

- Special dietary rules are observed on holidays – for example, fasting on Yom Kippur and eating only unleavened bread (matzos) during Passover.

For More Information

- Blau E, Deitsch T, Light C. *Spice and Spirit: The Complete Kosher Jewish Cookbook*. Brooklyn, NY: Lubavitch Women's Cookbook Publications; 1997.

- Marks, G. *Encyclopedia of Jewish Foods*. Hoboken, NJ: John Wiley & Sons; 2010.

- Nathan J. *Joan Nathan's Jewish Holiday Cookbook*. New York: Schoken Books, Random House; 2004.

- Orthodox Union, http://oukosher.org/index.php/common/article/ou_symbols

- Rich TR. *Kashrut: Jewish Dietary Laws*, www.jewfaq.org/kashrut.htm

- Roden C. *The Book of Jewish Food: An Odyssey from Samarkand to New York City*. New York: Penguin Books; 1999.

- Star-K Kosher Certification, www.star-k.org

- Wasserman T. *Entree to Judaism: A Culinary Exploration of the Jewish Diaspora*. New York: URJ Books and Music; 2010.

- Zeidler J. *The Gourmet Jewish Cook*. New York: William Morrow Cookbooks; 1999.

Chicken Fesenjan with Walnuts and Pomegranate Syrup

Tina Wasserman, Author, *Entree to Judaism: A Culinary Exploration of the Jewish Diaspora*, Dallas, Texas

Serves: 10

This dish holds well and can be prepared in advance. The combination of nuts and pomegranate syrup is a traditional Middle Eastern flavor profile. This dish is excellent for guests who keep kosher. Serve it with Basmati rice or Israeli couscous. Most of the fat in this recipe comes from the walnuts, which are high in heart-healthy fats.

Walnuts, pieces	1 ⅓	cup
Onions, diced	2	medium
Olive oil	5	tablespoons, divided
Tomato paste	¼	cup
Pomegranate molasses or syrup	¼	cup
Honey	¼	cup
Lemon juice	2	tablespoons
Kosher salt	½	teaspoon
Black pepper	¼	teaspoon
Cinnamon	1	teaspoon
Water	½	cup
Chicken stock	1 ½	cup
Chicken, breast or thighs, skinless	10	each

1. Toast the walnut pieces in a 350° F oven until fragrant. Remove from oven and cool. Reserve ⅓ cup for garnish.

2. Saute onion in 3 tablespoons olive oil. Chop onions and walnuts in a food processor to a coarse paste. Add the tomato paste, pomegranate molasses, honey, lemon juice, spices and water and process until mixed. Set aside.

3. Saute chicken in remaining 2 tablespoons of oil. Brown chicken on both sides. Remove and hold.

4. Deglaze the pan with chicken stock. Add walnut-onion sauce mixture and stir. If necessary, adjust seasonings by adding more honey or lemon juice to the mixture to get a balanced sweet/sour taste. Return chicken to pan. Cover pan.

5. Put in 350° F oven for 35 minutes or until meat is tender. Baste chicken several times while cooking.

6. When serving, garnish with reserved toasted walnuts.

Per Serving

Calories	370	Cholesterol	85	mg
Fat	18 g	Sodium	180	mg
Saturated Fat	2.5 g	Carbohydrates	17	mg
Trans Fat	0 g	Dietary Fiber	2	mg
Sugar	13 g	Protein	35	g

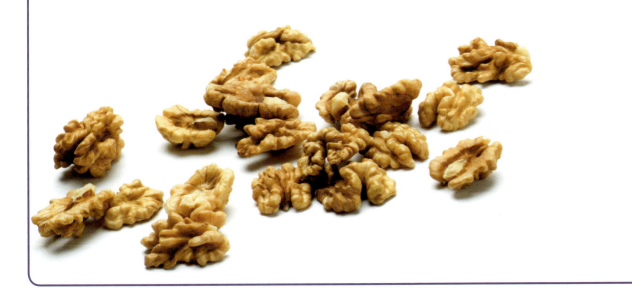

Halal

ESSENTIALS EXPERTS

Mariam Majeed is a food technologist who formerly worked for the Islamic Food and Nutrition Council of America, located in Park Ridge, Illinois.

Muhammad Munir Chaudry, PhD, is president of the Islamic Food and Nutrition Council of America. He estimates that there are 160 million people worldwide who follow Islamic dietary laws, 6 million to 8 million of whom live in the United States.

Because many chefs have limited knowledge of Islamic food practices and beliefs, our experts have explained them here in some detail.

Key Nutrition Points

Many Muslims are observant and adhere to the dietary restrictions that follow. Others of the Muslim faith, however, are far less stringent in adhering to dietary restrictions.

Requirements for Meat and Poultry

No pork is permitted in any form. Animals must be of an acceptable halal species, such as cattle and chicken. Animals and birds must be slaughtered by a Muslim of sound mind and blessed by pronouncing the name of Allah. A sharp knife must be used to severe the jugular vein, carotid arteries, trachea and esophagus, and blood must be drained out completely. The slaughtering must be done by hand with the complete removal of blood from the carcass.

Islam places great emphasis on humane treatment of all living things including animals. Meat that is not slaughtered in the Islamic manner is not suitable for Muslims. Because the rules for slaughter are similar, some Muslims eat kosher meat, although the rules of who does the slaughtering and the blessings differ. Any by-products of meat and poultry, such as beef fat or chicken broth, must come from an animal slaughtered in the Islamic way. Unlike those observing kosher rules, Muslims can eat meat and dairy together.

Vegetable soups that contain chicken or beef stock that are not halal are unsuitable for consumption by Muslims. Other ingredients that may be of animal origin include emulsifiers such as mono- and di-glycerides, which may be made from beef fat, lard or vegetable. If the source is not listed on the label as vegetable, the product is "mashbooh" (doubtful). Another ingredient of concern is glycerin or glycerol, which can be sourced from animals or plants; only the type from a vegetable source is permissible.

Those who observe the dietary tenets of Islam are usually aware which restaurants and grocery stores sell halal "zabihah meat." Some Muslims do not eat any meat or poultry when dining out, preferring instead to order vegetarian fare or seafood. Many halal meat products and other halal meat-based products are now available for foodservice and retail use. For information on how to obtain packaged halal-certified meat products, contact the Islamic Food and Nutrition Council of America at www.ifanca.org.

Requirements for Fish and Seafood

Due to the different schools of Islamic jurisprudence and certain cultural practices, some Muslims may not eat fish without scales such as catfish, while others will not eat mollusks and crustaceans, often referred to as "makrooh" (disliked). Various seafood flavors, such as shrimp flavors used in sauces, may be a concern.

Requirements for Eggs and Dairy Products

Milk and eggs from halal animals can be consumed without restrictions. The source of vitamins used in fortification can be questionable. Vitamin A sometimes includes gelatin as a carrier, which could be from pork or beef. If the source of the vitamin A is unknown, the vitamin is questionable, or mashbooh. Because gelatin is obtained after the animal is slaughtered, the animal must be Islamically slaughtered for that gelatin to be halal. Porcine gelatin can never be halal. Vitamin D is sometimes derived from lanolin; sheep's wool is an accepted source. Devout Muslims want to make sure that the source of vitamins, whether in milk or other products, is plant-based or synthetically produced. If synthetic, then the starting material should be non-animal.

Enzymes used during cheese making and whey products should be from microbial sources. Halal animal enzymes are rare; therefore, microbial enzymes used for cheese and whey are acceptable. Milk and egg products can become mashbooh if emulsifiers, mold inhibitors and other functional ingredients are from non-halal sources. For example, there may be vitamin A in butter or gelatin in sour cream. Some cheeses and other dairy products are certified as halal and carry a crescent M logo on the packaging.

Plants and Vegetables

This category is inherently halal except for alcoholic drinks or other intoxicants. In addition, vegetables that are processed using equipment also used for meat can be cross-contaminated. Certain ingredients derived from animal sources, such as mono- and diglycerides or cysteine, make these vegetables unacceptable choices.

L-cysteine is an amino acid used in commercial bakery products. L-cysteine derived from human hair is not acceptable; however, some Islamic certifying groups consider duck feathers an acceptable source for this amino acid ingredient. Others allow only vegetarian sources of l-cysteine. For observant Muslims, monitoring processing and production methods is necessary to keep halal status intact.

Key Terms

Halal – permissible and lawful

Haram – prohibited

Mashbooh – doubtful

Makrooh – disliked or detested

Zabihah – meat slaughtered by a Muslim according to Islamic law

Islam is a religion that is a complete way of life. Islam is often connected with the people of Middle Eastern origin, but it is for all Muslims. Commandments on how to live life are found in the Quran (divine book from Allah) and the Sunnah of Prophet Muhammad.

Followers of Islam are advised to eat moderately; to eat only permissible and pure foods; to eat with three or five fingers; to wash your hands prior to eating; to invoke Allah's bounties prior to eating; to thank Him after eating; and to drink water while sitting down.

Food is central to our lives and society because it brings people together, creates harmony and creates a sense of belonging. For a Muslim, food brings all these good things along with nourishment. Food becomes an act of worship and a way to attain good deeds in Islam. The goal of life is to be obedient to Allah. The life of a Muslim revolves around what is permissible (halal) and what is prohibited (haram).

Miriam Majeed
Formerly with the Islamic Food and
Nutrition Council of America

Sanitation and Cross Contamination

In food production, halal avoids cross-contamination of halal foods with non-halal or animal-based foods or ingredients. Certain equipment can be marked as "halal only." For non-meat products, equipment can be used for halal items after thorough washing. If meat items are being served in the same facility, it is best to use the same pans and equipment for halal and vegetarians, provided there is no alcohol or any other doubtful ingredients in the vegetarian dish.

Chemicals used for cleaning, including soaps and foams, should be checked to ensure they contain no animal products or alcohol. Check the Islamic Food and Nutrition Council of America, www.ifanca.org, for lists of food and cleaning products certified as halal.

Best Choices

- All fruits and vegetables
- Eggs
- Meat, poultry and dairy products, if certified as halal
- Vegetarian salads, soups and entrees
- Fish and seafood
- Grains
- Legumes
- Vegetable oils
- Sugar and sweeteners
- Herbs and spices

Foods to Limit

Foods that are "haram" (not permissible) include:

- Animals dead before slaughtering
- Blood or blood by-products
- Pork including all its by-products (for example, gelatin in any form)
- Animals not slaughtered according to halal rules
- Intoxicants of all types, including alcohol and drugs

- Carnivorous animals with fangs such as wolves, lions, dogs or tigers
- Birds with sharp claws (birds of prey) such as eagles, owls, falcons or vultures
- Certain land animals such as frogs or snakes

Alcohol is not permitted in any form, even if it may evaporate in cooking. Alcohol naturally present in fruits is acceptable in small amounts. Alcohol used for technical reasons, such as in vanilla or other flavor carriers, may be permitted if not derived from dates or grapes. Certain halal-certifying organizations, such as the Islamic Food and Nutrition Council of America, maintain that a product should contain less than 0.1% grain alcohol. A Muslim cannot buy, sell, raise, transport, slaughter or derive benefit from swine or alcohol.

Once something is haram it cannot be halal no matter what science may show, no matter how clean that animal might become and no matter what justifications anyone might suggest. In addition, there is a gray area between halal and haram called "mashbooh," which can involve a simple ingredient such as whey in a chocolate candy bar. If the source of enzyme used during the whey production for that candy bar is unknown, the food is considered doubtful and should not be eaten.

Tips for Chefs

- Sometimes customers will ask you to prepare foods in separate oil, change your gloves or use clean utensils to ensure that there has been no exposure to animal or non-halal products.

- Muslims may request a scrambled egg if they are unable to determine the halal status of other foods on the menu.

- To provide adequate information to customers, chefs who serve Muslim patrons should keep product specification sheets.

- If you have questions about how to prepare halal, contact a halal-certifying agency that works with foodservice operators to help accommodate halal in the kitchen.

Lentil Curry

Mariam Majeed, Food Technologist, formerly with the Islamic Food
and Nutrition Council of America, Park Ridge, Illinois

Yield: 7 cups
Serves: 10, ¾ cup

This recipe is suitable for halal, vegans, vegetarians and others. Serve over rice with pita or naan bread and a salad.

Red lentils	2 cups
Vegetable broth	6 cups
Oil, canola	¼ cup
Onions, diced	2 medium
Garlic cloves, diced or crushed	4 teaspoons
Ginger root, peeled and chopped	2 tablespoons
Curry powder	4 teaspoons
Red chili powder	½ teaspoon
Cumin, ground	2 teaspoons
Coriander, ground	2 teaspoons
Salt	1 teaspoon
Pepper	½ teaspoon
Tomatoes, chopped	1 can (14 ½ ounces)

1. Heat vegetable broth in pot until boiling. Add lentils and boil for one minute. Reduce heat to a simmer and simmer lentils until they resemble a thick paste.

2. While lentils are simmering, heat oil in frying pan. Add onion, garlic and ginger. Saute until soft. Add curry, chili, cumin, coriander, salt and pepper, saute for 2-3 minutes. Add tomatoes and cook for another 3-5 minutes.

3. Add fried spice mixture into lentil paste, stir and cook an additional 15-20 minutes over very low heat.

Per Serving

Calories	220	Cholesterol	0	mg
Fat	7 g	Sodium	370	mg
Saturated Fat	0 g	Carbohydrates	29	mg
Trans Fat	0 g	Dietary Fiber	7	mg
Sugar	4 g	Protein	12	g

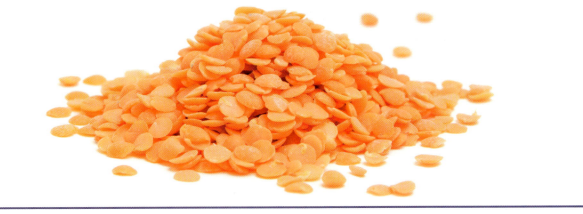

For More Information

- Hussaini MM. *Islamic Dietary Laws and Practices.* Bedford Park, IL: Islamic Food and Nutrition Council of America; 1983.

- Islamic Food and Nutrition Council of America, www.ifanca.org

- Riaz MN, Chaudry MM. *Halal Food Production.* Boca Raton, FL: CRC Press; 2003.

- Regenstein JM, T*he Cornell Kosher and Halal Food Initiative, 2007 Impact Statement.* Cornell University; 2007.

Opportunities for Chefs

Age, lifestyle and religious preference have a significant influence on the food people choose to eat. This chapter looked at the nutrition and basic menu planning requirements for children, aging adults, athletes, vegetarians, the weight-conscious, and people of the Jewish and Muslim faiths. Understanding the special needs of these groups gives you a head start in creating dishes and designing menus that appeal to the patrons you want to attract.

Learning Activities

1. Select a menu from a foodservice operation that you work in or visit frequently. Develop vegetarian options for each menu category.

2. You are catering a function for a religious group. Select a religion and plan the menu. Detail what type of function it is, how many people are attending and why you selected each menu item.

3. Develop five recipes for a spa. Include the following: breakfast item, appetizer, dessert, main course, salad and salad dressing.

CHAPTER 13
Serving Guests with Special Health Needs

LEARNING OBJECTIVES

After completing this chapter, you should be able to:

- Explain nutritional meal planning for guests with special health needs

- Plan menus for guests with special health needs

- Apply the American Heart Association nutrition recommendations in planning and preparing menu for patrons with cardiovascular disease

- Explain the DASH diet for the control of hypertension

- Discuss the relationship between cancer and diet

- Identify best food choices and poorest food choices for those with diabetes mellitus and explain why

- Describe the digestive process and contrast three digestive diseases

- Differentiate food allergies, intolerances and aversions

- Identify the most common allergens and at least 10 foods that include each of them

- Explain what gluten intolerance is and the dietary restrictions required to control it

Glance across a crowded dining room, a bustling hospital or school cafeteria, or an elegant catered event. Any time, any place a group of people gather for a meal, you can be sure there are some diners trying to prevent or manage a chronic disease or trying to skirt a food allergy or intolerance. The one thing all these people have in common is the desire to have a satisfying, flavorful meal.

This chapter focuses on serving guests with some common special health needs. Nutrition experts from around the country – our Essentials Experts – have come together here not only to give you a better understanding of how food affects these conditions (for better or worse), but also to share practical menu planning, preparation and presentation techniques that will make your foodservice operation seamlessly inclusive to all people who want to enjoy a good meal, whatever their special health needs may be.

While the chef sets the tone, he or she is not the only person who creates a winning atmosphere. Servers play a key role, too, by demonstrating the operation's commitment to accommodating a patron's special health needs, being knowledgeable about ingredients and cooking techniques, and carefully communicating guests' special requests and concerns to the chef.

Our Diet and our Health – How Big Is The Problem?

There is no question that food affects one's health – both in the short term and over a lifetime. As the chart on page 315 shows, diet plays a part in most of the top seven leading causes of death – heart disease, cancers, strokes and diabetes. Additionally, obesity is associated with increased risk of heart disease, stroke, diabetes, some cancers, hypertension, osteoarthritis and gallbladder disease. Some of the primary dietary risk factors associated with these diseases include high saturated fat and trans fat intake, low whole-grain, fruit and vegetable intake, high sugar intake, high refined-grain intake and excessive sodium intake. The foodservice industry can play an important role in providing all guests healthful menu options. For those guests with specific dietary needs, this is often a valuable service.

More than one-third of adult Americans (82 million) suffer from some form of cardiovascular disease, and more than 800,000 adults die each year from heart attacks or strokes. [1] Coronary heart disease is the number one killer of both men and women.

Approximately one-third of adult Americans have high blood pressure or hypertension. [2] Because hypertension is without symptoms, many people are unaware they have it. If uncontrolled, hypertension can lead to coronary heart disease, heart failure, stroke, kidney failure and other health problems.

While cancer is the second leading cause of death in America, rates of new diagnoses and rates of death from all cancers combined have declined significantly during the last decade for both men and women in the United States. This downward trend is driven largely by declines in the rate of new cases and lower rates of death for the three most common cancers in men (lung, prostate and colorectal) and for two of the three leading cancers in women (breast and colorectal). New diagnoses for all types of cancer in the United States decreased, on average, almost 1% per year from 1999 to 2006. Cancer deaths decreased 1.6% per year from 2001 to 2006. [3] These declines are surprising in light of the ongoing obesity epidemic and the relationship between weight and cancer.

According to the National Diabetes Information Clearinghouse, approximately 26 million people, or about 8% of the population, have diabetes and another 54 million have pre-diabetes. Diabetes is the seventh leading cause of death in the United States, and complications from the disease can lead to other very serious health problems. Potential complications include heart disease and stroke, high blood pressure, blindness, kidney disease, nervous system disease, amputations, dental disease and complications of pregnancy. Diabetes is also a financial drain on the healthcare system with estimated direct and indirect costs of about $174 billion annually. [4]

Leading Causes of Death in the United States

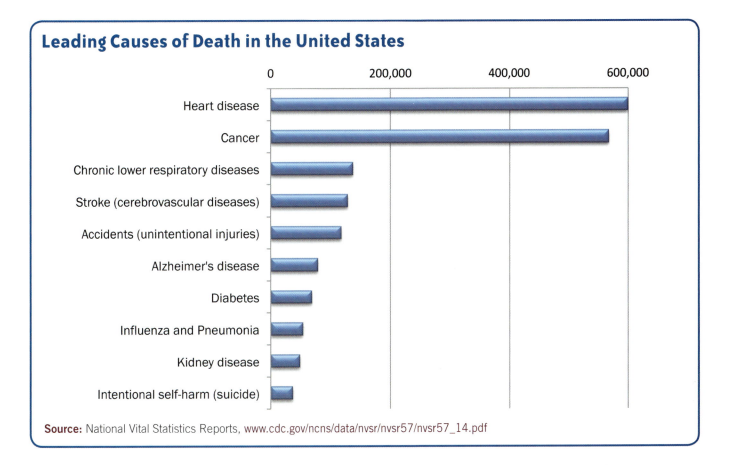

Source: National Vital Statistics Reports, www.cdc.gov/ncns/data/nvsr/nvsr57/nvsr57_14.pdf

Cardiovascular Disease

ESSENTIALS EXPERT

Penny M. Kris-Etherton, PhD, RD, FAHA, distinguished professor of nutrition at Pennsylvania State University, is a leading researcher on cardiovascular nutrition. Penny served on the 2005 Dietary Guidelines Advisory Committee and on the Institute of Medicine Committee of The National Academies of Science to establish macronutrient Dietary Reference Intakes. She is a recognized leader in the American Heart Association and the National Lipid Association.

Cardiovascular disease (CVD) is a group of diseases related to the heart and blood vessels. Many factors increase risk for cardiovascular disease, including heredity, cigarette smoking, physical inactivity, obesity, high blood pressure, and a diet high in saturated fat and trans fats and low in vegetables, fruits and whole grains. Guests, whether looking for foods that will help control cardiovascular diseases or wanting meals that will decrease risk of heart disease, appreciate foodservice operations that provide a wide range of flavorful, appealing foods that meet their unique dietary needs. Culinary professionals have a key role in developing foods that are lower in saturated

fat and trans fats and providing flavorful vegetables, whole grains and fruits.

Arteries become blocked due to a buildup of plaque on their inner walls. This process, known as ***atherosclerosis,*** affects almost everyone to varying degrees. The major dietary causes of plaque formation are saturated fats and trans fats. Obesity, diabetes and hypertension (related to high salt intake) also greatly increase risk factors for cardiovascular disease. Foodservice menu items are often high in calories, salt, saturated fat, trans fat and cholesterol – the very nutritional factors that individuals with cardiovascular disease need to limit. In addition, many foodservice menus offer few sources of soluble fiber, which is an important addition to diets low in saturated fat and cholesterol. Soluble fiber binds some of the cholesterol from food and digestive secretions and increases elimination of cholesterol from the body.

Key Nutrition Points

Patrons with cardiovascular disease, as well as those trying to prevent it, rely on the chef to create healthful dishes. Key menu-planning points for this audience are the same as those for planning a well-balanced diet in general.

- Include plenty of low-calorie menu items and fewer high-calorie items. People with cardiovascular disease are often overweight or obese and need fewer calories.

- Offer smaller portions. Portioning is the simplest way to manage calories. Be mindful of high-fat sauces and dressings.

- Use healthful cooking techniques for most offerings. Limit fried foods and reduce portion sizes of all fried foods offered.

- Use fat moderately throughout the menu. Substitute other cooking methods for frying wherever possible. If frying is necessary for some foods, serve a small portion as an accompaniment or garnish with foods prepared more healthfully.

- Use less heart-unhealthy fats and oils (butter, cream, bacon fat, meat drippings, saturated margarines and shortenings).

- Use only heart-healthy oils such as olive, grapeseed or canola oils. Use specialty oils (liquid at room temperature) such as nut, herb or spice-flavored oils to incorporate healthy fats in the diet and add flavor while decreasing salt. Other oils recommended by the Dietary Guidelines include safflower oil, sunflower oil, corn oil, soybean oil, peanut oil, and cottonseed oil.

- Unrefined whole-grain foods contain fiber that can help lower blood cholesterol and create a feeling of fullness that helps manage weight.

- Serve more and a greater variety of fruits and vegetables and higher-fiber foods. Pay particular attention to seasoning them without a lot of fat or salt.

- Provide more options for patrons to lighten up calories and fat – for example, light mayonnaise, light dressings or less dressing on salads, vegetable-based pasta sauces, and smaller main course options and dessert portions.

- Serve a bread basket with a variety of whole grain breads, bread sticks and rolls, including some that have vegetables, nuts and/or seeds in or on them.

- Use plenty of fat-free, 1% fat and low-fat dairy products.

- Use fruits and vegetables to increase the volume of the portions served without significantly increasing the calories.

Types of Cardiovascular Disease

Cardiovascular disease is an umbrella term for conditions that affect the heart (cardio) and the arteries (vascular).

- *Arteriosclerosis* is a chronic disease in which thickening, hardening and loss of elasticity of the arterial walls result in impaired blood circulation. It develops with age and with conditions such as hypertension, high blood cholesterol and diabetes.

- *Atherosclerosis* is a type of arteriosclerosis in which plaque causes the clogging or hardening of arteries or blood vessels. *Plaque* is an accumulation of substances including cholesterol, fibrous tissue and calcium.

- *Coronary heart disease*, the progressive reduction of blood supply to the heart muscle due to narrowing or blocking of a coronary artery, can lead to a heart attack.

- *Hypertension*, or high blood pressure, is the force of blood pushing against the walls of arteries as it flows through them.

- *Ischemic stroke* is the sudden death of brain cells in a localized area due to inadequate blood flow caused by pieces of plaque creating a blockage.

The American Heart Association's Life's Simple 7 Steps

For ideal cardiovascular health:

1. Don't Smoke
2. Maintain a Healthy Weight
3. Engage in Regular Physical Activity
4. Eat a Healthy Diet
5. Manage Blood Pressure
6. Take Charge of Cholesterol
7. Keep Blood Sugar at Healthy Levels

The American Heart Association recommends eating a wide variety of nutritious foods daily. Even simple, small changes can make a big difference in living a better life. As part of a healthy diet, an adult consuming 2,000 calories daily should aim for:

- **Fruits and vegetables:** At least 4 to 5 cups a day
- **Fish (preferably oily fish):** At least two 3.5-ounce servings a week
- **Fiber-rich whole grains:** At least three 1-ounce equivalent servings a day
- **Sodium:** Less than 1,500 milligrams a day (1 teaspoon salt contains 2,300 milligrams of sodium)
- **Sugar-sweetened beverages:** No more than 450 calories (36 ounces) a week

Other recommendations:

- **Nuts, legumes and seeds:** At least 4 servings a week
- **Processed meats:** No more than 2 servings a week
- **Saturated fat:** Less than 7% of total energy intake

Source: American Heart Association, http://mylifecheck.heart.org/Multitab.aspx?NavID=3&CultureCode=en-US

- Look for ways to increase food volume, such as incorporating air in recipes. Souffles, angel food cake, meringues and foams have volume without a lot of added calories.
- Include heart-healthy meatless dishes such as appetizers, entrees and side dishes.
- Find ways to include more legumes in the menu.
- Focus on nutrient-rich foods like sweet potatoes instead of white potatoes, berries instead of apples, and spinach salad instead of iceberg lettuce salad.

Best Choices

Moderation and variety are keys to planning, preparing and serving heart-healthy foods. Be creative when planning menu items for guests with cardiovascular disease. Remember that everyone benefits from heart healthy foods – not only those with heart disease. Prevention of heart disease should be a goal for everyone.

- Emphasize fruits and vegetables in menu planning. Make vegetables so scrumptious that patrons will order more. Add more grilled and roasted vegetables; they are delicious and colorful and open up a new world of options for patrons. Incorporate vegetables and fruits in appetizers, entrees, side dishes, breads and desserts. Experts at the 2010 Worlds of Healthy Flavors program at the Culinary Institute of America said that doubling produce usage should be a leading goal of the foodservice industry. [5]
- Serve a variety of whole grains that are naturally low in fat and high in fiber. Include whole-grain breads, rolls and crackers, brown rice, quinoa, barley and cereals. Use flaxseed, wheat germ and oatmeal as ingredients. Even a 50% or 75% whole grain is a better choice than a refined grain. Explore legume and nut flours for healthier crackers and flat breads.

- While fish and poultry are good lean proteins, they are not the only answer to keeping fat and calories under control. Also offer lean lamb, bison, beef and pork. Offer fish dishes (not fried). Use omega-3-rich fish such as salmon, mackerel and herring. Walnuts and flax seeds also are sources of omega-3 fatty acids.

- Serve moderate portions: 4-ounce entrees of lean meat cuts; 5 to 6 ounces of poultry; 6 to 8 ounces of fish. Portions of heart-healthy foods can be larger than less healthful items.

- Serve legumes, peas, beans, lentils and soy products as protein sources. They are low in fat and contain no cholesterol. Feature plant proteins prepared using high-flavor techniques from various world cuisines. These foods add health benefits including fiber and reduce food costs.

- Serve low-fat and nonfat dairy products and use them liberally as ingredients.

- As noted, use plant oils that are healthy and unsaturated, such as those from canola, soy, peanuts, olives, fish, nuts, seeds, avocados and whole grains.

- Shift the balance in composite salads by replacing or using only small amounts of croutons, cheese, bacon and dressings. Avocado is high in heart-healthy fat, so it can be used moderately.

- Serve balsamic vinegar, olive oil, marinara sauce, pesto, hummus or bean dips for bread, rather than butter.

- If ground meat or sausage is used, choose lower-fat, lower-salt varieties and use small portions.

- Use plenty of egg whites and moderate amounts of whole eggs. (Egg yolks are rich in cholesterol.) Pair eggs with healthful ingredients such as whole grains, low-fat dairy products, vegetables, nuts, seeds, legumes and healthful fats.

Foods to Limit

Calorie-dense foods should be served in small portions. Limit:

- All fried foods – chips, doughnuts, fried vegetables, fried chicken or fish, French fries, etc.

- Salad dressings. Offer dressing "on the side" so guests can control it. Make salad dressings with liquid vegetable oils. Use small amounts of cheese, croutons or fried anything on salads.

- Soups, dips and sauces made with cream or sour cream or roux-based thickeners

- Bacon, hot dogs and sausage. Substitute Canadian bacon, turkey sausage or lean pork to cut fat and sodium.

- Prime grade or high-fat cuts of meat such as short ribs, brisket, spare ribs and rib-eye

- Doughnuts, sweet rolls, croissants, biscuits and other high-fat breads

- Refined grains and added sugars, including table sugar, sweetened beverages and syrups

- Butter, lard, high-fat dairy products, hydrogenated oils or shortenings, and coconut, palm, cottonseed and palm kernel oils

- Organ meats, such as liver and especially foie gras

Sources of Soluble Fiber

Apples, pears, bananas, berries, prunes

Broccoli, carrots

Legumes, soy products, peas, beans

Oats, barley

Potatoes, yams and root vegetables

Tips for Chefs

Chefs have an important opportunity to make a difference in the cardiovascular health of Americans. Here are a few tips:

- Reduce unhealthy fats and salt to the lowest level that yields excellent flavor and functionality. Use healthy fats prudently so as not to markedly increase calories..

- Use reduced-sodium sauces (soy sauce) and bases routinely.

- Pay attention to sodium, saturated fat, trans fat and total calories. Offer more plant-based entrees with fruits and vegetables, whole grains and legumes.

- Don't be afraid of seasonings when preparing lean or low-fat food items. Boost flavors with aromatic herbs or spices that do not add salt.

- Encourage shared desserts or offer mini-desserts. Include fruit as a dessert option.

- Use a range of cooking techniques for fruits such as poaching, grilling and roasting.

- Use smaller plates, bowls and glasses to serve food and beverages so moderate portions do not look skimpy.

Larger colorful veggie portions show people how a plate can be full and the meal filling and pleasing with the same favorite foods in adjusted portions. Patients tell me they tire of yellow squash and zucchini and want to see more veggie options on menus. I believe red and green foods should be on every plate! I tell my patients, "Red and green keep your arteries clean." I also suggest delectable sharp cheeses in small amounts. If you use cheese creatively for flavor, you can use less and have a powerful taste!

Georgia Kostas, MPH, RD, LD
Georgia Kostas & Associates

For More Information

- American Heart Association, www.americanheart.org

- American Heart Association. *The New American Heart Association Cookbook, 8th Edition.* New York: Clarkson Potter/Publishers; 2010.

- Kostas G. *The Cooper Clinic Solution to the Diet Revolution: Step Up to the Plate!* Dallas: Good Health Press; 2009. www.georgiakostas.com

Hypertension

ESSENTIALS EXPERT

Georgia Kostas, MPH, RD, LD, is a consulting nutritionist, speaker, author and president of Georgia Kostas & Associates, Inc. in Dallas, Texas. She is a cardiovascular and preventive medicine registered dietitian who focuses on weight management, wellness and health promotion through nutrition and fitness. In her 25 years as director of nutrition at the Cooper Clinic, she has counseled more than 25,000 people. Georgia is an innovator who believes the chef–dietitian team is key to demonstrating that healthy can be delicious.

Blood pressure is the force of blood pushing against the walls of arteries as it flows through them. When blood pressure is measured, two numbers are reported: systolic and diastolic pressures. **Systolic** is the pressure created when the heart beats while pumping blood. **Diastolic** is the pressure created when the heart is at rest between beats. Blood pressure numbers are written with the systolic number above or before the diastolic – for example, 120/80 mmHg. (The mmHg stands for "millimeters of mercury," the units used to measure blood pressure.) Healthy resting blood pressure is 120 over 80 or below.

Blood Pressure Levels in Adults

Category	Systolic (top number)	Diastolic (bottom number)
Normal	Less than 120	Less than 80
Pre-hypertension	120 - 139	80 - 89
High blood pressure Stage 1 Stage 2	 140 - 159 160 or higher	 90 - 99 100 or higher

Source: American Heart Association, www.americanheart.org/presenter.jhtml?identifier=4450

High blood pressure can be caused by many factors including genetics, smoking, stress, weight, diet and inactivity. The body's sodium level is a major factor regulating blood pressure. Sodium helps maintain fluid and **electrolyte balance** in the body and also helps regulate heartbeat. While some dietary sodium (about 200 milligrams per day) is essential for life and health, dietary excesses create problems.

Reducing sodium in the diet generally reduces blood pressure, but the American public really enjoys sodium-rich foods. Culinary professionals are challenged to prepare lower-sodium, flavorful foods that can help diners control their sodium intake. Chefs are the experts on developing flavor in foods while reducing dependency on salt and high-sodium ingredients. Because much of our sodium comes from processed foods, chefs have an advantage when using less-processed foods and ingredients.

Key Nutrition Points

- The report of the *Dietary Guidelines for Americans, 2010* advises Americans to try to consume only 1,500 milligrams of sodium per day. Since average consumption is about three times the recommended level, a significant reduction is needed for optimal health. The American Heart Association also recommends 1,500 milligrams daily. [6]

- In 2006, the American Medical Association recommended a minimum 50% reduction in the amount of sodium in processed foods, fast food products and restaurant meals to be achieved over the next decade. [7]

- While some foods are naturally rich in sodium, most sodium in the typical diet comes from salt (sodium chloride) added during food processing or preparation. More than 75% of sodium in the American diet comes from processed food. [8]

- The DASH (Dietary Approaches to Stop Hypertension) eating plan is a heart healthy, nutrient-rich diet based on research supported by the National Heart, Lung and Blood Institute. Adherence to the DASH diet requires eating whole, fresh or frozen foods and only a few processed products, which provides a sodium intake of less than 2,300 milligrams/day. Research supporting the DASH diet shows that individuals can reduce blood pressure further if they limit sodium to 1,500 milligrams per day. Following the DASH diet for six weeks lowers systolic blood pressure 8 to 14 points (mm Hg) – as much as medications! [9]

- Some restaurant main courses contain more than 3,000 milligrams of sodium per serving, more than twice the recommended daily limit in one food item.

- Because high blood pressure increases the risk of chronic diseases that contribute to healthcare costs, reducing sodium has become a major public health issue. With research showing the benefits of reducing dietary sodium and with increased regulatory pressures, the foodservice industry needs to find ways to meet the challenge of reducing salt and other sodium sources in food. [10]

Daily Nutrient Goals Used in the DASH Studies
For a 2,100-Calorie Eating Plan

Total fat	27% of calories
Saturated fat	6% of calories
Protein	18% of calories
Carbohydrate	55% of calories
Cholesterol	150 milligrams
Sodium	2,300 milligrams*
Potassium	4,700 milligrams
Calcium	1,250 milligrams
Magnesium	500 milligrams
Fiber	30 grams

*1,500 mg sodium was a lower goal tested and found to be even better for lowering blood pressure. It was particularly effective for middle-aged and older individuals, African Americans, and those who already had high blood pressure.

Source: DASH Eating Plan, www.nhlbi.nih.gov/health/public/heart/hbp/dash/new_dash.pdf

National Salt Reduction Initiative

The National Salt Reduction Initiative (NSRI) is a partnership of more than 85 state and local health authorities and national health organizations coordinated by the New York City Health Department. This effort is committed to reducing population salt intake by at least 20% by 2014 by setting targets and monitoring progress through a transparent, public process. Voluntary targets for salt levels have been set in 62 categories of packaged food and 25 categories of restaurant food to guide salt reductions in 2012 and 2014.

The NSRI applauds the restaurants that have committed to reduce salt in their menu items to meet the NSRI restaurant food targets and encourages all restaurants and foodservice companies to follow their example. The following companies have agreed to work toward restaurant food targets:

- Au Bon Pain
- Bertucci's Italian Restaurant
- McCain Foods
- Starbucks Coffee Company
- Subway®
- Uno Chicago Grill

The following are a few of the companies that have agreed to pursue one or more NSRI targets for packaged food:

- Boar's Head Provisions Co.
- Butterball
- Campbell Soup Company
- Goya Foods
- Hain Celestial
- Heinz
- Kraft Foods
- McCain Foods
- Red Gold, Inc.
- Unilever

Targets for sodium levels in various food categories set for 2014. No menu item should be over 1,200 milligrams sodium/serving.

Soup	280 mg sodium/100 grams
Hamburgers	330 mg sodium/100 grams
Sandwiches	370 mg sodium/100 grams
Cheese pizza	390 mg sodium/100 grams

Source: National Salt Reduction Initiative. www.nyc.gov/health/salt

The DASH Diet: Dietary Approaches to Stop Hypertension

Foods	Recommended Servings
Whole grains	6 - 8 per day (each is ½ cup or 1 slice bread)
Fruits and vegetables	8 - 10 per day (4 - 5 cups total)
Fat-free or low-fat dairy	2 - 3 per day (2 - 3 cups total)
Lean meat, poultry, fish	6 ounces or less per day
Nuts, seeds and beans	4 - 5 per week (½ cup beans or 1 ounce of nuts is 1 serving)
Fats and oils	2 - 3 small servings per day (2 - 3 teaspoons)
Sweets	5 or fewer per week
Sodium	1,500 or 2,400 milligrams per day (1,500 milligrams recommended for individuals with hypertension)

Source: DASH Eating Plan, www.nhlbi.nih.gov/health/public/heart/hbp/dash/new_dash.pdf

Best Choices

- More unprocessed foods that are naturally low in sodium (fruits, vegetables, whole grains and dry beans)

- Fresh or frozen vegetables. Avoid canned vegetables with added salt.

- Desserts with fruits as the base. Fruits are naturally high in potassium and antioxidants, and low in saturated fat, trans fat, cholesterol and sodium. Use dried fruits, nuts and nut flour to add flavor and texture without a lot of added sugar.

- Plain rice or brown rice, noodles, and whole grains not seasoned with mixes that contain sodium but rather with sauteed mushrooms, onions, dried fruits, nuts and herbs

- Fresh and frozen fruits, including sorbets and fruit ices

- Most beverages, except vegetable juices and sports drinks

- Low-fat or nonfat dairy products

- High-fat foods and ingredients in moderation. Switch the balance from a rich dessert with a fruit garnish to bite-sized desserts or a fruit dessert with a small cookie, meringue or brownie.

- Fresh foods and packaged foods that are unsalted, no salt added, sodium-free or low-sodium

- Healthful cooking techniques

- Foods low or moderate in calories to assist with weight control

- Herbs, spices, aromatics, and lemon juice and zest to season foods without salt

Potassium and High Blood Pressure

The *Dietary Guidelines* report that potassium intake is low enough to be a public health concern for both adults and children. The guidelines recommend choosing foods that provide more potassium, which is found in vegetables, fruits, whole grains, beans and peas, and milk and milk products.

Dietary potassium can lower blood pressure by blunting the adverse effects of sodium. Other possible benefits of eating a diet rich in potassium include a reduced risk of developing kidney stones and decreased bone loss. The recommended intake for potassium for adults is 4,700 milligrams per day. Available evidence suggests that African Americans and individuals with hypertension especially benefit from increasing their intake of potassium.

Foods to Limit

- Salt and seasoned salts

- High-sodium ingredients such as spice blends, soy sauce, MSG (monosodium glutamate), anchovies, olives and capers, pickles, steak sauce, barbeque sauce, Worcestershire sauce, most Asian sauces, and any ingredient that is pickled, brined, smoked or cured

- All processed foods (including processed cheese) that are high in sodium. Choose natural sharp cheeses that can be used in smaller amounts.

- Salted or cured foods, such as ham, bacon, hot dogs, olives, corned beef and smoked salmon

- Breaded fish, poultry and meats

- Prepared mixes for stuffing and breading

- Broths or bases containing salt or sodium in any form

- Most cheeses (check labels), canned soups, snack foods, chips, crackers, salted nuts and popcorn

- Dried soup mixes and bouillon cubes

Tips for Chefs

- Omit or reduce salt used in food preparation. Pay particular attention to enhancing flavor without sodium-rich ingredients. Focus on flavors from spices, herbs and aromatics and on flavor-building techniques from world cuisines.

- Describe healthful foods in ways that stimulate the senses. Try the "stealth health" strategy – present healthful, full-flavored foods but don't label them as "healthy" on the menu. Have nutrition information available upon request.

- Use lots of fresh herbs, unsalted seasoning blends, spices and aromatic ingredients to boost flavor without salt, including Kitchen Bouquet® and Angostura Bitters®.

- Prepare food with olive oil or canola oil when possible. Corn, peanut and other oils are also unsalted.

- Have oil and vinegar, fruit juice, or fruit infusions available for making an unsalted salad dressing.

- Always read labels and check for listed sodium content.

For More Information

- How to Understand and Use the Nutrition Facts Label, www.fda.gov/Food/LabelingNutrition/ConsumerInformation/ucm078889.htm

- National Heart Lung and Blood Institute, www.nhlbi.nih.gov

- Your Guide to Lowering Blood Pressure with DASH, www.nhlbi.nih.gov/health/public/heart/hbp/dash/new_dash.pdf

- Your Guide to Lowering Blood Pressure, www.nhlbi.nih.gov/health/public/heart/hbp/hbp_low/hbp_low.pdf

- *American Heart Association Low-Salt Cookbook*, 3rd edition. New York: Clarkson-Potter Publisher; 2006.

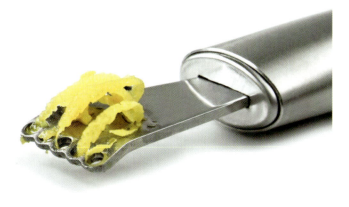

Cancer

ESSENTIALS EXPERT

Donna L. Weihofen, MS, RD, *is senior clinical nutritionist at the University of Wisconsin Carbone Cancer Center in Madison, Wisconsin. Her main areas of expertise are the role of food and nutrition in the prevention of cancer and nutritional care as part of cancer treatment. Donna is the author of five books and has done hundreds of broadcast and print interviews throughout the country. She says, "One of my favorite activities is creating new recipes for my television programs and testing them out on family and friends. I appear to practice what I teach concerning good nutritional habits, although I am known for my 'sweet tooth.' Being a practical nutritionist, I know that depriving oneself of chocolate can lead to deviant behavior, so I have learned to budget certain essential sweets into a healthy diet."*

Cancer is actually many different diseases caused by many different types of abnormal cells. Thus, it requires many different treatments. Because there are so many types of cancer, it is difficult to predict necessary dietary modifications. In addition, nutrition issues can change during treatment or recovery, after recovery, or while living with advanced cancer. Maintaining good nutritional status is important in all phases of cancer, and chefs can help guests with cancer to enjoy their meals.

"After people are told they have cancer, they are often confused by all the advice they get from the media and well-meaning family and friends," says Donna Weihofen. "They become extremely interested in choosing a healthful diet that will help in dealing with the challenges of fighting cancer and any side effects from cancer treatment. It is important to note that it has not been proven that any special diet or any single food cures cancers, but we do know that healthful diets can keep individuals with cancer in good nutritional status so they can fight cancer and decrease the risk of recurrence."

Many people with cancer adhere to vegetarian, vegan or raw diets. Vegetarian diets include many healthful features and tend to be low in saturated fats and high in fiber, vitamins and phytochemicals. The American Cancer Society states that, "It is not possible to conclude at this time . . . that a vegetarian diet has any special benefits for the prevention of cancer." [11]

For the cancer patient, maintaining a healthy weight is extremely important. Being overweight or gaining excess weight during treatment increases the risk of recurrence, especially for those with breast and prostate cancer. Being underweight or losing weight is also a serious problem during cancer treatment. The patient's goal should be to maintain normal weight. That may mean eating higher-calorie foods and eating small meals more frequently. When dining out, people with cancer may want to order small portions, share their food or take some food home for another meal.

The many side effects of cancer treatment can cause a variety of problems. One issue is early satiety – getting full fast or being able to eat only a few bites at a time. Some cancer patients also have problems with nausea, dry mouth and sores in the mouth. Taste changes can be an issue as well. Food may taste like cardboard or metal due to medications that change the composition of saliva and alter the flavor of food. Radiation and other treatments can alter taste perception and the ability to swallow.

American Cancer Society Guidelines on Nutrition and Physical Activity for Cancer Prevention

Achieve and maintain a healthy weight throughout life.

- Be as lean as possible throughout life without being underweight.
- Avoid excess weight gain at all ages. For those who are overweight or obese, losing even a small amount of weight has health benefits and is a good place to start.
- Get regular physical activity and limit intake of high-calorie foods and drinks as keys to help maintain a healthy weight.

Be physically active.

- Adults: Get at least 150 minutes of moderate intensity or 75 minutes of vigorous intensity activity each week (or a combination of these), preferably spread throughout the week.
- Children and teens: Get at least 1 hour of moderate or vigorous intensity activity each day, with vigorous activity on at least 3 days each week.
- Limit sedentary behavior such as sitting, lying down, watching TV, and other forms of screen-based entertainment.
- Doing some physical activity above usual activities, no matter what one's level of activity, can have many health benefits.

Eat a healthy diet, with an emphasis on plant foods.

- Choose foods and drinks in amounts that help you get to and maintain a healthy weight.
- Limit how much processed meat and red meat you eat.
- Eat at least 2½ cups of vegetables and fruits each day.
- Choose whole grains instead of refined grain products.

If you drink alcohol, limit your intake.

- Drink no more than 1 drink per day for women or 2 per day for men.

Source: American Cancer Society, www.cancer.org

Key Nutrition Points

- Eating a diet rich in fruits and vegetables may reduce a person's risk for cancer because these foods are rich in antioxidants that protect cells from cellular changes and damage. Studies suggest that people who eat lots of vegetables and fruits have lower risk of developing some types of cancer.

- Antioxidants in pill form do not convey the same benefits as food sources of antioxidents.

- Folate is a B vitamin that is thought to reduce cancer risk. Folate is found in fruits, vegetables, whole grains and enriched grain products. Getting enough folate is especially important for people who drink alcoholic beverages.

- The health benefits of allium compounds found in garlic and some other vegetables have been widely publicized. Garlic is being studied for its ability to reduce cancer risk, but there is not enough evidence at this time to support a specific recommendation.

- There is some controversy about the role of soy foods in relation to cancer, particularly breast cancer. The scientific evidence is inconsistent. Most experts agree that women with breast cancer should eat only moderate amounts of soy foods because of its estrogenic/hormonal effects.

- Studies have found a link between alcohol and increased risk of cancer of the mouth, throat, larynx, esophagus, liver, breast and colon. Generally, people living with cancer are advised to limit or avoid alcohol. Moderate consumption is 1 drink per day for women, and no more than 2 for men.

- There is little solid scientific evidence that total fat, type of fat, cholesterol, sugar, fluoride, organic foods, approved food additives or irradiated food has any specific effect on cancer incidence or re-occurrence. These substances may be positive or negative for other health reasons but are statistically unrelated to cancer risk.

- Maintaining a healthy weight may reduce the risk for cancer and is considered a key to preventing cancer recurrence. Being overweight or obese substantially raises the risk for endometrial (uterine), breast, prostate and colorectal cancers.

- Other ways to reduce cancer risk include avoiding tobacco, limiting alcohol use, and avoiding excessive exposure to ultraviolet rays from the sun and tanning beds.

- Physical activity is very important both in preventing many cancers and decreasing risk of cancer reoccurrence.

- A healthful diet may help the person with cancer fight the disease and survive, but this is not the time to be overly concerned about dietary restrictions. Serve whatever will please the guest and meet his/her unique needs.

- Common vitamin and mineral deficiencies experienced by cancer patients include magnesium, potassium, calcium and vitamin D.

Best Choices

A person with cancer may have a limited appetite, so serve as many nutrient-rich foods as possible. Fruits and vegetables are an excellent choice because they contain antioxidants that may help prevent or slow down cancer by protecting cells from abnormal changes. Fruits and vegetables with the most antioxidant power include:

Fruits: blueberries, blackberries, strawberries, cranberries, grapes, cherries, apples, melon, oranges and pomegranates

Vegetables: broccoli, cauliflower, cabbage, Brussels sprouts (all cruciferous vegetables are considered cancer fighters), onions, garlic, spinach, asparagus, peppers, peas, beets, squash, pumpkin, sweet potatoes and tomatoes

The person with cancer who is having difficulty maintaining weight needs nutrient-rich fluids with calories, such as fruit juice, smoothies, milkshakes or lattes made with whole milk. Any liquid counts toward fluid intake. For example, tea (particularly green tea) and coffee are good fluids and also contain antioxidants. Both caffeinated and decaffeinated teas and coffee are fine. Tea has been shown to decrease risks of some cancers and may even slow some cancer cell growth. The suggestion that coffee promotes pancreatic cancer has not been confirmed by new research. In fact, coffee is actually a plant and provides a rich source of antioxidants that may decrease risk of some cancers.

Nutrition-Related Problems of the Cancer Patient

Individuals with cancer may have some of these problems:

- Weight loss and loss of appetite
- Weight gain
- Diarrhea
- Constipation
- Nausea
- Vomiting
- Sore mouth, tongue and throat
- Dry mouth
- Difficulty swallowing
- Feeling full quickly
- Taste changes
- Fluid retention
- Milk or lactose intolerance
- Fatigue

Adapted from: American Cancer Society, Managing Eating Problems Caused by Certain Treatment, www.cancer.org/Treatment/SurvivorshipDuringandAfterTreatment/NutritionforPeoplewithCancer/index

Some people with cancer need very mild foods with very few spices because they have mouth sores. Others who have damaged taste buds may enjoy more spice in their foods. Serve foods with a variety of spice-level options. Offer a balsamic vinegar reduction and a balsamic vinegar/sugar reduction to drizzle on vegetables and other dishes to add flavor and cut through the bad taste in the mouth caused by many cancer medications.

Some medications cause dry mouth, which makes it difficult to chew and swallow. Guests taking these medications need moist, semi-pureed or very soft foods with gravies or sauces. Soups, puddings, custards and flans, eggs, risotto, mashed potatoes and ice cream are easy to chew and swallow. Offer some high-calorie options for those who need to gain or maintain their weight.

The Sugar Myth

A common myth in cancer treatment is that "sugar feeds cancer." In fact, the constant supply of sugar in the blood stream is available to all cells, including cancer cells. Cancer cells will not grow faster if you eat a chocolate chip cookie. When a person with cancer has little appetite, some sugar may help increase caloric intake.

Limit your intake of high sugar foods, but it is not necessary to completely eliminate all sugars from your diet. It is best to eat a food high in sugar within a meal to prevent insulin levels from surging. High sugar food when eaten alone can increase insulin levels and increasing circulating insulin on a regular basis may promote cancer cell growth. Remember, a diet with lots of sugar is not a healthful diet. High sugar foods are usually low in important nutrients and full of empty calories. Choose foods with higher level of nutrients.

Artificial Sweeteners and Cancer

There is no clear evidence that the artificial sweeteners commercially available in the United States are associated with increased cancer risk in humans. Questions about artificial sweeteners and cancer arose when early studies showed that cyclamate, in combination with saccharin and given in huge amounts, caused bladder cancer in laboratory animals. Results from subsequent studies of these sweeteners, however, have not provided evidence of increasing cancer in humans. Similarly, studies of other Food and Drug Administration approved sweeteners have not demonstrated evidence of any association with cancer in humans.

Source: Weihrauch MR, Diehl V. Artificial sweeteners – do they bear a carcinogenic risk? *Ann Oncol.* 2004;15:1460-65.

Foods to Limit

- Some studies have suggested that an increased colorectal and stomach cancer risk is associated with eating lots of red or processed meats.

- The burnt proteins on charred meat can form cancer-promoting compounds called heterocylic amines.

- Processed meats and lunchmeats are made with nitrates, smoke and salt. It is not clear which of these ingredients is a potential cancer-causing agent, so it is wise to limit salt-cured, smoked and nitrate-cured foods.

- Although sweets are not good sources of nutrients and may contribute to unwanted weight gain, it is not necessary for cancer patients to avoid all sugar.

- Eggs served to guests with cancer must be fully cooked. Do not serve foods with uncooked eggs (soft boiled, poached or in salad dressings or soft meringues) unless the eggs are pasteurized.

- Raw meat, seafood, shellfish, sushi or any food that is likely to carry bacteria should be avoided.

Tips for Chefs

- Provide higher-calorie, nutrient-rich foods for cancer patients who are trying to maintain their weight.

- Offer smaller portions. Many cancer patients experience early satiety – getting full quickly or being able to eat only a few bites at a time.

- Provide foods with a range of flavors. Medications may change a cancer patient's taste and alter the flavor of food.

- Serve high-protein foods as a first course, when the guest's appetite is strongest.

- Odors are often bothersome to people with cancer. Try serving foods cold or at room temperature. Hot fragrant foods can sometimes aggravate nausea.

- Serve soft-textured foods. Mouth, tongue and throat sores can result from cancer therapy.

- Adding sugar to some foods can help decrease salty, bitter or unpleasant tastes.

- Tart foods and beverages such as oranges and grapefruit, lemon sorbet, yogurt or lemonade may be appealing.

- Some people with cancer are on raw or juice diets. Although most scientific research does not support this practice, as with all guests, try to provide foods acceptable to their wishes.

- Be particularly careful to avoid serving any food that carries increased risk of bacteria or other contaminants because cancer patients often have compromised immunity.

For More Information

- Center for Disease Control, Division of Cancer Prevention and Control, www.cdc.gov/cancer

- Katz R, Edelson M. *The Cancer-Fighting Kitchen: Nourishing, Big-Flavor Recipes for Cancer Treatment and Recovery.* Berkeley, CA: Celestial Arts; 2009.

- Kushi LH, Byers T, Doyle C, Bandera EV, McCullough M, Gansler T, Andrews KS, Thun MJ, The American Cancer Society 2006 Nutrition and Physical Activity Guidelines Advisory Committee. American Cancer Society Guidelines on Nutrition and Physical Activity for Cancer Prevention. *Cancer Journal for Clinicians.* 2006: 56:254-281. http://caonline.amcancersoc.org/cgi/reprint/56/5/254

- National Cancer Institute, National Institutes of Health, www.cancer.gov

- University of Wisconsin Carbone Cancer Center recipes, www.uwhealth.org/donnasdish

- Weihofen DL. *The Easy-to-Swallow & Easy-to-Chew Cookbook.* New York: John Wiley & Sons; 2002.

Panna Cotta

Donna Weihofen, MS, RD, Senior Clinical Nutritionist,
University of Wisconsin Comprehensive Cancer Center, Madison, Wisconsin

Serves: 6, ½ cup servings

Here is a base recipe for a dessert that can be adapted to varied nutritional needs. Changing ingredients will change the calorie, fat and sugar content according to the needs of your guests. Sugar, Splenda® or Splenda® Sugar Blend can be used for the sweetener. Dairy products range from fat-free half-and-half to heavy cream. The calories in the panna cotta can be as low as 80 or as high as 410 per serving.

Panna cotta is Italian for "cooked cream." It is very similar to the Scandinavian Swedish Cream. This smooth and creamy dessert can be served with nutrient-rich fruits such as blueberries, strawberries, cherries, peaches, plums or citrus fruit or with a simple fruit coulis.

Panna Cotta, base recipe

Unflavored gelatin	1	envelope
Water	2	tablespoons
Dairy	2	cups
Sugar	½	cup
Sour cream	1	cup
Vanilla extract	2	teaspoons

Reduced calorie

Unflavored gelatin	1	envelope
Water	2	tablespoons
Whole milk	2	cups
Sugar or Splenda®	½	cup
Fat-free sour cream	1	cup
Vanilla extract	2	teaspoons

Reduced calorie, fat-free

Unflavored gelatin	1	envelope
Water	2	tablespoons
Fat-free half & half	1	cup
Nonfat milk	1	cup
Sugar or Splenda®	½	cup
Fat-free sour cream	1	cup
Vanilla extract	2	teaspoons

Moderate calorie

Unflavored gelatin	1	envelope
Water	2	tablespoons
Half & half	2	cups
Sugar	½	cup
Sour cream	1	cup
Vanilla extract	2	teaspoons

High calorie

Unflavored gelatin	1	envelope
Water	2	tablespoons
Heavy cream	2	cups
Sugar	½	cup
Sour cream	1	cup
Vanilla extract	2	teaspoons

1. In a medium heavy saucepan, combine gelatin powder and water. Stir to soften gelatin. Add 2-3 tablespoons of dairy and stir to mix.

2. Add remaining dairy and sugar or Splenda®

3. Cook over medium heat while stirring constantly until mixture comes to a boil. Remove from heat and cool until mixture comes to room temperature and just begins to set.

4. Add sour cream and vanilla. Stir to mix well.

5. Portion into individual ramekins or custard cups.

6. Cover and refrigerate until set and ready to serve.

Per Serving

	Calories	Fat (gm)	Sat fat (gm)	Trans fat (gm)	Cholesterol (mg)	Sodium (mg)	Carbohydrates (gm)	Dietary Fiber (gm)	Sugar (gm)	Protein (gm)
Base recipe	180	9	5	0	25	65	22	0	22	4
Reduced calorie with sugar	150	2.5	1.5	0	10.0	100	28	0	21	5
Reduced calorie with Splenda®	100	2.5	1.5	0	10	100	13	0	6	5
Reduced calorie, fat free with sugar	140	0.5	0	0	5	135	29	0	21	5
Reduced calories, fat free with Splenda®	80	0.5	0	0	5	135	14	0	6	5
Moderate calorie	240	16	9	0	45	60	21	0	18	4
High calorie	410	36	22	1	125	60	20	0	18	3

Diabetes

ESSENTIALS EXPERTS

Maggie Powers, PhD, RD, CDE, is a research scientist at the International Diabetes Center at Park Nicollet, in Minneapolis. The author of Handbook of Diabetes Medical Nutrition Therapy, Guide to Eating Right When You Have Diabetes, The American Diabetes Association's Forbidden Foods Cookbook, and many other publications, Maggie is an internationally known diabetes educator. She is a leader in the American Diabetes Association, the American Association of Diabetes Educators and The Academy of Nutrition and Dietetics. Maggie has always been concerned about the "food" side of nutrition therapy. She says that "the best nutrition therapy recommendations don't mean a thing if someone cannot obtain healthy food and enjoy it. Nutrition therapy is based on one's ecology, the system they live in and all of its influences on behaviors. There is a science and art to providing nutrition therapy."

Carolyn Leontos, MS, RD, CDE, is professor emeritus retired, University of Nevada Cooperative Extension in Las Vegas. She is the author of What to Eat When You Get Diabetes and The Diabetes Holiday Cookbook and has been active in the culinary education community. Carolyn loves to cook and travel and continually expand her repertoire of international cuisine.

Diabetes mellitus is a chronic metabolic disease characterized by high blood glucose, also called blood sugar, and insufficient or ineffective insulin. By knowing what persons with diabetes want and need, foodservice professionals can help 26 million people enjoy better health. A primary goal of diabetes care is to help people with the disease attain and maintain a blood glucose level as close to normal as possible. Because carbohydrate is the food component that raises blood glucose levels, people with diabetes need to monitor the amount of carbohydrates they eat by balancing food intake with physical activity and insulin – either their own or injected insulin. Experts recommend distributing carbohydrates fairly evenly thoughout the day – some at each meal and with snacks. People with diabetes should not skip breakfast and lunch and then eat a very large dinner. A quick, appetizing and easy-to-consume snack may be substituted for breakfast or lunch.

When foods, particularly carbohydrates, are eaten, they are digested and absorbed as glucose. Glucose is the energy source for all cells in the body. The body needs the hormone insulin to move glucose from the bloodstream into cells. Individuals with diabetes can increase or decrease blood sugar levels with more or less food and exercise. When blood sugar levels are too low, an individual with diabetes needs a quick source of sugar – often fruit juice. If blood sugar levels are too high, insulin may be injected to prevent medical emergencies.

The person with diabetes either makes too little insulin or is resistant to insulin produced. As a result, blood glucose levels get too high (**hyperglycemia**). This condition can be controlled with medications that boost insulin production, with injections of insulin or with medications that help control blood glucose levels. Early in the development of diabetes, some people can manage their blood glucose by food and exercise alone. Even when medications are added, food and exercise are still important parts of the diabetes management plan. Near-normal blood glucose levels help people feel better and may reduce or prevent the complications of diabetes.

Too much insulin, too little food or unplanned exercise can cause a low blood glucose level (**hypoglycemia**). When blood glucose is too low, a person may be hungry, irritable and feel very weak. This condition can be avoided by having a treatment plan that has been individualized for them so it fits into their food habits, meal times and exercise schedule.

Diabetes is a chronic disease that has several forms based on how much insulin is produced and the level of insulin resistance. Generally, **type 1 diabetes** occurs earlier in life and requires daily insulin injections or an insulin pump. **Type 2 diabetes** is much more common and, until recently, generally occurred later in life. It is reported that one in three children born today will develop type 2 diabetes. This type of diabetes may be controlled by diet, by diet and pills, or by diet and insulin injections. Being overweight and inactive increases the likelihood of developing type 2 diabetes. Early in the condition, small amounts of weight loss and improved food choices are sometimes enough to control blood glucose without medication.

Many people with diabetes use *Choose Your Foods: The Exchange Lists for Diabetes* (6th edition, 2008) developed by the American Diabetes Association and The American Dietetic Association. (See Appendix F: Exchange Lists.) There are seven exchange lists, with foods grouped according to similar numbers of calories, carbohydrates, proteins and fats. The portion size of each food varies so that foods can be exchanged for each other in a predetermined meal plan. The exchange lists are very useful for chefs as a resource for nutrient content and information about food for guests with diabetes.

Another popular resource, *My Food Plan* (4th edition, 2008) developed by the International Diabetes Center, focuses primarily on carbohydrate counting, which some find easier to use than planning for all seven exchange groups. (See Appendix G: Carb Counting.) The list of carbohydrates includes single foods, mixed dishes, snacks and desserts. Portions (choices) are similar; each contains about 15 grams of carbohydrates. *My Food Plan* includes guidance for determining how many carbohydrate choices are best for each meal and snack. Food plans based on a vegetarian diet and several ethnic diets can be found on the International Diabetes Center website, http://www.idcpublishing.com/testimonials.asp.

Many people with diabetes have 2 to 4 more carbohydrate choices (servings) at each meal. One cup of berries (1 choice) and a sandwich made with 2 slices of bread (2 choices) equals 3 carbohydrate choices. A large bagel counts as 4 carbohydrate choices. Self-monitoring of blood glucose (or blood sugar) helps people with diabetes know if they are eating the right amount of carbohydrate.

Key Nutrition Points

- The overall emphasis is on healthful eating. Those with diabetes benefit from eating a variety of food with a basic healthful food plan emphasizing whole grains, fresh food and moderate serving sizes. Their diet should be low in saturated and trans fat since people with diabetes are at a higher risk for developing cardiovascular disease.

- People with diabetes need to manage their carbohydrate intake – how much they consume and when they consume it. Amount and types of food and eating at regular mealtimes are important.

- Healthy eating for people with diabetes is the same as healthful eating for all people and does not necessarily require special "diet" foods. Carbohydrate is the nutrient requiring particular attention. To assist those with diabetes, chefs should offer lower-carbohydrate alternatives, such as spaghetti squash (instead of pasta) with marinara or Bolognese sauce and sandwiches on bread rather than on oversized buns.

- Each person with diabetes should have a meal plan tailor-made to his/her individual needs, food preferences, medications and lifestyle -- preferably planned with a registered dietitian, who may also be a certified diabetes educator. Some professionals recommend counting carbohydrates. Others use the exchange system with certain types and amounts of foods from various food groups at each meal and snack.

- In addition to controlling carbohydrates, people with diabetes should limit sweet, salty and high-fat food. People with diabetes are especially prone to cardiovascular disease and kidney disease.

- Generally, there is relatively little room for added sugar in a diet for a person with diabetes; sweetened food products should be limited because they take the place of more nutrient-rich carbohydrates.

- Sugar substitutes may be useful, especially in beverages. People with diabetes and those controlling their weight expect packets of sugar substitute to be available and appreciate desserts low in sugar. See Chapter 3 for information about sugar substitutes.

- Portions of food for those with diabetes should be quite modest. For those using food exchanges or carbohydrate counting, 1 serving is equal to 15 grams of carbohydrates, which is 1 ounce of bread, ½ English muffin, ½ tortilla, or ⅓ cup of rice or pasta. A modest 1 cup of plain pasta counts as 3 servings for someone with diabetes. The typical serving of meat should be a 3 to 4 ounce portion.

- People with diabetes can consume a delicious-looking dessert or have jelly on their toast and be well within their eating guidelines. Unfortunately, some people judge what someone with diabetes is eating based on outdated information.

- Some guests will decline a bread basket or ask for an open-faced sandwich to avoid consuming extra carbohydrates. Offering a salad with the dressing on the side or a steamed or grilled vegetable in place of potatoes is a thoughtful substitution. Including a broth-based soup on the menu gives the person with diabetes a food option when others are having a high-fat, high-carbohydrate appetizer.

Best Choices

There are very few differences between a diabetic diet and the healthy diet of someone without diabetes. Food for patrons with diabetes should be as enjoyable as food for any guest. Just be sure to have a variety of items on the menu that are low in calories, carbohydrates and fat so that guests with diabetes have a full range of choices. Generally, foods promoted in *MyPlate* are best choices for those with diabetes.

- Several food items or dishes that are low in carbohydrates should be available so guests with diabetes can manage their intake and still have choices within each menu category.

- The best food choices are those that don't have hidden fat or carbohydrate and thus allow the guest to make an informed choice. For example, many restaurants will make mashed potatoes with lots of added fat. A little extra fat is acceptable, but too often it can be quite high. It is helpful to offer simple foods – vegetables with no added fat (or less than 1 teaspoon per serving) and desserts with no added sugar such as fresh cut fruit. If the clientele includes many diners with diabetes, offering sugar-free gelatin with some berries would be a good menu addition.

- Foods prepared without added fat or with just enough fat to maintain a flavorful presentation are best. Because total calories are an important issue for them, people with diabetes are encouraged to eat plenty of low-carbohydrate vegetables in salads, side dishes, entrees and soups. Fill the plate with low-carbohydrate vegetables such as green beans, broccoli or asparagus simply steamed, roasted or grilled.

- Because individuals with diabetes are frequently seeking a 3- to 4-ounce protein source, appetizers such as crab cakes or chicken skewers are good entree choices.

Foods to Avoid

Virtually all foods can be worked into a diabetes food plan, even if in a small amount. There are some foods, however, that people with diabetes should avoid because they are easy to overeat and very high in carbohydrates. These foods include sugared beverages such as sodas, punches, ades, juices and sweet tea (containing regular sugar). People with diabetes are encouraged to avoid high-calorie foods and foods high in fat, especially saturated and trans fat.

People with diabetes who want to eat high-sugar foods such as regular jam, regular syrup or a dessert, can certainly do so and enjoy it, but they also must be aware of how much carbohydrate they are consuming and adjust for it in the same or other meals or snacks.

Tips for Chefs

- Be creative! Help your customers savor the taste of fresh food that blends textures and taste using lot of vegetables, legumes, fruit and whole grains. Offer "fillers" that don't add carbohydrates and fat.

- One of the most important steps you can take to help people with diabetes and anyone seeking healthful food is to reduce portion sizes. List the size or ounces of the piece of meat, chicken or fish so that guests know how much they are getting. Offer low-fat, low-calorie side dishes and salad dressings and sauces on the side so that guests can control the amount they use. Remember that people who have diabetes do not need special foods; however, they do need reasonable options from which to choose.

- Cook with as little fat and sugar as possible.

- Offer at least one green salad with interesting vegetables, fresh fruit, and herbs but without croutons, bacon and other high-fat ingredients. Have a low-fat dressing or oil and vinegar available. Dress salads lightly.

- Have fresh berries, sliced melon or other fresh, ripe, delicious fruits available as a dessert option. Fresh fruit is a good menu addition for those on almost any special diet, for those watching their weight and for kids.

- An appetizer of hummus with crudités – fairly low in carbohydrate and fat, crunchy, and tasty – helps decrease hunger.

- Provide packets of a calorie-free sweetener so guests can sweeten beverages without adding sugar.

- If a hostess or server is told that a guest with diabetes must eat soon, react quickly. Bring a glass of fruit juice and ask what else to bring to avoid an emergency caused by low blood sugar.

For More Information

- American Diabetes Association, www.diabetes.org
- Leontos C. *What to Eat When You Get Diabetes*. New York: John Wiley & Sons; 2000.
- Mills, J. *1000 Diabetes Recipes*. Hoboken, NJ: John Wiley & Sons, Inc., 2011.
- National Center for Chronic Disease Prevention and Health Promotion, www.cdc.gov/diabetes
- National Institute of Diabetes and Digestive and Kidney Diseases, www2.niddk.nih.gov
- Powers M. *American Dietetic Association Guide to Eating Right When You Have Diabetes*. New York: John Wiley & Sons; 2003.
- Powers M, Hendley J. *Forbidden Foods Diabetes Cooking*. Alexandria, VA: American Diabetes Association; 2000.
- Smith C. *The Diabetic Chef's Year Round Cookbook*. Alexandria, VA: American Diabetes Association; 2008.
- Warshaw H. *Diabetes Meal Planning Made Easy*, 4th ed. Alexandria, VA: American Diabetes Association; 2010.

Blueberry Cobbler

Carolyn Leontos, MS, RD, CDE, Professor Emeritus Retired,
University of Nevada Cooperative Extension, Las Vegas, Nevada

Yield: 12 servings

To accommodate individuals with diabetes who want fewer calories, bake with Splenda® or another non-nutritive sweetener that withstands heat. Splenda® Sugar Blend adds some calories, but the sugar in the blend enhances the texture and color of the crust.

Blueberries, fresh or frozen	2 pounds
Flour, all-purpose	2 tablespoons
Splenda® or Splenda® Sugar Blend or the equivalent amount of other non-nutritive sweetener	⅜ cup ... ¾ cup
All purpose flour	1 ½ cups
Baking powder	1 tablespoon
Salt	¾ teaspoon
Splenda® or Splenda® Sugar Blend or the equivalent amount of other non-nutritive sweetener	3 tablespoons
1% milk	1 ¼ cups
Oil, vegetable	5 tablespoons

1. Preheat oven to 400° F.

2. Let blueberries thaw, if frozen. Mix 2 tablespoons flour and ¾ cup sweetener into the blueberries. Put blueberry mixture into individual ramekins sprayed with non-stick spray. Do not overfill, as mixture will bubble up in oven.

3. Mix 1 ½ cups flour, baking powder, salt and 3 tablespoons sweetener. Add milk and oil to flour mixture and mix just until dry ingredients are moistened. Mixture will be thin and lumpy. Spoon dough onto berry mixture. Bake 30-35 minutes until crust is golden brown.

Blueberry Cobbler made with Splenda®

Carb Choices: 1 ½

Diabetic Exchanges: ½ starch + 1 fruit + 1 fat

Blueberry Cobbler made with Splenda® Blend

Carb Choices: 2

Diabetic Exchanges: 1 starch + 1 fruit + 1 fat

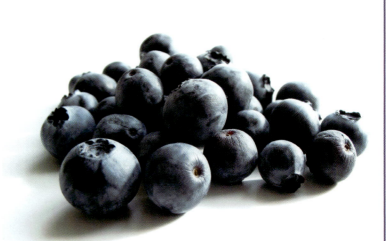

Per Serving

	Calories	Fat (gm)	Sat fat (gm)	Trans fat (gm)	Cholesterol (mg)	Sodium (mg)	Carbohydrates (gm)	Dietary Fiber (gm)	Sugar (gm)	Protein (gm)
with Splenda®	170	7	1	0	0	280	25	3	9	3
with Splenda® blend	190	7	1	0	0	280	30	3	14	3

Breakfast Spinach Strata

Maggie Powers, PhD, RD, CDE, Research Scientist,
International Diabetes Center at Park Nicollet, Minneapolis, Minnesota

Serves: 10

The breakfast strata is a way to add a variety of vegetables to the morning meal. This strata uses spinach. Other vegetables that would work well include asparagus, portabello mushrooms, red peppers, onions, broccoli, kale or butternut squash. Serve with a red pepper coulis if desired.

Olive oil . . . . .1 tablespoon

Spinach, fresh, chopped . . . . .10 ounces

Garlic clove, minced. . . . . .1 each

Eggs . . . . .10 each
OR egg substitute . . . . .2 ½ cups

Low-fat milk . . . . .2 cups

Whole grain bread, cubed,
day old . . . . .10 slices

Pepper Jack cheese,
shredded . . . . .4 ounces

1. Spray individual ramekins with nonstick cooking spray. Alternatively use an 8 cup baking pan.

2. Heat olive oil in a pan. Saute spinach and garlic until spinach is wilted.

3. In a medium bowl, whisk the eggs until frothy. Add the milk and bread. Let stand for 5 minutes. Add the spinach and cheese and stir to blend. Pour into the prepared ramekins. Cover and refrigerate 8 hours or overnight.

4. Preheat the oven to 350° F.

5. Bake the strata, uncovered, until the top is lightly browned, about 30 minutes. Serve hot or at room temperature.

Carb choices: 1

Diabetic Exchanges: 1 medium fat meat + ½ starch

Per Serving			
Calories	210	Cholesterol	190 mg
Fat	10 g	Sodium	250 mg
Saturated Fat	4 g	Carbohydrates	16 mg
Trans Fat	0 g	Dietary Fiber	5 mg
Sugar	5 g	Protein	13 g

Adapted from: Powers, M and Hendley J. *Forbidden Foods Diabetic Cooking*. Alexandria, VA : American Diabetes Association; 2000.

Digestive Disorders

ESSENTIALS EXPERT

Leslie Bonci, MPH, RD, LDN, CSSD, director of sports nutrition at the University of Pittsburgh Medical Center, is the dietitian for the Pittsburgh Steelers, Pittsburgh Penguins, Pittsburgh Pirates, Pittsburgh Ballet Theatre and Milwaukee Brewers. Leslie is a board-certified specialist in sports nutrition and consults for both the Women's National Basketball Association and the National Collegiate Athletic Association. Leslie has also contributed to The American Dietetic Association's Sports Nutrition Manual and is a veteran textbook author.

Digestion is the process by which food and drink are reduced to smaller nutrient units that can be absorbed into the bloodstream and carried throughout the body to build and nourish cells and to provide energy. **Absorption** is the passage of these molecules through the walls of the digestive tract so the substances can enter the bloodstream and then enter cells. **Metabolism** is the chemical activity within cells that breaks down nutrients to provide energy, uses nutrients to build necessary compounds and tissues, and releases the end products.

Organs that make up the digestive tract are the mouth, esophagus, stomach, small intestine, large intestine (or colon), rectum and anus. Inside these hollow organs is a lining called the **mucosa**. In the mouth, stomach and small intestine, the mucosa contains tiny glands that produce digestive juices to help break down the food. The digestive tract also contains a layer of smooth muscle that helps break down food and move it along the tract. Two solid digestive organs, the liver and the pancreas, produce digestive juices that reach the intestine through small tubes called ducts. The gallbladder stores the liver's digestive juices until they are needed in the intestine. Parts of the nervous and circulatory systems also play major roles in the digestive system.

Digestive disorders include diseases such as diverticulitis, celiac disease, ulcers, gastric reflux (GERD), irritable bowel syndrome, hepatitis, ulcerative colitis, Crohn's disease, dyspepsia, functional heartburn and chronic constipation. Each affects different parts of the digestive system. In ulcerative colitis for example, the colon is inflamed but the small intestine works normally. Crohn's disease affects the small intestine, making it difficult to digest and absorb nutrients.

In all digestive disorders, alterations in taste, poor nutrient utilization, pain, decreased appetite and the inflammatory process can lead to weight loss and malnutrition. With recurrent diarrhea, the risk for anemia and vitamin deficiencies rises. Small, frequent meals of foods that can be tolerated minimize symptoms. Gastrointestinal problems tend to reduce the efficiency of nutrient absorption, so a nutrient-dense diet is advisable. Adequate liquids are necessary to prevent dehydration.

The Digestive Tract

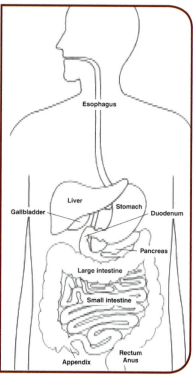

Source: National Institute of Diabetes and Digestive and Kidney Diseases, http://digestive.niddk.nih.gov/ddiseases/pubs/yrdd/index.htm

Diverticulitis is an inflammation of small pouches in the lining of the large intestine. Fecal matter becomes trapped in these pouches if the diet does not have adequate fiber. Symptoms include abdominal cramping, painful spasms, distention, nausea and fever. The treatment is bowel rest with a temporary low-residue liquid diet followed by a low-fiber, low-residue diet. When symptoms disappear, high-fiber foods are introduced and lots of water is generally recommended.

Irritable Bowel Syndrome (IBS) is a common disorder causing abdominal pain, bloating and changes in bowel habits. Crohn's disease and ulcerative colitis are two types of IBS. In IBS, the colon is very sensitive and may contract causing pain and diarrhea, or it may fail to contract causing severe constipation and pain. Sometimes bacterial infections cause IBS.

Crohn's disease is an inflammation of the small intestine that makes digestion and the absorption of key nutrients difficult and painful. It causes bloating, diarrhea, abdominal pain and cramping and can lead to malnutrition, anemia and low levels of certain vitamins and folic acid. Although the disease is an immune reaction in the intestinal tract, avoiding certain foods that "trigger" the painful symptoms is important. With Crohn's disease, eating regular meals and additional snacks throughout the day ensures that an ample supply of key nutrients is getting into the digestive tract. Doctors usually recommend vitamin and mineral supplements to replenish losses. Once a person determines what foods cause symptoms to flare up, the troublesome foods can be avoided or prepared in a different manner.

People with *ulcerative colitis* (ulcerations in the colon/large intestine) should eat at regular times and eliminate alcohol, carbonated beverages, caffeine, dairy products and other foods that trigger reactions. Probiotics, such as yogurt, and adjusting levels of dietary fiber may be recommended, depending on symptoms.

Acid reflux, also called heartburn, or GERD (gastroesophageal reflux disease), occurs when the sphincter between the esophagus and stomach relaxes and food comes back up after it has been mixed with stomach acids. Foods that tend to stimulate stomach acid production and increase heartburn

Antibiotics and Gut Health

During and after taking antibiotics, many people experience some gastrointestinal distress. Oral antibiotics destroy the normal bacteria in the digestive tract that promote proper digestion and absorption. Eating probiotics, such as yogurt and foods with live active cultures (living microorganisms), helps repopulate the gut with "friendly bacteria." As a result, symptoms subside. Many people eat yogurt and other probiotics daily to promote gut health and avoid digestive disorders. Yogurts needs to have live active cultures to be beneficial - frozen yogurt and yogurt candies do not have live active cultures.

include caffeinated and carbonated beverages, alcohol, spicy foods, black pepper, citrus fruits and juices, and tomato juice. All high-fat foods and chocolate tend to relax the sphincter, often causing heartburn. Eating small frequent meals and not eating close to bedtime can help reduce heartburn.

An *ulcer* is a sore, an open painful wound. *Peptic ulcers* occur in the stomach or upper part of the small intestine. For almost 100 years, it was believed that ulcers were caused by spicy foods, stress and alcohol. Now we know that peptic ulcers are caused by a particular bacterial infection *(Helicobacter pylori)*, by certain medications or by smoking. Physicians Barry Marshall and Robin Warren received a Nobel Prize for this discovery in 1982. The formation of ulcers seems to require both *H. pylori* and over-secretion of stomach acids, which irritate the lining of the stomach. The treatment is typically antibiotics and antacids. Any food that specifically causes distress may be eliminated, but a bland diet is no longer the recommended treatment for peptic ulcers.

Key Nutrition Points

- Often foods that are too rich or very high in fat will cause digestive distress because there are not enough digestive enzymes or bile to break down the fat to molecules that can be absorbed.

- Very spicy foods can cause discomfort when they irritate the lining of the digestive tract.

- Too much acid, as in raw or lightly cooked tomatoes, can be a problem for some people. Using a tomato sauce instead of raw tomatoes may alleviate this problem.

- Individuals vary greatly in their ability to digest different types of food. This variability has to do with the amount of secretions (particularly digestive enzymes), the condition of the membranes within the digestive tract, and the presence of normal bacteria that help break down foods for absorption.

- When the amount of food eaten exceeds the digestive tract's ability to break it down efficiently, the result is gastrointestinal distress. Bloating, burping or belching, cramping and abdominal pain, gas and diarrhea are common symptoms of gastrointestinal distress.

- Getting enough fiber in the diet is important to promote regular elimination and also to help rid the body of excess cholesterol. If the body has difficulty breaking down food for any reason, gastrointestinal distress results and nutrients are poorly absorbed.

- Certain high-fiber foods, such as bran or flax seeds, may increase gas production and bloating. Gas-producing fiber is usually insoluble (mainly found in cereals or whole grains). Soluble fiber, mainly found in vegetables and fruits, is less likely to cause gastrointestinal distress. Certain foods, such as beans, cabbage, legumes (peas, peanuts and soybeans), and sometimes apples, melons, grapes and raisins may produce gas in the lower bowel. Bacteria in the colon ferment undigested particles of food, which causes flatulence (gas) and distress.

Best Choices

- Most Americans do not eat enough fiber. Adding high-fiber vegetables, fruits, grains, legumes, seeds and nuts to the menu is desirable – unless fibers cause distress.

- People with gastrointestinal diseases have especially sensitive digestive tracts. Small meals are usually best for them because large portions of food can trigger symptoms. Adequate protein intake is important; lean proteins are preferred.

- Live active cultures in buttermilk, yogurt and other foods promote gastrointestinal health and generally aid digestion. Use these foods as ingredients in cooking and when making smoothies, dips, sauces and salad dressings.

- Ginger is a gut-friendly spice and ginger tea is a soothing beverage that can alleviate nausea for many people with gastrointestinal problems. Freshly grated ginger and crystallized ginger add a lot of flavor and are versatile ingredients.

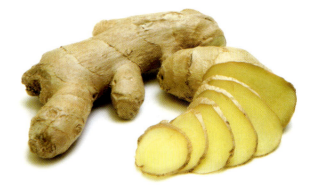

Foods to Avoid

- There is no scientifically proven diet for inflammatory bowel disease. Each person with IBS has his/her own trigger foods. The guest will know what foods he or she must avoid and should be able to order accordingly. Often-reported trigger foods include:

  - Alcohol-containing beverages

  - Butter, oil and other fats

  - Carbonated beverages

  - Coffee and tea

  - Chocolate

  - Cornhusks

  - Gas-producing foods

  - High-fiber foods such as raw fruits and vegetables and bran

  - Red meat and pork

  - Spicy foods

  - Nuts and seeds

- If a primary digestive disorder symptom is flatulence that causes pain, it helps to limit gas-causing foods. People with this problem generally know which foods to avoid – for example, cruciferous vegetables and legumes, specifically mature beans and peas.

- For some people, flaxseeds are an irritant. Other seeds and nuts can also irritate the villi in the lining of the intestines.

- Large volumes of food in the gastrointestinal tract can trigger symptoms such as bloating, abdominal discomfort and diarrhea.

Tips for Chefs

Guests with irritable bowel syndrome, Crohn's disease, celiac disease and other gastrointestinal disorders usually know which foods trigger symptoms and order foods accordingly. They may ask if foods have specific ingredients that they must avoid. Servers should be prepared to answer these questions.

For More Information

- Bonci L. *American Dietetic Association Guide to Better Digestion.* Chicago: The American Dietetic Association; 2003.

- International Foundation for Functional Gastrointestinal Disorders (IFFGD), **www.iffgd.org**

- Magge E. *Tell Me What to Eat If I Have Irritable Bowel Syndrome.* Franklin Lakes, NJ: Career Press; 2000.

- *Mayo Clinic on Digestive Health,* 2nd ed. Rochester, MN: Mayo Clinic Trade Publishing; 2004.

- The National Institute of Diabetes and Digestive and Kidney Diseases, **www2.niddk.nih.gov**

- Raman M, Sirounis A, Shrubsole J. *The Complete IBS Health and Diet Guide.* Toronto, Canada: Robert Rose, 2011.

Wild Rice Salad

Provided by **Leslie Bonci, MPH, RD, LDN, CSSD,**
Director of Sports Nutrition,
University of Pittsburgh Medical Center
Recipe from Chefs Kevin Watson and Denise Pierchalski

Yield: 8 cups
Serves: 10 servings, ¾ cup each

This side dish or salad is colorful and has a variety of flavors and textures. The sweetness of the dried cherries balances nicely with the sourness of the salad dressing. The toasted pecans and sweet peppers add just the right crunch. This salad is perfect for most diets, including vegan, kosher and halal.

Vegetable broth	5 cups
Wild rice, rinsed	⅔ cup
Short grain organic brown rice	1 cup
Pecans, toasted, chopped	½ cup
Dried cherries or sweetened cranberries	¾ cup
Scallions, light and dark green parts only, sliced thin	1 bunch
Red pepper, diced	1 each
Yellow pepper, diced	1 each
Zest of one orange	2 tablespoons

Dressing:

Dijon mustard	1 tablespoon
Shallot, minced	2 teaspoons
Garlic, minced	1 teaspoon
Brown sugar	1 tablespoon
Cider vinegar	¼ cup
Basil, fresh, chopped	2 teaspoons
Salt	½ teaspoon
Pepper	¼ teaspoon
Olive oil	⅓ cup

1. Bring 2 ½ cups of vegetable broth to a boil, add wild rice and simmer covered for about 40 minutes, stirring occasionally until rice starts to break open and becomes tender, add more liquid if needed. Remove rice to a sheet pan to cool.

2. Bring 2 ½ cups of vegetable broth to a boil, add brown rice and simmer about 30 minutes until liquid is absorbed, and remove rice to a sheet pan to cool.

3. In a large bowl combine pecans, cherries, scallions, peppers and orange zest. Add cooked wild and brown rice and mix well.

Dressing

1. Combine Dijon mustard, shallot, garlic, brown sugar, vinegar, basil, salt and pepper in a bowl. Slowly whisk in olive oil. Pour dressing over salad and toss well. Refrigerate until needed, serve at room temperature.

Per Serving

Calories	240	Cholesterol	0	mg
Fat	10 g	Sodium	170	mg
Saturated Fat	1.5 g	Carbohydrates	32	mg
Trans Fat	0 g	Dietary Fiber	3	mg
Sugar	8 g	Protein	4	g

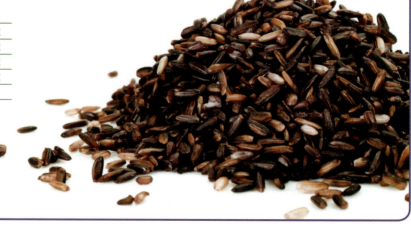

Food Allergies and Intolerances

ESSENTIALS EXPERT

Margaret Condrasky, EdD, RD, CCE, is associate professor of food science and human nutrition at Clemson University. She has written extensively and designed culinary nutrition seminars and refreshers, particularly for the American Culinary Federation. Marge works with industry chefs and product developers. At the university she directs the CU CHEFS® (Clemson University's Cooking and Healthy Eating Food Specialists) instructional program and, in the academic arena, she focuses on the culinary sciences for undergraduates and graduate students.

In 2009, the Food Channel identified allergen free, gluten free and casein free as important food trends. Food allergies are relatively uncommon, affecting only about 5% of children and about 3% to 4% of adults. All told, only about 12 million Americans have food allergies, but the number is increasing. During the last decade, food allergies have become more common in children. Fortunately, most children outgrow them, especially allergies to milk, eggs and soy. Although only eight foods account for 90% of all food-related allergic reactions – milk, eggs, peanuts, tree nuts, fish, shellfish, wheat and soy – a growing allergen-consciousness is evidenced by the introduction of many new products created and labeled as allergen-free. [12]

A **food allergy** occurs when a food protein is attacked by the immune system. This attack triggers a sudden release of histamine, among other chemicals, and results in allergic reaction symptoms. These symptoms may be relatively mild (rashes, hives, itching, runny nose, watery eyes, headache, cramping, swelling, etc.) or severe (trouble breathing, wheezing, loss of consciousness, etc.). A severe or life-threatening allergic reaction – when the airways swell closed and breathing is blocked – is called **anaphylaxis** or **anaphylactic shock** and can cause death if not treated immediately. Symptoms usually occur immediately but may appear up to two hours after ingesting an allergen.

If there is any indication that a guest is having an allergic reaction, call 911 immediately. Also check to see if the person is carrying the prescription drug epinephrine, typically as a pen-like device (EpiPen®). If so, administer the drug immediately. The device contains a spring-loaded needle that exits the tip of the pen. The medication should be injected into the person's outer thigh.

Since chefs know so much about ingredients, they can equip themselves with awareness and techniques to help guests with food allergies enjoy wonderful meals. Individuals with food allergies or intolerances who would potentially enjoy dining away from home compose a virtually untapped market segment in the restaurant world. Chefs and foodservice establishments can and should work to gain the trust and patronage of this group who will bring family and friends to places where they can dine safely.

Margaret Condrasky, EdD, RD, CCE
Clemson University

Because of the potential danger associated with an allergic reaction, people with food allergies must assess and evaluate their food choices carefully. They may ask a lot of questions about ingredients and cooking techniques. These are not idle queries. Servers should convey all of these concerns to the chef, and both serving staff and chefs should be prepared to answer all questions completely.

Even tiny traces of an allergen can trigger reactions in susceptible individuals. The only way to assure diners that a dish is safe to eat is to know what is in it. Often, a potential allergen is not obvious or not recognizable in foods. Sometimes allergens are in food processing ingredients, such as stabilizers or thickeners.

Cross contamination is one of the leading causes of food allergy reactions in restaurants. Clean utensils and work surfaces thoroughly before using them to prepare food for an allergic guest. Be especially careful of cutting boards, slicers and other kitchen equipment that may have been used before for an allergen-containing food. Traces of egg, flour or nuts may adhere to rubber gloves, parchment paper or a spatula. Garnishes or salad bowls with traces of crushed nuts, pasta water that was used to boil cheese-filled pasta, tongs used to turn fish then used to turn beef – all of these can lead to severe reactions in allergic guests who have carefully ordered foods they assume to be safe. Consider having a separate "allergy-free" station with dedicated equipment, a dedicated pot of boiling water to be used for gluten-free cooking, and cutting boards, mixers, etc., that are used only for allergy-free orders. Evaluate your menu and train servers to know which menu items are free of major allergens.

As part of an allergy response plan, maintain a looseleaf notebook with ingredient lists of all menu items, including ingredients in outsourced foods. Make a list of menu items suitable for guests with specific allergens or intolerances. Include text on your menu that encourages guests to notify the serving staff about food allergies. During hours of operation, a restaurant should have at least one person on duty, ideally the manager, who can handle questions and special requests from guests with food allergies. Because so many ingredients may contain allergens, guests may request to read the list for themselves, rather than having a staff member interpret ingredients for them. This involvement places some of the responsibility for ascertaining the safety of foods on the customer.

Food Intolerance and Aversion

A food intolerance and food aversion are not the same. A **food intolerance** is characterized by unpleasant symptoms, such as stomach cramps or diarrhea that occur after consuming certain foods. People with a food intolerance can eat minimal amounts of the food in question without experiencing major symptoms. The amount of food tolerated varies greatly from person to person.

A **food aversion** is neither an allergy nor intolerance. It is an intense dislike that may cause a biological response (usually nausea). Aversions usually have psychological and/or physiological causes or effects. Many aversions are based on what foods are acceptable within one's culture. Sometimes aversions occur because a food made that person ill at an earlier time.

Key Nutrition Points

- For the person with a food allergy, complete avoidance of the allergenic ingredient is critical.

- Reading labels, particularly ingredient lists, is essential.

- Encourage diners with special needs to call ahead to make sure you can accommodate them and encourage them to pre-order so the chef can check ingredients and use appropriate equipment for food preparation.

- Avoid cross contamination. Use clean equipment and clean spoons and measures for adding ingredients. For example, is the wok you are using to stir-fry vegetables the same wok just used for a stir-fry containing shrimp?

- Be sure the chef understands that foods for guests with allergies must be prepared using only the ingredients in the recipe directions. Creative adjustments such as adding a bit of flour to thicken or butter to enrich can cause a dangerous reaction in an allergic guest.

Milk Allergy

A *milk allergy* is an immune system response to the protein in milk. People with a milk allergy are likely to be allergic to goat, sheep and cows' milk and products made from them. Soymilk, rice milk and nut (almond) milk are useful alternatives if no other allergies are present. Each of these "milks" has a different nutrient profile and cooking and flavor characteristics.

Milk allergy is different from the more common lactose intolerance. People with **lactose intolerance** lack the enzyme lactase, which is required to digest lactose, a sugar in milk. They experience gas, bloating and abdominal pain. Many lactose-intolerant people drink dairy products with added lactase or take lactase tablets before they drink milk or eat foods containing milk or milk products. Individuals who do not drink milk early in life can stop making lactase and may become lactose intolerant later.

Many lactose-intolerant people can handle some but not much lactose without ill effects. They can enjoy cultured milk products like yogurt or kefir; hard aged cheeses like Cheddar, Colby, Swiss or Parmesan; and milk products found in very small quantities in food additives or preservatives.

Allergens Listed on the Food Label

The Food Allergen Labeling and Consumer Protection Act (FALCPA), which took effect January 1, 2006, mandates that the labels of foods containing major food allergens (milk, eggs, fish, crustacean shellfish, peanuts, tree nuts, wheat and soy) declare the allergen in plain language, either in the ingredient list or by one of these two statements:

- The word "Contains" followed by the name of the major food allergen – for example, "Contains milk, wheat"

- A parenthetical statement in the list of ingredients – for example, "albumin (egg)"

Allergenic ingredients must be listed if they are present in any amount, even in colors, flavors or spice blends. Additionally, manufacturers must list the specific nut (for example, almond, walnut, cashew, etc.) or seafood (for example, tuna, salmon, shrimp, lobster, etc.) used. Unfortunately, gluten is not included in FALCPA.

Source: U. S. Food and Drug Administration, www.fda.gov/Food/LabelingNutrition/FoodAllergensLabeling/GuidanceCompliance-RegulatoryInformation/ucm106187.htm

Dairy Products to Avoid

All milk products must be excluded from the diet when there is a milk allergy.

Acidophilis milk	Margarine containing milk solids
Butter	Milk chocolate
Buttermilk	Puddings
Cheese	Sour cream
Cheese food	Whipped cream
Coffee creamer	Whole, skim and low-fat milk
Condensed milk	Yogurt
Creamed soups	
Custards	
Evaporated milk	
Ice cream	

Ingredients to Avoid

Ammonium caseinate

Binding agents

Butter flavorings

Calcium caseinate

Caramel or caramel flavorings

Carob

Casein

Casein hydrolysate

Ghee

Lactalbumin

Lactate

Lactic acid

Lactoferrin

Lactoglobulin

Lactulose

Malted milk

Milk protein

Non-dairy creamer (may contain casein)

Nougat

Protein hydrolysate

Rennet casein

Simplesse™

Skim milk solids

Sodium caseinate

Whey

Whey protein hydrolysate

Tips for Chefs

- Have soymilk, rice milk or almond milk in the kitchen to substitute for cow's milk.

- Use vegetable oil instead of butter when possible.

- Offer a tapenade or hummus as a spread for bread instead of butter.

- Kosher foods marked pareve contain no milk or dairy products; therefore they are acceptable for those with milk allergy or lactose intolerance.

Foods Commonly Containing Milk or Milk Products

Baked goods, cakes and cookies

Biscuits

Bread

Breakfast cereals

Butter, alone, in or on foods

Candy, fudge, milk chocolate and caramels

Canned tuna (some brands contain casein)

Cheese

Cocoa mixes

Crackers and cereals

Cream sauces

Custard

Deli meats and cold cuts with casein as binder

Egg substitutes

Foods fried in batter

Gravies

Ice cream, gelato and sherbet

Instant drink mixes

Instant potatoes

Hot dogs (unless kosher)

Margarine

Mayonnaise

Pancakes and waffles

Salad dressings

Sausages

Soups

Sour cream

Soy/vegetarian cheese

Specialty coffees, latte, cappuccino

Tofu

Vegetables in cream or cheese sauces

Whipped toppings

Yogurt

Egg Allergy

Egg allergy, especially an allergy to egg whites, is more common in children than in adults and is likely to be outgrown over time. Strictly avoiding eggs and food containing eggs and egg products is the only way to prevent a reaction. It is not always easy to avoid these foods because many unexpected products contain eggs. For example, egg yolks are sometimes used to glaze baked items like pretzels or bagels. Eggs also may be used as a foaming agent in beer, lattes or cappucinos.

Always check the label for ingredients before you use a product. In addition, check the label each time you use the product; manufacturers occasionally change recipes, and a trigger food may be added to the new recipe. Several terms indicate that egg products have been used in manufacturing processed foods. Terms that imply egg protein is present include:

Albumin

Globulin

Lecithin

Livetin

Lysozyme

Simplesse™

Vitellin

Words starting with "ova" or "ovo," such as ovalbumin or ovoglobulin

Foods and Ingredients to Avoid

Angel food cake

Cholesterol-free egg substitutes (usually contain egg whites)

Cream pies

Custard

Eggs, egg whites and egg yolks

French toast

Hollandaise sauce

Mayonnaise

Meringue

Pancakes

Phosvitin

Puddings

Silicalbuminate

Soufflés

Surimi

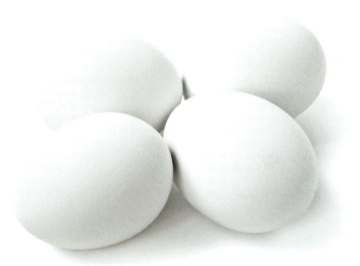

Foods Commonly Containing Eggs

- Baked goods, muffins, rolls and cakes
- Bearnaise sauce and hollandaise sauce
- Beer
- Breaded or battered foods
- Breads, such as challah or others with egg in the dough or an egg glaze
- Broth (clear), consomme or stock clarified with eggs
- Casseroles made with eggs
- Cream-filled chocolates
- Cookies
- Custard
- Divinity and fondant
- Foam in milk toppings on specialty coffee drinks
- Fried food (with eggs used in the batter)
- Fudge
- Ice cream
- Jelly beans (some)
- Marshmallows
- Marzipan
- Mayonnaise and mayonnaise-containing products, such as deli salads
- Meat loaf, meatballs
- Newburgh sauce
- Nougat
- Pastas including those in prepared foods such as soup (non egg pastas may be made on equipment also used for making egg-containing pasta)
- Pretzels
- Root beer
- Salad dressings
- Sausages (some)
- Sherbet
- Sweet rolls and pie crusts (with egg glaze)
- Tartar sauce
- Wine (some are clarified with egg)

Tips for Chefs

- Substitute mashed avocado, mustard, hummus, red pepper spread or tapenade for mayonnaise on sandwiches.
- Use tofu instead of eggs for a breakfast scramble.

Replacing Eggs in Recipes

If the eggs are used for leavening:

- 1½ tablespoons liquid + 1½ teaspoons oil + 1 teaspoon baking powder
- 1 teaspoon baking powder + 1 tablespoon liquid + 1 tablespoon vinegar
- 1 teaspoon yeast + ¼ cup warm water
- ½ teaspoon baking powder + 2 tablespoons liquid
- 2 tablespoons flour + 1 ½ tablespoons shortening + ½ teaspoon baking powder + 2 tablespoons liquid

If the eggs are used as a binder:

- 1 packet of plain gelatin + 2 tablespoons warm water
- 1 tablespoon of fruit puree
- 1/3 cup of water blended with 1 tablespoon of flax seeds (for 1 egg)
- Soft tofu

Peanut Allergy

Peanuts are not actually nuts; they are legumes. Also known as groundnuts or monkey nuts, peanuts pose a unique problem because many children love peanut butter and peanut snacks. Some schools ban peanuts when a few children are allergic to them. Exposure can occur in three ways:

- **Direct contact:** The most common exposure is eating peanuts or peanut-containing foods. Sometimes direct skin contact with peanuts can trigger an allergic reaction.

- **Cross contact:** The unintended introduction of peanuts into a product is generally the result of exposure during processing or handling of a food product. Cross contact could come from serving a fruit sherbet with an ice cream scoop that had been previously used for ice cream with nuts.

- **Inhalation:** An allergic reaction may occur if dust or aerosols containing peanuts is inhaled – for example, peanut flour or peanut oil cooking spray.

Ingredients to Avoid

- Peanuts
- Peanut oil

Foods Commonly Containing Peanuts

- African, Chinese, Indonesian, Thai, Vietnamese and Mexican dishes (Thai dipping sauces, salads, pad Thai, etc.)

- Sauces, such as pesto, gravy, mole sauce and peanut sauce

- Artificial nuts (peanuts reflavored as pecans or walnuts)

- Nuts roasted in peanut oil

- Baked goods

- Chocolate candy, peanut brittle and candy bars

- Egg rolls

- Foods that contain extruded, cold-pressed or expelled peanut oil, which may contain some peanut protein

- Ice cream

- Salad dressing

- Seeds, such as sunflower seeds and soy nuts made or processed on equipment shared with peanuts

- Some vegetarian and vegan food products, especially those sold as meat substitutes

- Sweets, such as puddings, cookies and hot chocolate

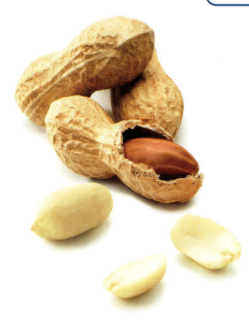

Tree Nut Allergy

Most people allergic to tree nuts are also allergic to peanuts. Water chestnuts are actually part of a plant root and are not nuts. They, like nutmeg, are safe for someone allergic to tree nuts.

Tree Nuts

Almonds	Coconuts	Macadamia nuts
Beech nuts	Gingko nuts	Pecans
Brazil nuts	Hazelnuts/filberts	Pinenuts
Cashews	Hickory nuts	Pistachios
Chestnuts	Lychee nuts	Walnuts

Foods Commonly Containing Tree Nuts

- Barbecue sauce
- Breading for chicken or fish
- Cereals
- Chocolate candies, nougat, macaroons, marzipan
- Cookies and desserts
- Crackers
- Foie gras (sometimes pistachios)
- Honey and chestnut honey
- Mandelonas (peanuts soaked in almond flavoring)
- Meat-free burgers
- Mexican coffee (uses piñon)
- Mortadella (may contain pistachios)
- Natural flavorings and extracts (pure almond extract)
- Nut butters, nut oils
- Nut-flavored coffee/liqueurs (Amaretto®, Frangelico®)
- Pancakes
- Piecrust, some pies and tarts
- Salads and salad dressings
- Spreads, such as almond paste, chocolate nut, nougat, Nutella® and nut paste

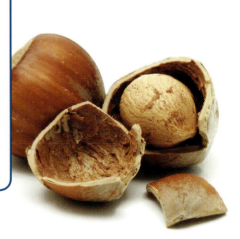

Fish Allergy

Fish and shellfish allergies tend to be severe. People who are allergic to fish should avoid seafood restaurants because of the risk of contamination of non-fish meals. Fish protein can become airborne during cooking.

Foods to Avoid

- All fish with fins and scales
- All products made with fresh, canned, processed or frozen fish

Foods Commonly Containing Fish

- Asian fish-based sauces
- Barbecue sauce (some are made from Worcestershire)
- Bouillabaisse, chowder, gumbo, Jambalaya and cioppino
- Caesar salad (may contain anchovies in the salad dressing)
- Caponata and sweet/sour relishes that may contain anchovies
- Imitation fish or shellfish (surimi)
- Meatloaf and meatballs (may contain Worcestershire sauce)
- Salad dressings
- Steak sauce
- Surimi
- Sushi
- Worcestershire sauce

Shellfish Allergy

Shellfish allergy is one of the most common and severe food allergies. Those with shellfish allergy may have an allergic reaction to only certain kinds of shellfish or may be allergic to all varieties. People with shellfish allergies are often sensitive to iodine as well. Nori rolls and other seaweeds contain high levels of iodine.

Common Allergy-Causing Shellfish

Crustaceans	Bivalves	Gastropods	Cephalopods
Crabs	Clams	Limpets	Squid
Crayfish	Mussels	Periwinkles	Cuttlefish
Lobster	Oysters	Snails (escargot)	Octopus
Langoustines	Scallops	Abalone	
Prawns			
Shrimp			
Mollusks			

Wheat Allergy

People who are allergic to wheat have a specific intolerance to wheat protein. This allergy is not the same as gluten intolerance (celiac disease). Many wheat-allergic children outgrow this allergy. For those with wheat allergy, alternative grains such as quinoa and rice should be offered. See the following section on gluten-free for grains to use.

Foods and Ingredients to Avoid

All-purpose flour

Bran

Bread (unless wheat-free)

Breadcrumbs

Bulgur

Cake flour

Cracked wheat

Durum flour

Enriched flour

Gelatinized starch

Gluten

Graham flour

Kamut®

Miller's bran

Modified food starch

Pastry flour

Semolina

Spelt

Starch

Vegetable gum

Wheat germ

Whole-wheat flour

Foods Commonly Containing Wheat

Beer

Bouillon base and cubes

Breads (many corn or rye breads also contain some wheat flour) and rolls

Breakfast bars

Breakfast cereals

Candy

Cakes and muffins

Coffee substitutes

Condiments, such as catsup

Couscous

Cookies, doughnuts

Dairy products, such as ice cream

Deli meat products, cold cuts and sausages

Farina

French fries

Gelatinized starch

Hot dogs

Hydrolyzed vegetable protein

Ice cream

Imitation crabmeat

Malt

Meat, crab or shrimp substitutes

Modified food starch

Natural flavorings

Noodles

Pancakes, pancake and waffle mixes

Pasta

Processed meats

Sausage

Soup mixes

Soy sauce

Tempura batter

Vegetable gum

Waffles

Wheat germ

Wheat starch

Tips for Chefs

When baking with wheat-free flours, a combination of flours usually works best. Experiment with different blends to find one that will give you the texture you are trying to achieve. Blends composed of high proportions of white rice flour, potato starch, arrowroot and tapioca flour and lower proportions of sorghum, millet, gar-fava and/or brown rice flour yield the best baked items. Gluten-free blends and mixes are available.

Adapting a recipe to be wheat- and dairy-free comes down to four considerations: solutions and proportions of ingredients, acid, protein and a gum. Generally more leavening is needed in wheat-free products.

Baker's Asthma

Baker's asthma is an allergic reaction to wheat flour and other types of flour. As the name of the disorder suggests, it's a particular problem for bakers or anyone who works with uncooked wheat flours. Inhaling flour rather than eating it causes the allergic reaction. Baker's asthma primarily results in problems breathing. The allergy-causing substance that triggers baker's asthma may be wheat protein or another substance such as a fungus.

Saffron Buckwheat Pilaf & Three-Bean Relish with a Spicy Tomato Vinaigrette

Provided by **Margaret Condrasky, EdD, RD, CCE,**
Associate Professor of Food Science and Human Nutrition,
Clemson University, Clemson, South Carolina
Recipe by Joel Schaefer, President & Chef, Allergy Chefs, Inc.,
Dawsonville, Georgia

Yield: 8 cups
Serves: 10 (some dressing remains for another use)

This dish is excellent as an entree or appetizer. Its many healthy components can be used separately with other items on your menu. The spicy tomato vinaigrette is a good reduced-calorie salad dressing and makes a zesty dip for crudités. It is great for vegans or anyone who wants a healthful option.

Saffron Buckwheat Pilaf (yield: 8 cups)

Herb oil or olive oil	2	tablespoons
Diced onions	½	cup
Garlic, minced	2	cloves
Vegetable stock	4	cups
Whole buckwheat groats	2	cups
Bay leaves	2	each
Saffron	⅛	teaspoon
Salt	½	teaspoon
Black pepper, freshly ground	¼	teaspoon

Three-Bean Relish (yield: 4 ¾ cups)

Black beans	1	15 ounce can
Great northern beans	1	15.5 ounce can
Red beans	1	15.5 ounce can
Sweet onions, caramelized	½	cup
Red bell peppers, diced	½	cup
Green bell peppers, diced	½	cup
Champagne vinaigrette	½	cup

Champagne Vinaigrette (yield: ¾ cup)

Champagne vinegar	¼	cup
Extra virgin olive oil	⅜	cup
Garlic cloves	2	each
Italian flat parsley	1	tablespoon
Salt	½	teaspoon
Black pepper, freshly ground	¼	teaspoon

Spicy Tomato Vinaigrette (Yield: 2 cups)

Diced tomatoes, no salt added, undrained	1	14.5 ounce can
Sambal oelek	1	teaspoon
Olive oil	¼	cup
Oregano, fresh, chopped	2	tablespoons
Salt	1	teaspoon
Balsamic vinegar	1	tablespoon

Garnish

Italian flat leaf parsley, fresh, springs	¼	cup

Saffron Buckwheat Pilaf:

1. In a large saucepan, saute onions and garlic in oil until onions are translucent.

2. Add the vegetable stock and bring to a boil over high heat; quickly stir in the buckwheat, reduce heat to low, add bay leaves and saffron and cover pan tightly.

3. Simmer 15 minutes or until groats are tender and liquid is absorbed. Add salt and pepper to taste. Let sit for 5 minutes and fluff with a fork. Remove bay leaves.

Champagne Vinaigrette:

1. Blend the champagne vinegar, olive oil, garlic cloves and Italian parsley in a blender. Set aside.

Three-Bean Relish:

1. Drain and rinse the beans. Combine the beans, caramelized onions, bell peppers and ½ cup of the champagne vinaigrette. Toss to combine.

Spicy Tomato Vinaigrette:

1. Place all ingredients in a blender and puree.

Assembly:

1. Mold the buckwheat pilaf in 10 3-inch rings or greased ramekins. Unmold on plate. Pour the spicy tomato vinaigrette around the buckwheat. Drizzle remaining dressing lightly around plates. Portion the three-bean relish over the buckwheat. Garnish with fresh Italian parsley.

Per Serving

Calories	360	Cholesterol	0	mg
Fat	15 g	Sodium	575	mg
Saturated Fat	2 g	Carbohydrates	48	mg
Trans Fat	0 g	Dietary Fiber	9	mg
Sugar	6 g	Protein	10	g

Soy Allergy

Read labels carefully. Soybeans have become a major part of processed food products such as baked goods, canned items, cereals, crackers, sauces and soups. Avoiding products made with soybeans can be difficult. Check for soy as an ingredient in anything labeled as vegetarian or vegan; soy products are often added to boost nutrient value. MSG (monosodium glutamate) may be made from corn or soy.

Ingredients to Avoid

Artificial flavorings

Asian flavoring

Bouillon cubes (beef, chicken, vegetable, etc.)

Canned chicken broth

Canned vegetable broth

Edamame

Emulsifier

Glycine max

Hydrolyzed plant protein

Hydrolyzed protein

Hydrolyzed soy protein

Hydrolyzed vegetable protein (HVP)

Lecithin

Miso

Mono- and diglycerides

Monosodium glutamate (MSG)

Natto (fermented soybeans)

Natural flavoring

Plant protein

Protein extender

Protein filler

Shoyu

Sobee® and other soy formulas

Soy albumin

Soy fiber

Soy flour

Soy grits

Soy meal

Soymilk

Soy nut butter

Soy nuts

Soy protein isolate

Soy sauce

Soy sprouts

Soya

Soybeans

Soybean butter

Soybean granules or curds

Tamari

Tempeh

Texturized vegetable protein (TVP)

Tofu

Vegetable gum

Vegetable starch

Worcestershire sauce

Foods Commonly Containing Soy

Baked goods

Bread

Butter substitutes

Candies

Canned broths

Canned soups

Canned tuna

Cereal

Condiments

Crackers

Desserts

Energy bars

Gravies

High-protein energy bars and snacks

Ice cream

Infant formulas

Liquid meal replacements

Low-fat peanut butter

Margarine

Meat substitutes

Salad dressings

Soups

Veggie burgers

Vegetarian sausages and meat substitutes

Foods to Avoid for Corn Allergy

Corn is not on the list of the eight top allergens. It affects less than 1% of the American population. Although a rare allergy, it is difficult because a corn derivative, high-fructose corn syrup, is ubiquitous. Corn-containing foods to avoid include:

- Corn chips and tortillas
- Corn flakes and other breakfast cereals containing corn
- Corn grits, corn flour and cornmeal
- Corn oil, alone or in salad dressings or fried foods
- Corn syrup and high fructose corn syrup
- Fresh or frozen corn, alone or as an ingredient
- Frostings and icings
- Instant coffee and drinks
- Catsup, jams, gums and candy with corn syrup
- Popcorn and corn snacks
- Sorbitol and maltodextrin
- Yogurt and other foods sweetened with corn syrup
- Pizza crust dusted with cornmeal
- Soft drinks and sweetened beverages

Tips for Chefs

- Try using paneer (pressed Indian cheese) instead of tofu.
- Substitute rice or cow's milk for soymilk.

For More Information

- *Chef Card Template*. Fairfax, VA: The Food Allergy & Anaphylaxis Network, www.foodallergy.org
- Food Allergies Challenges & Opportunities for Food Service, www.ciaprochef.com/foodallergies
- Food Allergy Initiative, www.faiusa.org/
- Mayo Clinic, Food Allergies: Watch Food Labels for These Top 8 Allergens, www.mayoclinic.com/health/food-allergies/AA00057
- *Welcoming Guests with Food Allergies*. Fairfax, VA: The Food Allergy & Anaphylaxis Network; 2008. www.foodallergy.org

Non-Food Products Made from Corn

Aspirin

Cosmetics

Crayons and chalks

Envelope and stamp glue

Lotions and ointments

Penicillin

Shaving creams

Soaps and cleansers

Toothpastes

Gluten Intolerance

ESSENTIALS EXPERT

Renee Zonka, CEC, RD, CHE, MBA, is managing director and dean of Kendall College in Chicago. She became interested in gluten-free cooking while attending a seminar given by a celiac disease organization at the Culinary Institute of America and when she was an evaluator for a gluten-free cooking class. Her background in science, medicine and healthcare helped her realize how important it is for culinarians to meet this need for their guests. Renee writes extensively and teaches many classes to culinary students, chefs, dietitians and the public on celiac disease and gluten-free recipe development.

Gluten is the protein part of all forms of wheat (including durum, semolina and spelt), rye, barley and grain hybrids such as triticale and kamut. Gluten intolerance is an inherited autoimmune condition also known as **celiac disease**. People with this condition cannot tolerate gluten when it comes in contact with the small intestine. In fact, gluten will eventually destroy their small intestine.

According to a study by the University of Maryland Center for Celiac Research, nearly one of every 133 Americans suffers from celiac disease. [13] Some of them can tolerate small amounts of gluten without reaction. Others have severe symptoms from any contact with gluten. Gluten intolerance is not a wheat allergy, but wheat is the key food to avoid in order to control gluten intolerance. Symptoms of gluten intolerance are abdominal bloating, pain, diarrhea, weight loss and fatigue. Wheat allergy has respiratory and other severe symptoms.

More and more diners are requesting gluten free food, and the demand for gluten-free retail products is growing. Some food laws, however, make it difficult to know whether or not a food is truly gluten free. For example, if a snack food contains wheat, it must be labeled, but if it contains vinegar that was derived from wheat, no label is required. So although gluten-free foods have improved dramatically in quantity and quality, people on a gluten-free diet should rely more on whole foods and less on packaged and prepared foods. Gluten free foods are abundant in nature.

Websites such as www.allergyeats.com and others provide listss of restaurants that offer gluten-free menu options or are entirely gluten free.

Key Nutrition Points

- People with gluten intolerance must avoid all foods containing gluten, a protein in many grains.

- A person can develop intolerance to gluten at any time. It can be triggered by physical trauma, pregnancy, infection, severe emotional stress or surgery.

- In people with gluten intolerance, as gluten is ingested, it destroys the finger-like projections (**villi**) of the small intestine. The villi are essential for the absorption of vitamins and minerals and other nutrients.

- Absorption of calcium and lactose are most affected by the change in the lining of the small intestines. Everyone with gluten intolerance should also be tested for osteoporosis and lactose intolerance. Over time, other allergies may occur including soy, corn and dairy.

- When someone with gluten intolerance strictly follows a gluten-free diet, the villi return to normal function. The gluten intolerance remains but can be managed by diet. If the person consumes gluten, the villi will be destroyed once again. Thus, the gluten-free diet is a lifetime commitment.

- Some people with gluten intolerance have no symptoms; others have bloating, cramping, stomachache, diarrhea, weight loss, lactose-intolerance, anemia and fatigue. When gluten is consumed in even minuscule amounts, it can trigger these symptoms.

Best Choices

Food staples of the gluten-free diet include:

- Fruits and vegetables, fresh, frozen and dried

- Meat, fish, poultry (without wheat breading) and eggs

- Potatoes, corn and beans

- Rice, quinoa, buckwheat, millet, flax, sorghum and teff

- Dairy products

- Cereals made without wheat or barley malt

- Lentils and other legumes

- Seeds, such as amaranth, flax, sesame and sunflower

- Specialty foods, such as pasta, bread, crackers, pancakes, pastries and chips made with permitted grains (rice, tapioca, arrowroot, potato, soy or corn flours and starches)

Chef Renee Zonka advises, "When diners indicate they are gluten intolerant, you must be direct and honest if you do not have gluten-free items on the menu." Here are a few things you can offer:

- Salads made with fresh vegetables and fruits can be served with homemade vinaigrette. Use distilled vinegar. The distilling process destroys and filters out any gluten. Skip the croutons.

- Broth-based soups without noodles are a good alternative to cream or roux-based soups.

- Meat or fish can be broiled, roasted, sauteed, braised, stewed or pan-fried. The most important thing to remember is preparation. No wheat flour can be used for dusting meats when braising or stewing. Sauce cannot be made with a wheat-flour roux. If meat or fish is sauteed, use a clean pan and tongs.

- Sauces that are reduced from liquids are ideal. If the sauce must be thickened, use arrowroot, potato flour, cornstarch or tapioca flour instead of wheat flour.

- Vegetables can be steamed with butter. Tortilla chips or French fries can be prepared in a clean pot with fresh oil. Rice is a gluten-free food, even glutinous (sticky) rice. Many unusual grains are exciting to experiment with for a creative plate, such as amaranth, quinoa, teff, Jobs tears, millet and buckwheat.

- Many desserts have a wheat component. Even the famous flourless chocolate cake should be offered with caution. It is usually baked in a floured pan, and some recipes do contain a tablespoon of flour. A cheese course with dried fruits and nuts is a welcomed treat. Avoid offering bleu cheese from Europe because it may have gluten particles due to the fermentation and aging process.

- Breakfast items include eggs prepared in a variety of ways, homemade hash browns, fresh fruit and 100% juice.

Grains and Starches Allowed in the Gluten-Free Diet

Amaranth

Arrowroot

Beans and bean flours

Buckwheat

Corn, corn flour, popcorn, corn tortillas, cornmeal

Grits, polenta

Taco shells, unseasoned corn tortilla chips

Couscous

Garfava

Millet

Nut flours

Potato flour

Puffed rice, corn or millet

Pure gluten-free oats and oat flour

Quinoa and quinoa flour

Rice (plain), including brown rice, rice flour, rice noodles, rice crackers

Sorghum, sorghum flour

Soy, soy flour

Tapioca, tapioca flour

Teff, teff flour

Wild rice

Foods to Avoid

The gluten-free diet eliminates all foods, beverages and medications made from the ingredients that contain gluten, including items made with any type of wheat flour (all purpose, white or whole wheat).

Many ingredients contain hidden gluten. Gluten or wheat is used as a flavoring agent, fermenting agent and stabilizer. As more ready-made foods become available for foodservice, it will be imperative to know all the components. Here is a list of foods that always or usually contain gluten. Some will be obvious, some not.

- Alcohol: beer, ale and lager (usually made from malted barley, though some gluten-free beer is now available); some wines, gin, whiskey and vodka

- Artificial vanilla (pure vanilla is fine)

- Baked beans thickened with flour

- Cooking sprays for baking (may contain wheat flour or starch)

- Breading

- Breads, muffins, biscuits and flour tortillas

- Broths

- Brown rice syrup (frequently made from barley)

- Buckwheat and buckwheat pasta (soba noodles) made with wheat flour

- Cake icings and frostings (made with small amounts of wheat flour or starch)

- Cakes, pies, cobblers and cookies

- Caramel color made from barley

- Cereals and products made from cereal

- Cheese spreads and sauces thickened with wheat starch or protein

- Chocolates and licorice containing wheat flour

- Coating mixes

- Communion wafers

- Crackers

- Croutons

- Dextrin made from wheat

- Flavored coffee mixes that contain a chip-like ingredient made from cookie crumbs

- Flour (products that are primarily an allowed flour but have small amounts of prohibited flours)

- Gravies and sauces

- Hydrolyzed vegetable protein (HVP), texturized vegetable protein (TVP) or hydrolyzed plant protein (HPP), unless made from soy or corn

- Imitation bacon

- Imitation seafood

- Malt products such as malt flavoring, malt vinegar and malt beverages made from barley

- Marinades

- Meat loaf and frozen burgers with breadcrumbs or fillers

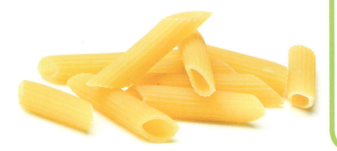

Gluten free doesn't mean bland. In a fine-dining restaurant, chefs take doing gluten-free meals as a creative challenge. Fortunately, gluten-free products are becoming more mainstream. As a dietitian who has gluten intolerance, I pick my restaurants carefully. One place lets me bring in my own brown rice pasta and charges me half price for pasta dishes. I bring my own gluten-free soy sauce when I go out for sushi. Another chef I know keeps a collection of gluten-free ingredients on hand for his regulars. Still another has an area in his kitchen devoted only to gluten-free cooking. This is the kind of commitment it takes – and you will be building a loyal clientele.

Diane Barrera, MPH, RD
Chicago, Illinois

- Modified starch or modified food starch (unless arrowroot, corn, potato, tapioca, waxy maize or maize as the grain source)
- Mono- and diglycerides
- Pastas
- Processed meats with fillers or seasoning containing hydrolyzed wheat protein
- Rice cakes and crackers containing some flour
- Rice mixes containing hydrolyzed wheat protein or soy sauce
- Roux and sauces made with roux
- Sauces
- Self-basting poultry
- Snack foods such as seasoned chips, taco chips and soy nuts containing wheat products in seasonings
- Soup bases
- Soy sauce fermented with wheat, and sauces that are made from soy sauce, such as dumpling and teriyaki sauce
- Specialty mustards with wheat flour
- Stuffing
- Tempeh seasoned with soy sauce
- Thickeners
- Vegetarian burgers or meat substitutes (may have wheat gluten, wheat proteins or barley malt)
- Vegetable gum (unless carob bean gum, locust bean gum, cellulose gum, guar gum, gum arabic, gum aracia, gum tragacanth, xanthan gum or vegetable starch)

Grains Containing Gluten

- Wheat in all forms: wheat starch, wheat bran, wheat germ, cracked wheat, hydrolyzed wheat protein
- Barley (all forms including malt)
- Kamut®
- Oats, unless grown and processed without contact with other grains. Pure oats are fine.
- Rye
- Spelt
- Triticale, a cross between wheat and ryes
- Wheat flours (durum, semolina, etc.)

Oats or No Oats

Oats do not contain gluten, but most have been grown, harvested, transported or processed on equipment used for other grains. Assume there has been cross contact and that most oats carry traces of gluten. Some companies, however, have dedicated fields and processing equipment and produce pure oats that are gluten free. See www.glutenfreediet.ca/oats.php.

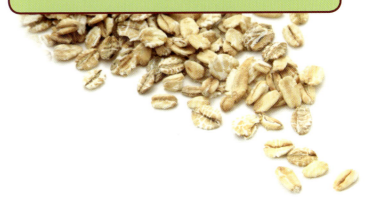

Tips for Chefs

Gluten-free foods that routinely appear on menus include plain, unsauced steaks, fish fillets, grilled meats, and vegetables that are cooked whole. Fish and meats can be "breaded" with nut meal instead of bread crumbs. Guests who want to eat gluten free usually will ask a lot of questions of the server about method of preparation, cooking liquids and sauces. Servers should be educated on menu items and method of preparation.

Be very careful of cross contamination. Items that are naturally gluten free may share transportation, a production line, a knife, a fryer, a toaster, a strainer or a grill with a **gluten-containing** grain. This contact will contaminate an item that would otherwise be gluten free. Utensils that have touched bread or bread baskets, spoons that have stirred roux-based soups, and spatulas that have flipped toasted cheese sandwiches will carry some residual gluten. Ovens can be used for gluten-free cooking if the temperature has been raised to 500° F and held for 15 minutes before cooking the gluten-free item.

If you decide to prepare gluten-free food on a regular basis, the kitchen and all equipment should be thoroughly cleaned and allowed to rest for 24 hours. Baking and mixing equipment should be specific for gluten-free items and cordoned off from the rest of the equipment to avoid cross contact. When not in use, equipment should be covered in plastic wrap. Ideally, a specific area should be identified for gluten-free food preparation. [14]

In the front of the house, create a special menu to help guide diners to appropriate choices, or develop a list that service staff can use to make appropriate suggestions. Encourage diners to call ahead to alert the chef to their special needs. Some restaurants ask these diners to make reservations for a time when the kitchen is less busy.

For More Information

- Be Free for Me, www.befreeforme.com/blog
- Bowland S. *The Living Gluten-Free Answer Book.* Naperville, IL: Sourcebooks, Inc.; 2008.
- Case S. *Gluten-Free Diet, A Comprehensive Resource Guide.* Saskatchewan, Canada: Case Nutrition Consulting; 2008.
- Celiac Disease Center at Columbia University, www.celiacdiseasecenter.columbia.edu
- Celiac Disease Foundation, www.celiac.org
- Celiac Sprue Association/USA, Inc., www.csaceliacs.org
- Celiac Sprue Research Foundation, www.celiacfoundation.org
- Duane J. *Bake Deliciously! Gluten and Dairy Free Cookbook.* Centennial, CO: Alternative Cook, LLC, www.alternativecook.com.
- Gluten Intolerance Group, www.gluten.net
- Kafka, B. *The Intolerant Gourmet.* Glorious Food Without Gluten & Lactose. New York: Artisan; 2011
- Keller M. Free of Gluten, Full of Flavor. *Today's Dietitian.* 2009;11(6):28-32.
- National Foundation for Celiac Awareness (NFCA), www.celiacfoundation.org
- Russel, LB. *The Gluten-Free Asian Kitchen.* Berkeley, CA: Celestial Arts; 2011.
- Thompson T. *Celiac Disease Nutrition Guide,* 2nd ed. Chicago: The American Dietetic Association; 2006.
- University of Maryland Center for Celiac Research, www.celiaccenter.org

Everyone in the kitchen and front of the house should be educated on gluten intolerance. Eating out is a profound social event that makes us feel good in spirit and mind. People who are gluten intolerant have a difficult time dining out because they are afraid of eating something that will make them ill. A restaurant must remain sustainable. Servicing a group with special needs will develop trust and long-lasting relationships.

Renee Zonka, CEC, RD, CHE, MBA
Kendall College

A Word from the Chef
A Vegetarian and a Person with Celiac Disease Walk into a Restaurant ...

"I am gluten intolerant and my girlfriend is a vegetarian. We're a nightmare for restaurants," quips Brian J. Karam, chef instructor at Le Cordon Bleu College of Culinary Arts in Chicago.

Brian was already an adult when he discovered that he had celiac disease. "Eating's not as enjoyable as it used to be," he admits. "I used to hate it when customers asked for substitutions. Now I am that person! Although more wait staff are aware of celiac disease, the burden is still on the customer to figure out what he can eat."

In his work with students, Brian teaches the classic techniques. "That means butter, cream and salt," he says. "But you need that grounding to evolve as a chef and master healthier techniques that are becoming more and more important, like using reductions for flavor." Brian says that he is always experimenting with new ideas. Gluten-free and vegetarian are at the top of his list.

casebycase
Ina's: The Good Taste of Gluten-Free

Ina Pinkney, owner of the legendary Ina's on Chicago's Near West Side, has always been ahead of the curve and a firm believer in doing the right thing on behalf of her loyal patrons – people who, since 1991, have come from all over the Chicagoland area to enjoy the food and ambience of her establishment.

Ina has never been one to sit on the sidelines when the public's health is at stake. She led the coalition to ban smoking in Chicago restaurants and hers was the first eatery in the city to go trans fat free. She uses only cage-free eggs that have been pasteurized and co-founded the Green Chicago Restaurant Co-op that now has more than 250 members.

"It's important that my customers trust me," Ina says. "We serve healthy, safe food in a healthy, safe environment. Feeding people is a very important responsibility." At Ina's, that responsibility extends to customers with food allergies and intolerances. On the second Wednesday of the month, Ina's offers gluten-free fried chicken cooked in a trans fat free omega-9 canola oil. Many customers have thanked her for the opportunity to enjoy some fried food, which requires a coating of flour to develop a crispy golden crust.

Fried food is always the first to go from wheat- and gluten-free diets. Ina's flour blend includes brown rice flour, rice flour, tapioca flour and potato starch to mimic the traditional flour-based coating. "We clean the fryer and start with fresh oil," she explains. As a special accompaniment to the fried chicken, Ina's also serves gluten-free **dinner rolls.** Gluten-free pita bread – good for sandwiches – and a gluten-free chicken sausage are also on the menu.

"People are thrilled with our gluten-free fried chicken and other choices," says Ina. "They could never eat out safely before and always felt marginalized due to their restrictions. Some guests are so happy they cry."

Gluten-Free Fried Chicken

Chef Ina Pinkney, Ina's, Chicago, Illinois   **Yield: 10 pieces**

Dry mix coating:

White rice flour	1	pound
Brown rice flour	4	ounces
Tapioca flour or tapioca starch	2	ounces
Potato starch (not potato flour)	1 ½	ounces
Kosher salt	1	teaspoon
Black pepper	½	teaspoon
Garlic powder	1	teaspoon

Marinade:

Buttermilk	2	cups
Kosher salt	1	teaspoon
Black pepper	½	teaspoon
Garlic, minced	2	cloves
Chicken pieces (thighs, legs or breasts)	10	each
Egg whites	3	each
Transfat free canola oil		

Note: For recipes using deep fat frying, nutritional analysis is more accurate than calculated values.

1. Combine white rice flour, brown rice flour, tapioca flour, potato starch, salt, pepper, and garlic powder.

2. Combine buttermilk, salt, black pepper and minced garlic. Soak chicken pieces overnight. Drain the chicken thoroughly before coating.

3. Dredge the chicken pieces in the flour mixture, then dip into lightly beaten egg whites and then back into the flour mixture. It is good to "pack" the mixture on the second dip and shake off any excess.

4. Heat a trans fat-free commercial canola oil to 275° F in a heavy deep pot. Gently place the chicken into the pot (chicken must be completely covered in the oil). Do not overload the pot and do not move the chicken around for at least ten minutes for the crust to set up. At this temperature, a breast will take 20-25 minutes, legs and thighs will take 20 minutes. Remove the chicken and set it on a rack to drain for about 5 minutes.

Per Piece

Calories	250		Cholesterol	85	mg
Fat	13	g	Sodium	170	mg
Saturated Fat	2	g	Carbohydrates	5	mg
Trans Fat	0	g	Dietary Fiber	0	mg
Sugar	0	g	Protein	27	g

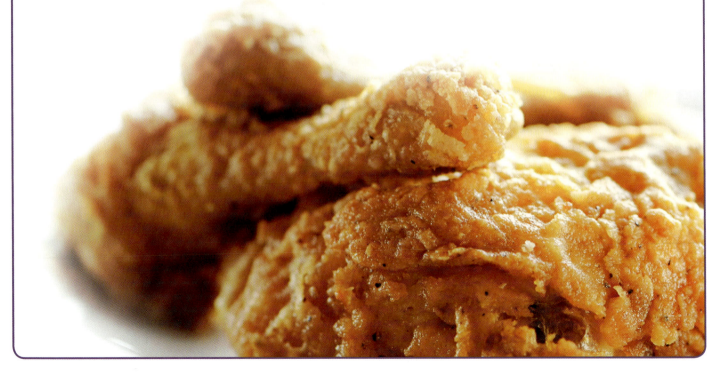

Christmas Beer Cake

Renee Zonka, CEC, RD, CHE, MBA
Managing Director and Dean, Kendall College, Chicago, Illinois

Yield: 10 inch bundt cake
Serves: 16

Sorghum flour	1 ½	cups
Tapioca flour	½	cup
Potato starch	½	cup
Baking powder	2	teaspoons
Baking soda	1	teaspoon
Salt	½	teaspoon
Xanthan gum	2	teaspoons
Butter, softened	¾	cup
Sugar	1 ½	cup
Eggs, large	3	each
Sour cream	1 ½	cup
Beer, gluten-free*	½	cup
Vanilla	1 ½	teaspoons

Filling and Topping:

Sugar	½	cup
Cinnamon	2	teaspoons
Walnuts, chopped	⅔	cup

1. Preheat oven to 350° F. Prepare a 10-inch tube pan or large bundt pan with nonstick spray.

2. Sift the flours, baking powder, baking soda, salt and xanthan gum in large bowl. Mix well.

3. In a mixing bowl, cream together butter and sugar. Add eggs, sour cream, beer and vanilla. Mix for about 2 minutes. Add dry ingredients and mix until all ingredients are well blended.

4. In a separate bowl, mix sugar, cinnamon and walnuts.

5. Spoon one-third of cake batter into greased pan. Sprinkle on one-third of cinnamon-nut mixture. Spoon on another third of cake batter and again sprinkle on a third of cinnamon-nut mixture.

6. Spoon on remaining third of batter. The cake will expand during baking so do not fill bundt pan to the top.

7. Bake 55-65 minutes until brown and cake tester comes out clean.

8. Cool and turn out of pan. Sprinkle remaining cinnamon-nut mixture on top of cake.

*Note: If beer is not desired, substitute sparkling water.

Per Serving

Calories	340	Cholesterol	70	mg
Fat	17	g	Sodium	310	mg
Saturated Fat	9	g	Carbohydrates	45	mg
Trans Fat	0	g	Dietary Fiber	2	mg
Sugar	26	g	Protein	4	g

Gluten-Free Brownies

Jean Duane, Alternative Cook, LLC, Centennial, Colorado   **Yield: 24 brownies**

Jean Duane, Alternative Cook, is known for her gluten-free cooking. She wrote Bake Deliciously! Gluten and Dairy Free Cookbook. *Jean maintains an active website, www.alternativecook.com, and blog, www.askjeanduane.com, with much information on gluten-free cooking. She shared this delicious recipe for gluten-free brownies.*

Sunflower oil	1	cup
Sugar	1 ½	cups
Eggs, large	4	each
Vanilla	2	teaspoons
Cider vinegar	1	teaspoon
Guar gum	2	teaspoons
Cocoa powder	⅔	cup
Sorghum flour	½	cup
Potato starch	¼	cup
Protein flour (soybean)	¼	cup
Baking powder	¾	teaspoon
Instant coffee crystals	2	teaspoons

1. Beat together the oil, sugar, eggs, vanilla and vinegar.
2. Whisk together the dry ingredients. Mix in the wet ingredients.
3. Put batter into an oiled 9 inch by 12 inch pan and bake at 350° F for 25 minutes.
4. Cool. Cut into 24, 2-inch squares.

Per Serving

Calories	170	Cholesterol	30	mg
Fat	10	g	Sodium	30	mg
Saturated Fat	1.5	g	Carbohydrates	18	mg
Trans Fat	0	g	Dietary Fiber	2	mg
Sugar	13	g	Protein	2	g

Used with permission from: Duane, Jean (2010) *Bake Deliciously! Gluten and Dairy Free Cookbook.* Centennial, CO: Alternative Cook, LLC. www.alternativecook.com.

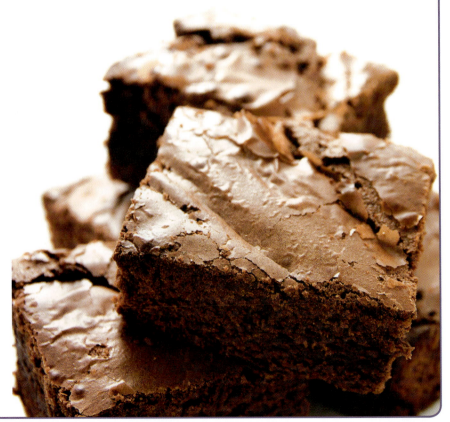

Opportunities for Chefs

Chefs and foodservice professionals prepare foods in a variety of operations, from healthcare facilitates to schools to fine-dining establishments. People with special dietary needs are dining every day in all of these settings. This chapter looked at key nutrition points, best food choices, foods to limit and tips for chefs to serve guests who are living with cardiovascular disease, hypertension, cancer, diabetes, digestive disorders, food allergies and celiac disease (gluten intolerance). Being prepared to serve these guests requires that you plan your meals and menus around healthful principles, offer a variety of choices, keep portions reasonable, and be open and willing to train staff to serve guests with special health needs.

Learning Activities

1. Select a menu from a foodservice operation that you work in or visit frequently. Select a particular food allergy. Identify items on the menu that would be appropriate for someone with that food allergy.

2. Develop a weeklong school lunch menu for children on a gluten-free diet.

3. You are catering a function for the local chapter of a diabetes support group (or cardiovascular disease or hypertension). Develop a menu and recipes for this event.

4. Collect two labels of foods from each basic food group. Using the ingredient lists, identify all sources of each of the eight common allergens.

Appendices

Appendix A

The American Institute of Wine & Food
Resetting the American Table:
Creating a New Alliance of Taste and Health

Reprinted with permission from the AIWF, **www.aiwf.org**

Standards for Food and Diet Quality

I.   **Nutrition**

II.   **Physical Activity**

III. **Food Availability, Quality and Preparation**

IV.   **Food Safety**

V.   **Education**

Umbrella Tenet

In matters of taste consider nutrition and in matters of nutrition consider taste. And in all cases consider individual needs and preferences.

Core Values

- Taste is the first determinant of consumer food choices in America. Along with taste comes a multitude of psychological, physiological, social, cultural, ethnic and economic influences that help shape our food preferences.

- Dietary recommendations should respect culinary traditions that reflect and support our cultural and ethnic heritages. At the same time, they must recognize individual needs to achieve nutritional adequacy and a sense of well-being.

- Nutrition and good health, as well as the cultural importance of food preparation and the enjoyment of eating, begin around the table at home with a healthy, positive attitude.

- There are no "good" or "bad" foods in isolation. It's the overall diet that counts.

The chefs, food journalists, nutrition scientists, physicians, exercise scientists, registered dietitians, public health professionals, anthropologists, psychologists, education specialists, food marketers and retailers who participated in this conference support the following statements, which define the relationship between food and diet quality and provide the link between taste and health.

I. Nutrition

- Emphasize the principles of moderation, variety, balance and choice as delineated in "The 1990 Dietary Guidelines for Americans," U.S. Department of Agriculture and U. S. Department of Health and Human Services.

  1. Eat a variety of foods.
  2. Maintain healthy weight.
  3. Choose a diet low in fat, saturated fat and cholesterol.
  4. Choose a diet with plenty of vegetables, fruits and grain products.
  5. Use sugars only in moderation.
  6. Use salt and sodium only in moderation.
  7. If you drink alcoholic beverages, do so in moderation.

- Evaluate diet quality by the total consumption of food over a period of several days, rather than by individual foods and/or meals. All foods can be part of a healthful diet.

- Encourage restaurants, retailers and food producers to offer choices for decreasing fat and increasing fruits, vegetables and grains in the diet.

  - Realize that the overconsumption of foods high in fat, often at the expense of foods high in complex carbohydrates and fiber, is the major nutrition concern in this country.

  - Recognize that a diet can include foods of high, as well as moderate or low fat content and still meet dietary guidelines. But in making higher fat choices, it is important to consider how often and how much.

- Consider individual and physiological needs and differences in food choices. Different people can achieve their nutritional needs in different ways.

- Support improved, truthful food labeling in a standardized format that facilitates planning a total diet and communicates nutritional information in accordance with dietary guidelines.
- Obtain recommended levels of nutrients primarily by eating a variety of foods rather than by relying on dietary supplements.

II. Physical Activity

- Recognize that physical activity enhances quality of life, overall health and a sense of well-being.
- Encourage regular and moderate levels of physical activity.
  - Realize that physical activity helps achieve and maintain healthy weight.
  - Realize that physical activity increases energy expenditure and expands the amount and variety of foods that can be consumed in a nutritious and satisfying diet.

III. Food Availability, Quality and Preparation

- Encourage the use of high-quality raw materials and ingredients that are made available at the point of maximum flavor, optimum condition and nutritive value. Flavor and texture are more crucial than appearance.
- Encourage a plentiful, conveniently available and affordable supply of raw materials and ingredients in peak flavor and in excellent condition.
- Encourage use and availability of an increasing diversity of ingredients, both in numbers of different foodstuffs and varieties of particular foods.
- Encourage the cultivation of varieties that yield optimal flavors, textures and nutrients.
- Prepare raw materials and ingredients with care to produce healthful foods that taste good.
- Enhance ingredients by conserving the quality of raw materials and ingredients during preparation.
- Reserve the use of fat for preparations where its presence makes a considerable difference in flavor and texture.
- Preserve culinary traditions from regional and ethnic cuisines.

- Encourage preparation of enjoyable food consistent with the nutrition recommendations cited earlier in this document.
  - Prepare foods at home from basic ingredients to gain more control over the quality and composition of what is eaten.
  - Use nutrition labeling to select foods consistent with the Dietary Guidelines for Americans.
- Encourage the food service industry, including restaurants and schools, to prepare meals consistent with the recommendations cited in this document.

IV. Food Safety

- Encourage a safe and well-inspected food supply.
- Encourage more careful handling, better preparation and more efficient storage procedures throughout the food distribution chain and in home and commercial kitchens to reduce the potential for food-borne illnesses.
- Encourage the reduction of microbiological contaminants in the food supply.
- Encourage efforts to lower levels of potentially harmful environmental and natural substances, including undesirable residues of drugs and pesticides.
- Seek international cooperation on all of the above.

V. Education

- Encompass the main elements of this document in education efforts to peers, consumers and broader audiences.
- Educate consumers and commercial food preparers and planners on how to identify and locate affordable, high-quality ingredients.
- Educate consumers and commercial food preparers and planners in the cooking skills necessary to prepare healthful, flavorful dishes practically, easily and safely.

Appendix B

Dietary Reference Intakes (DRIs): Recommended Intakes for Individuals, Macronutrients, Vitamins and Mineral Elements

Food and Nutrition Board, Institute of Medicine, National Academies

	Children 9-18	Males 19-70 years	Females 19-70 years	Males over 70 years	Females over 70 years
Total water (L/day)	2.1 -3.3	3.7	2.7	3.7	2.7
Carbohydrate (g/day)	130	130	130	130	130
Total fiber (g/day)	26-38	30-38	21-25	30	21
Protein (g/day)	34-52	56	46	56	46
Vitamin A (µg/day)	600-900	900	700	900	700
Vitamin C (mg/day)	45-75	90	75	90	75
Vitamin D (µg/day)	5	5-10	5-10	15	15
Vitamin E (mg/day)	11-15	15	15	15	15
Vitamin K (µg/day)	60-75	120	90	120	90
Thiamin (mg/day)	.9-1.2	1.2	1.1	1.2	1.1
Riboflavin (mg/day)	.9-1.3	1.3	1.1	1.3	1.1
Niacin (mg/day)	12-16	16	14	16	14
Vitamin B_6 (mg/day)	1.0-1.3	1.3-1.7	1.3-1.5	1.7	1.5
Folate (µg/day)	300-400	400	400	400	400
Vitamin B_{12} (µg/day)	1.8-2.4	2.4	2.4	2.4	2.4
Pantothenic acid (mg/day)	4-5	5	5	5	5
Biotin (µg/day)	20-25	30	30	30	30
Choline (mg/day)	375-550	550	425	550	425
Calcium (mg/day)	1300	1000-1200	1000-1200	1200	1200
Chromium (µg/day)	21-35	30-35	20-25	30	20
Copper (µg/day)	700-890	900	900	900	900
Fluoride (mg/day)	2-3	4	3	4	3
Iodine (µg/day)	120-150	150	150	150	150
Iron (mg/day)	8-15	8	8-18	8	8
Magnesium (mg/day)	240-410	400-420	310-320	420	320
Manganese (mg/day)	1.6-2.2	2.3	1.8	2.3	1.8
Molybdenum (µg/day)	34-43	45	45	45	45
Phosphorus (mg/day)	1250	700	700	700	700
Selenium (µg/day)	40-55	55	55	55	55
Zinc (mg/day)	8-11	11	8	11	8
Potassium (g/day)	4.5-4.7	4.7	4.7	4.7	4.7
Sodium (g/day)	1.5	1.3-1.5	1.3-1.5	1.2	1.2
Chloride (g/day)	2.3	2.0-2.3	2.0-2.3	1.8	1.8

Adapted from **Dietary Reference Intakes (DRIs): Recommended Intakes for Individuals, Vitamins, Dietary Reference Intakes (DRIs): Recommended Intakes for Individuals, Elements** and **Dietary Reference Intakes (DRIs): Recommended Intakes for Individuals, Macronutrients**, Food and Nutrition Board, Institute of Medicine, National Academies

Appendix C

Daily Values

Food Component	Daily Value
Total fat	65 grams (g)
Saturated fat	20 g
Cholesterol	300 milligrams (mg)
Sodium	2,400 mg
Potassium	3,500 mg
Total carbohydrate	300 g
Dietary fiber	25 g
Protein	50 g
Vitamin A	5,000 international units (IU)
Vitamin C	60 mg
Calcium	1,000 mg
Iron	18 mg
Vitamin D	400 IU
Vitamin E	30 IU
Vitamin K	80 micrograms (µg)
Thiamin	1.5 mg
Riboflavin	1.7 mg
Niacin	20 mg
Vitamin B_6	2 mg
Folate	400 µg
Vitamin B_{12}	6 µg
Biotin	300 µg
Pantothenic acid	10 mg
Phosphorus	1,000 mg
Iodine	150 µg
Magnesium	400 mg
Zinc	15 mg
Selenium	70 µg
Copper	2 mg
Manganese	2 mg
Chromium	120 µg
Molybdenum	75 µg
Chloride	3,400 mg

Source: Food Labeling Guide, U. S. Food and Drug Administration, www.fda.gov/Food/GuidanceComplianceRegulatoryInformation/ GuidanceDocuments/FoodLabelingNutrition/FoodLabelingGuide/ucm064928.htm

Appendix D

MyPlate and Physical Activity

MyPlate illustrates the five food groups that are the building blocks for a healthy diet using a familiar image – a place setting for a meal. The five food groups are:

Fruits: Focus on fruits.

Vegetables: Vary your veggies.

Grains: Make at least half your grains whole.

Protein: Go lean with protein.

Dairy: Get your calcium-rich foods.

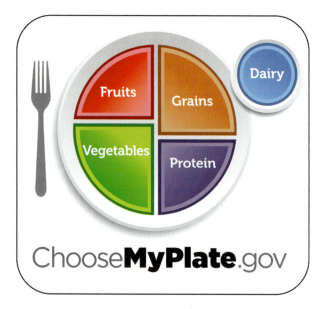

In addition to guiding food choices, *MyPlate* also emphasizes physical activity. Physical activity simply means movement of the body that uses energy. Walking, gardening, briskly pushing a baby stroller, climbing the stairs, playing soccer, or dancing the night away are all good examples of being active. For health benefits, physical activity should be moderate or vigorous intensity.

Moderate physical activities include:

- Walking briskly (about 3 ½ miles per hour)
- Bicycling (less than 10 miles per hour)
- General gardening (raking, trimming shrubs)
- Dancing
- Golf (walking and carrying clubs)
- Water aerobics
- Canoeing
- Tennis (doubles)

Vigorous physical activities include:

- Running/jogging (5 miles per hour)
- Walking very fast (4 ½ miles per hour)
- Bicycling (more than 10 miles per hour)
- Heavy yard work, such as chopping wood
- Swimming (freestyle laps)
- Aerobics
- Basketball (competitive)
- Tennis (singles)

You can choose moderate or vigorous intensity activities, or a mix of both each week. Activities can be considered vigorous, moderate, or light in intensity. This depends on the extent to which they make you breathe harder and your heart beat faster.

Only moderate and vigorous intensity activities count toward meeting your physical activity needs. With vigorous activities, you get similar health benefits in half the time it takes you with moderate ones. You can replace some or all of your moderate activity with vigorous activity. Although you are moving, light intensity activities do not increase your heart rate, so you should not count these toward meeting the physical activity recommendations. These activities include walking at a casual pace, such as while grocery shopping, and doing light household chores

Being physically active can help you:

- Increase your chances of living longer
- Decrease your chances of becoming depressed
- Sleep well at night
- Move around more easily
- Have stronger muscles and bones
- Stay at or get to a healthy weight
- Enjoy yourself and have fun

When you are not physically active, you are more likely to:

- Get heart disease
- Get type 2 diabetes
- Have high blood pressure
- Have high blood cholesterol
- Have a stroke

Physical activity and nutrition work together for better health. Being active increases the amount of calories burned. As people age their metabolism slows, so maintaining energy balance requires moving more and eating less.

Some types of physical activity are especially beneficial:

Aerobic activities make you breathe harder and make your heart beat faster. Aerobic activities can be moderate or vigorous in their intensity. Vigorous activities take more effort than moderate ones. For moderate activities, you can talk while you do them, but you can't sing. For vigorous activities, you can only say a few words without stopping to catch your breath.

Muscle-strengthening activities make your muscles stronger. These include activities like push-ups and lifting weights. It is important to work all the different parts of the body - your legs, hips, back, chest, stomach, shoulders and arms.

Bone-strengthening activities make your bones stronger. Bone strengthening activities, like jumping, are especially important for children and adolescents. These activities produce a force on the bones that promotes bone growth and strength.

Balance and stretching activities enhance physical stability and flexibility, which reduces risk of injuries. Examples are gentle stretching, dancing, yoga, martial arts, and t'ai chi.

Source: www.ChooseMyPlate.gov

Appendix E

Body Mass Index Table

BMI	Normal weight						Overweight					Obese					
Height (inches)	19	20	21	22	23	24	25	26	27	28	29	30	31	32	33	34	35
											Body Weight (pounds)						
58	91	96	100	105	110	115	119	124	129	134	138	143	148	153	158	162	167
59	94	99	104	109	114	119	124	128	133	138	143	148	153	158	163	168	173
60	97	102	107	112	118	123	128	133	138	143	148	153	158	163	168	174	179
61	100	106	111	116	122	127	132	137	143	148	153	158	164	169	174	180	185
62	104	109	115	120	126	131	136	142	147	153	158	164	169	175	180	186	191
63	107	113	118	124	130	135	141	146	152	158	163	169	175	180	186	191	197
64	110	116	122	128	134	140	145	151	157	163	169	174	180	186	192	197	204
65	114	120	126	132	138	144	150	156	162	168	174	180	186	192	198	204	210
66	118	124	130	136	142	148	155	161	167	173	179	186	192	198	204	210	216
67	121	127	134	140	146	153	159	166	172	178	185	191	198	204	211	217	223
68	125	131	138	144	151	158	164	171	177	184	190	197	203	210	216	223	230
69	128	135	142	149	155	162	169	176	182	189	196	203	209	216	223	230	236
70	132	139	146	153	160	167	174	181	188	195	202	209	216	222	229	236	243
71	136	143	150	157	165	172	179	186	193	200	208	215	222	229	236	243	250
72	140	147	154	162	169	177	184	191	199	206	213	221	228	235	242	250	258
73	144	151	159	166	174	182	189	197	204	212	219	227	235	242	250	257	265
74	148	155	163	171	179	186	194	202	210	218	225	233	241	249	256	264	272
75	152	160	168	176	184	192	200	208	216	224	232	240	248	256	264	272	279
76	156	164	172	180	189	197	205	213	221	230	238	246	254	263	271	279	287

Appendix F

Exchange Lists for Diabetic Menu Planning

The following chart shows the amounts of nutrients in 1 serving from each food list.

Food List	Carbohydrate (grams)	Protein (grams)	Fat (grams)	Calories
Carbohydrates				
Starch: breads, cereals and grains, starchy vegetables, crackers, snacks, beans, peas and lentils	15	0-3	0-1	80
Fruits	15	0	0	60
Milk Fat-free, low-fat, 1% Reduced-fat, 2% Whole	12 12 12	8 8 8	0-3 5 8	100 120 160
Sweets, desserts and other carbohydrates	15	Varies	Varies	Varies
Nonstarchy vegetables	5	2	0	25
Meat and Meat Substitutes				
Lean Medium-fat High-fat Plant-based proteins	0 0 0 Varies	7 7 7 7	0-3 4-7 8+ Varies	45 75 100 Varies
Fats	0	0	5	45
Alcohol	Varies	0	0	100

Adapted from: *Choose Your Foods: Exchange Lists for Diabetes*, American Diabetes Association and The American Dietetic Association, 2008

Appendix G

Carb Counting

Carb counting (also called "*carbohydrate counting*") is estimating the number of carbohydrate grams in a given meal or snack. Total carbs are tallied on a running basis to ensure that the total doesn't exceed a predetermined dietary goal for the meal and/or day.

An alternative form of carb counting is called "carbohydrate choice" or "simple carb counting." With this method, every 15 grams of carbs are counted as one carbohydrate choice, with a predetermined number of choices allotted daily. While not as precise as carb gram counting, simple carb counting may be preferred by those who like the simplicity.

Both types of carb counting are useful for people with type 1 diabetes who use fast-acting insulin to cover the carb content in their meals. Carb counting allows them to calculate the right amount of insulin to counteract the corresponding blood sugar rise from their meal.

Check food labels for carbohydrate values and to convert to carb choices.

Quick Carb Counting Guide

1 carb choice	=	15 grams carbohydrate
2 carb choices	=	30 grams carbohydrate
3 carb choices	=	45 grams carbohydrate
4 carb choices	=	60 grams carbohydrate
5 carb choices	=	75 grams carbohydrate

1 carb choice = 15 grams carbohydrate	2 carb choices = 30 grams carbohydrates	3 carb choices = 45 grams carbohydrates
⅓ cup cooked rice	⅔ cup cooked rice	1 cup cooked rice
1 slice of bread (1 ounce)	1 small sandwich bun (2 ounces)	1 medium-sized bagel (3 ounces)
1 small piece of fruit	1 large banana	½ cup dried apricots
½ cup fruit juice	1 cup fruit juice	
1 cup milk or ⅔ cup low-fat yogurt, plain	1 cup chocolate milk	1 cup fruit yogurt

Adapted from: *Count Your Carbs: Getting Started*, American Diabetes Association and The American Dietetic Association, 2010

Carbohydrate Counting List

The following foods contain about 15 grams of carbohydrates.

Group	Measure
Breads	1 slice of bread 2 slices of light bread ½ hamburger or hot-dog bun ½ of an English muffin 1 pancake or waffle (4-inch size) 1 corn or flour tortilla (6-inch size)
Cereal and Grains	⅓ cup rice ⅓ cup pasta ⅓ cup bread stuffing ½ cup cooked cereal ½ cup bran cereal ½ cup sugar-frosted cereal 1½ cup puffed cereal ¾ cup unsweetened cereals
Fruit	1 small orange, apple, pear, kiwi, peach, nectarine or banana ⅓ cup baked apple slices 2 small plums or tangerines ½ cup unsweetened applesauce ⅓ of a cantaloupe 1 slice of watermelon or honeydew melon ½ cup fruit cocktail 17 grapes 2 tablespoons of raisins 1¼ cup whole strawberries 1 cup raspberries ½ cup apple, pineapple, grapefruit or orange juice ⅓ cup grape juice, prune juice or cranberry cocktail
Non-starchy vegetables	3 cup raw vegetables 1½ cup cooked of any vegetable not listed on the starchy vegetable list
Starchy vegetables	½ cup corn 1 cup mixed vegetables containing corn or peas ½ cup peas ½ cup mashed potatoes 1 small baked or sweet potato ½ cup winter squash ½ cup cooked dry beans ⅔ cup lima or butter beans
Dairy foods	1 cup milk 1 cup buttermilk 1 cup plain yogurt

Source: American Diabetes Association, www.diabetes.org

Appendix H

Recipe Index: Carb Choices and Exchanges

Recipe Name	Carb Choices	Exchanges
Asian Ratatouille, pg. 46	1	1 starch + 1 fat
Banana Bread, pg. 289	2	1 starch + 1 fruit
Black Bean Quinoa Burgers, pg. 301	1	1 lean meat + 1 starch
Blueberry Cobbler made with Splenda®, pg. 334	1 ½	½ starch + 1 fruit + 1 fat
Blueberry Cobbler made with Splenda® Blend, pg. 334	2	1 starch + 1 fruit + 1 fat
Breakfast Spinach Strata, pg. 335	1 ½	1 medium fat meat + ½ starch
Butternut Squash Ginger Cheesecake, pg. 3	3	3 starch
Butternut Squash Soup with Fried Sage Leaves, pg. 265	1	1 starch
Chicken Fesenjan with Walnuts and Pomegranate Syrup, pg. 307	1	5 lean meat + 1 fruit
Christmas Beer Cake, pg. 361	3	3 starch + 3 fat
Cold Watermelon Ginger Soup, pg. 295	1	1 fruit
Cucumber Lemon Refresher, pg. 128	0	free
Fruit and Nut Granola with Agave Syrup, pg. 64	2	2 starch + 3 fat
Gluten-Free Brownies, pg. 362	1	1 starch + 2 fat
Gluten-Free Fried Chicken, pg. 360	0	4 medium fat meat
Green Goddess Dressing, pg. 86	0	1 fat
Grilled Eggplant Steak with Roasted Red Pepper Salad, pg. 199	1	1 starch + 2 fat
Lentil Curry, pg. 311	2	1 medium fat meat + 2 starch
Morning Glory Muffins, pg. 65	1 ½	1 starch + ½ fruit + 1 fat
Oven Roasted Cod with Three Colored Peppers and Baby Potatoes, pg. 182	1 ½	4 lean meat + 1 starch + 1 nonstarch vegetable
Oven-Crisp Chicken, pg. 85	½	5 lean meat + ½ starch
Panna Cotta, base recipe, pg. 329	1 ½	½ whole milk + 1 starch + 1 fat
Panna Cotta, high-calorie, pg. 329	1	1 starch + 7 fat
Panna Cotta, moderate-calorie, pg. 329	1 ½	½ whole milk + 1 starch + 2 fat
Panna Cotta, reduced-calorie, pg. 329	1	½ 2% milk + ½ starch
Panna Cotta, reduced-calorie, fat-free, pg. 329	1	½ fat-free milk + ½ starch
Peanutty Energy Bars, pg. 289	2	1 medium fat meat + 2 starch
Poached Chicken Breast with Root Vegetables, pg. 246	2	4 lean meat + 2 starch
Saffron Buckwheat Pilaf and Three-Bean Relish with Spicy Tomato Vinaigrette, pg. 351	3	1 medium fat meat + 3 starch + 1 fat
Seared Beef Tenderloin with Tomato Confit, Kale and Sage Polenta, pg. 296	1	5 lean meat + ½ starch + 1 nonstarch vegetable
Slow Roasted Glazed Salmon, pg. 94	0	4 lean meat
Spinach Salad with Green Goddess Dressing, pg. 86	1	2 nonstarch vegetable + 2 fat
Sweet Potato and Pineapple Salad, pg. 135	2	1 starch + 1 fruit + 1 fat
Turkey Meatloaf, pg. 264	½	3 lean meat + ½ starch
Vegetarian Posole Soup, pg. 219	2	1 medium fat meat + 2 starch
Wild Mushroom Farroto, pg. 206	2	2 starch + 1 nonstarch vegetable + 3 fat
Wild Rice Salad, pg. 340	2	1 starch + 1 fruit + 2 fat

References

Chapter 1

1. Mintel Group. Press release. Five foodservice trends from Mintel set to shape restaurant menus in 2012. Available at www.mintel.com/press-centre/press-releases/783/five-foodservice-trends-from-mintel-set-to-shape-restaurant-menus-in-2012. Accessed May 30, 2012.

2. Mozaffarian D, Ludwig D. Dietary guidelines in the 21st century – a time for food. *J Am Med Assoc.* 2010;304(6):681-82.

3. Ogden CL, Carroll M. Prevalence of Overweight, Obesity, and Extreme Obesity Among Adults: United States, Trends 1976–1980 Through 2007–2008. Available at www.cdc.gov/NCHS/data/hestat/obesity_adult_07_08/obesity_adult_07_08.pdf. Accessed September 1, 2012.

4. Ogden CL, Carroll M, Curtin LR, Lamb MM, Flegal KM. Prevalence of high body mass index in US children and adolescents, 2007-2008. *J Am Med Assoc.* 2010;303(3):242-49.

5. Academy of Nutrition and Dietetics. *Nutrition and You: Trends 2011.* Available at www.eatright.org/Media/content.aspx?id=7639. Accessed September 1, 2012.

6. Caranfa M, Morris D. Putting health on the menu. *Food Technology.* 2009;June:29-36.

7. Atwater WO. *Principles of Nutrition and Nutritive Value of Food.* U.S. Department of Agriculture, Farmers' Bulletin 1902; No.142.

8. Centers for Disease Control. Chronic Diseases and Health Promotion. Available at www.cdc.gov/chronicdisease/overview/index.htm. Accessed September 1, 2012.

9. Report of the Dietary Guidelines Advisory Committee on the Dietary Guidelines, 2010. Available at www.cnpp.usda.gov/DGAs2010-DGACReport.htm. Accessed September 1, 2012.

10. Eheman C, Henley SJ, Ballard-Barbash R, Jacobs EJ, Schymura MJ, Noone AM, Pan L, Anderson RN, Fulton JE, Kohler BA, Jemal A, Ward E, Plescia M, Ries LAG, Edwards BK. Annual report to the nation on the status of cancer, 1975–2008, featuring cancers associated with excess weight and lack of sufficient physical activity. CANCER; Published Early Online: March 28, 2012. Available at http://www.cdc.gov/features/dscancerannualreport/index.html. Accessed September 1, 2012.

11. Cordain L, Eaton SB, Sebastian A, Mann N, Lindeberg S, Watkins BA, O'Keefe JA, Brand-Miller J. Origins and evolution of the Western diet: health implications for the 21st century. *Am J Clin Nutri.* 2005;81:341-45.

12. International Food Information Council Foundation. 2012 Food & Health Survey: Consumer Attitudes Toward Food Safety, Nutrition, & Health. Available at http://www.foodinsight.org/foodandhealth2012.aspx. Accessed September 1, 2012.

13. Mackenzie M. Is the family meal disappearing? *Journal of Gastronomy.* 1993;7(1):35-45.

14. Condrasky M, Hegler. M. Bridging the nutrition gap for chefs. *The National Culinary Review.* 2009;Feb:54-56.

15. Schwartz J, Byrd-Bradbenner C. Portion distortion: typical portion sizes selected by young adults. *J Am Diet Assoc.* 2006;106:1412-1418.

16. Mintel Group. Healthy Dining Trends – US – May 2012. Scope and Themes. Available at http://oxygen.mintel.com/sinatra/oxygen/display/id=623040/display/id=622993. Accessed May 30, 2012.

Chapter 2

1. Front-of-Package Nutrition Rating Systems and Symbols: Promoting Healthier Choices, IOM Report Brief, October 2011. Available at www.iom.edu/frontofpackage2. Accessed September 5, 2012.

2. Food and Drug Administration, *Background Information on Point of Purchase Labeling,* October 2009. Available at www.fda.gov/Food/LabelingNutrition/LabelClaims/ucm187320.htm. Accessed September 5, 2012

Chapter 3

1. Sugar and Sweeteners Outlook, SSS-M-286, Economic Research Service, U.S. Department of Agriculture. June 18, 2012. Available at http://usda01.library.cornell.edu/usda/current/SSS/SSS-06-18-2012.pdf. Accessed July 9, 2012.

2. US Departments of Agriculture and Health and Human Services. Dietary Guidelines for Americans, 2010, Foods and Food Components to Reduce. 7th ed. Washington, DC: US Government Printing. Available at http://www.cnpp.usda.gov/Publications/DietaryGuidelines/2010/PolicyDoc/Chapter3.pdf. Accessed July 9, 2012.

3. Position of the American Dietetic Association: Use of Nutritive and Nonnutritive Sweeteners. Available at http://www.eatright.org/About/Content.aspx?id=8363. Accessed July 18, 2012

4. Bellisle F. Effects of diet on behaviour and cognition in children. *Br J Nutr.* 2004; 92(suppl 2):S227-S232.

5. Corwin RL, Grigson PS. Symposium overview—Food addiction: Fact or fiction? *JNutr.* 2009;139(3):617-619.

6. McGinnis JM, Gootman JA, Kraak VI, Ed. Food Marketing to Children and Youth: Threat or Opportunity? Committee on Food Marketing and the Diets of Children and Youth. Available at http://www.nap.edu/catalog.php?record_id=11514. Accessed July 9, 2012

Chapter 4

1. National Academy of Sciences and Institute of Medicine. *Dietary Reference Intakes for Energy, Carbohydrate, Fiber, Fat, Fatty Acids, Cholesterol, Protein and Amino Acids.* Washington, DC: National Academy Press; 2002.

Chapter 5

1. Apolzan JW, Carnell NS, Mattes RD, Campbell WW. Inadequate dietary protein increases hunger and desire to eat in younger and older men. *J Nutr.* 2007;137(6):1478-82.

2. Johnston, CS, Tionn SL, Swan PD. High-protein, low-fat diets are effective for weight loss and favorably alter biomarkers in healthy adults. *J Nutr.* 2004; 134: 586-91.

Chapter 6

1. National Research Council. Dietary Reference Intakes: The Essential Guide to Nutrient Requirements. Washington, DC: The National Academies Press, 2006. Available at http://www.nap.edu/catalog.php?record_id=11537#toc. Accessed August 27, 2012.

2. National Research Council. Dietary Reference Intakes for Water, Potassium, Sodium, Chloride, and Sulfate. Washington, DC: The National Academies Press, 2005. Available at http://www.iom.edu/Reports/2004/Dietary-Reference-Intakes-Water-Potassium-Sodium-Chloride-and-Sulfate.aspx. Accessed August 27, 2012.

3. Salleh A. Athletes caffeine use reignites scientific debate. ABC Science Online. August 2, 2008. Available at www.abc.net.au/news/stories/2008/08/02/2322263.htm. Accessed August 27, 2012.

4. NCAA Banned Drugs List. Available at http://www.ncaa.org/wps/wcm/connect/public/ncaa/health+and+safety/drug+testing/resources/ncaa+banned+drugs+list. Accessed August 27, 2012.

5. Chen L, Appel LJ, Loria C, Lin P, Champagne CM, Elmer PJ, Ard JD, Mitchell D, Batch BC, Svetkey LP, Caballero B. Reduction in consumption of sugar-sweetened beverages is associated with weight loss: The PREMIER trial. *Am J Clin Nutr.* 2009; 89:1299-06.

6. Marcus K. Research and findings: A User's Guide to Wine Science. *Wine Spectator.* Available at www.winespectator.com/wssaccess/show/id/40815. Accessed August 27, 2012.

Chapter 7

1. US Departments of Agriculture and Health and Human Services. *Dietary Guidelines for Americans, 2010*, Foods and Nutrients to Increase. 7th ed. Washington, DC: US Government Printing. Available at http://www.cnpp.usda.gov/Publications/DietaryGuidelines/2010/PolicyDoc/Chapter4.pdf Accessed July 18, 2012.

2. Kushi LH, Doyle C, McCullough M, Rock CL, Demark-Wahnefried W, Bandera EV, Gapstur S, Patel AV, Andrews K, Gansler T, and The American Cancer Society 2010 Nutrition and Physical Activity Guidelines Advisory Committee (2012). American Cancer Society guidelines on nutrition and physical activity for cancer prevention. CA: A Cancer Journal for Clinicians, 62: 30–67. doi: 10.3322/caac.20140. Available at http://onlinelibrary.wiley.com/doi/10.3322/caac.20140/full. Accessed July 18, 2012.

3. U.S. Department of Agriculture, Agricultural Research Service. 2011. USDA National Nutrient Database for Standard Reference, Release 24. Nutrient Data Laboratory Home Page. Available at http://www.ars.usda.gov/Services/docs.htm?docid=8964. Accessed July 18, 2012.

4. Rickman JC, Barrett DM, Bruhn CM. Nutritional comparison of fresh, frozen and canned fruits and vegetables. *J Sci Food Agric.* 2007; 87(7):1185-96.

Chapter 8

1. Restaurant menus to focus on quality, not just cost, in 2010 press release. Available at http://www.mintel.com/press-centre/press-releases/432/restaurant-menus-to-focus-on-quality-not-just-cost-in-2010. Accessed July 18, 2012.

2. US Departments of Agriculture and Health and Human Services. Dietary Guidelines for Americans, 2010, Helping Americans Make Healthy Choices. 7th ed. Washington, DC: US Government Printing. Available at http://www.cnpp.usda.gov/Publications/DietaryGuidelines/2010/PolicyDoc/Chapter6.pdf. Accessed July 18, 2012.

3. National Restaurant Association. Chef Survey: What's Hot in 2012. Available at http://www.restaurant.org/pressroom/social-media-releases/images/whatshot2012/What's_Hot_2012.pdf. Accessed July 18, 2012.

4. Crawford D. Managing and reporting sustainability. *CMA Management Magazine.* February 2005. Available at http://www.environmental-expert.com/resulteacharticle.aspx?cid=20851&codi=3815. Accessed July 18, 2012.

5. Rolls BJ, Hermann M. *The Ultimate Volumetrics Diet: Smart, Simple, Science-Based Strategies for Losing Weight and Keeping It Off.* New York: William Morrow Cookbooks; 2012.

6. Bellisle F. Effects of diet on behaviour and cognition in children. *Brit J Nutri.* 2004;92(Suppl 2):S227-32.

7. Wesnes KA, Pincock C, Richardson D, Helm G, Hails S. Breakfast reduces declines in attention and memory over the morning in school children. *Appetite.* 2003;41(3):329-31.

8. Wilson NC, Parnell WR, Wohlers M, Shirley P. Eating breakfast and its impact on children's daily diet. *Nutrition & Dietetics.* 2006;63:15-20.

9. Young LR, Nestle M. The contribution of expanding portion sizes to the US obesity epidemic. *Am J Public Health.* 2002;92(2):246-49.

10. Young LR, Nestle M. Expanding portion sizes in the US marketplace: Implications for nutrition counseling. *J Am Diet Assoc.* 2003;103:231-34.

11. Food, Agriculture, Conservation and Trade Act of 1990. Available at http://www.csrees.usda.gov/about/offices/legis/25fact.html. Accessed July 18, 2012.

12. University of California Sustainable Agriculture Research and Education Program. Available at http://www.sarep.ucdavis.edu/. Accessed July 18, 2012.

13. 2012 Restaurant Industry Forecast, National Restaurant Association. Available at http://www.restaurant.org/research/forecast. Accessed July 18, 2012

14. The American Dietetic Association Sustainable Food System Task Force. *Healthy Land, Healthy People: Building a Better Understanding of Sustainable Food Systems for Food and Nutrition Professionals.* Available at http://www.hendpg.org/docs/Sustainable_Primer.pdf. Accessed July 18, 2012.

15. Hartman Group. *The Many Faces of Organic 2008.* Bellevue, WA: Hartman Group, Inc.; 2008.

16. Organic Trade Association, 2011 Organic Industry Survey. Available at http://www.ota.com/pics/documents/2011OrganicIndustrySurvey.pdf/. Accessed July 18, 2012

17. Dangour AD, Dodhia SK, Hayter A, Allen E, Lock K, Uauy R. Nutritional quality of organic foods: A systematic review. *Am J Clin Nutri*. 2009;90:680-85.

18. Benbrook C, Zhao X, Yanez J, Davies N, Andrews P. *New evidence confirms the nutritional superiority of plant-based organic foods*. The Organic Center. Available at http://www.organic-center.org/reportfiles/NutrientContentReport.pdf. Accessed September 13, 2010.

19. Institute of Food Technologists. Functional foods: Opportunities and challenges. Available at www.ift.org/knowledge-center/read-ift-publications/science-reports/expert-reports/functional-foods.aspx. Accessed July 18, 2012.

20. Position of the Academy of Nutrition and Dietetics: Functional Foods. *J Am Diet Assoc*. 2009;109:735-46.

Chapter 9

1. International Food Information Council Foundation. *2012 Food & Health Survey: Consumer Attitudes toward Food Safety, Nutrition and Health*. Available at: www.foodinsight.org/Resources/Detail.aspx?topic=2012_IFIC_Foundation_Food_Health_Survey_Media_Resources. Accessed August 5, 2012.

2. 2010 Mintel Healthy Dining Trends Survey press release.

3. Mintel Group. Healthy Dining Trends – US – May 2012. Scope and Themes. Available at http://oxygen.mintel.com/sinatra/oxygen/display/id=623040/display/id=622993. Accessed May 30, 2012.

4. Hartman Group. *Reimagining Health + Wellness Lifestyle and Trends Report 2010*. June 2010. Available at http://hartman-group.com/publications/reports/reimagining-health-wellness-lifestyle-and-trends-report-2010. Accessed September 1, 2012.

5. Librairie Larousse's Gastronomic Committee. Larousse Gastronomique. Updated. New York: Clarkson Potter Publishers; 2009.

6. Mattes RD. The taste for salt in humans. *Am J Clin Nutr*. 1997;65(suppl):692S-97S.

7. Beauchamp GK. Sensory and receptor responses to umami: An overview of pioneering work. *Am J Clin Nutr*. 2009;90(3):723S-27S.

8. Mattes RD, Hollis J, Hayes, D, Stunkard J., Appetite: measurement and manipulation misgivings, *J Am Diet Assoc*. 2005;105:S87-S97.

9. Nasser J. Taste, food intake and obesity. *Obes Rev*. 2001;2:213-18.

10. Rolls BJ, Barnett RA. *Volumetrics: Feel Full on Fewer Calories*. New York: Harper Collins; 1999.

11. Gerstein DE, Woodward-Lopez G, Evans AE, Kelsey K, Drewnowski A. Clarifying concepts about macronutrients' effects on satiation and satiety. *J Am Diet Assoc*. 2004;104(7):1151-53.

12. Page K, Dorenburg A. T*he Flavor Bible: The Essential Guide to Culinary Creativity, Based on the Wisdom of America's Most Imaginative Chefs*. New York: Little Brown & Co.; 2008.

13. Report of the Dietary Guidelines Advisory Committee on the Dietary Guidelines, 2010. Available at www.cnpp.usda.gov/DGAs2010-DGACReport.htm. Accessed September 1, 2012.

14. Dickinson BD, Havas S. For the Council on Science and Public Health, American Medical Association. Reducing the population burden of cardiovascular disease by reducing sodium intake. *Arch Intern Med*. 2007;167(14):1460-68.

15. The Salt Institute. Available at www.saltinstitute.org. Accessed August 9, 2012.

Chapter 10

1. FDA Food Code, Chapter 3: Food. Available at http://www.fda.gov/Food/FoodSafety/RetailFoodProtection/Food01Code/FoodCode2009/default.htm. Accessed July 22, 2102.

2. Gil MI, Aguayo E, Kader AA. Quality changes and nutrient retention in fresh-cut versus whole fruits during storage. *J Agril Food Chem*. 2006;54(12):4284-96.

3. U.S. Department of Agriculture, Agricultural Research Service. 2009. Table of Nutrient Retention Factors, Release 6. Nutrient Data Laboratory. Available at www.nal.usda.gov/fnic/foodcomp/Data/retn6/retn06.pdf. Accessed August 4, 2012.

Chapter 11

1. Patient Protection and Affordable Care Act. Public Law 111-148. Available at www.gpo.gov/fdsys/pkg/PLAW-111publ148/content-detail.html. Accessed August 4, 2012.

2. 2010 Mintel Healthy Dining Trends Survey press release. Available at www.mintel.com/press-centre/press-releases/556/menu-transparency-takes-effectand-consumers-eat-it-up-reports-mintel. Accessed August 4, 2012.

3. U.S. Food and Drug Administration. Food Labeling Guide. Available at http://www.fda.gov/Food/GuidanceComplianceRegulatoryInformation/GuidanceDocuments/FoodLabeling-Nutrition/FoodLabelingGuide/default.htm. Accessed August 4, 2012.

4. National Restaurant Association. New Restaurant Operator Research Reveals Opportunities for Produce in Foodservice. July 27, 2009. Available at www.restaurant.org/pressroom/pressrelease/?id=1829. Accessed August 4, 2012.

Chapter 12

1. State of the Plate: 2010 Study on America's Consumption of Fruits and Vegetables, 2010. Produce for Better Health Foundation. Available at http://www.pbhfoundation.org/pdfs/about/res/pbh_res/stateplate.pdf. Accessed August 2, 2012.

2. Centers for Disease Control and Prevention, National Center for Chronic Disease Prevention and Health Promotion. Youth Risk Behavior Surveillance System-United States, 2011. Available at http://www.cdc.gov/mmwr/pdf/ss/ss6104.pdf. Accessed August 2, 2012.

3. Gleason P, Suitor S. Children's Diet in the Mid 1990s:Dietary Intake and its Relationship with School Meal Participation. Available at http://www.fns.usda.gov/ora/MENU/Published/CNP/FILES/ChilDietsum.htm. Accessed August 2, 2012.

4. Burns JS, Dockery DW, Neas LM, Schwartz JS, Coull BA, Raizenne M, Speizer FE. Low dietary nutrient intakes and respiratory health in adolescents. Available at http://journal.publications.chestnet.org/article.aspx?articleid=1085242. Accessed August 2, 2012.

5. Weng FL, Shults J, Leonard MB, Stallings VA, Zemel BS. Risk factors for low serum 25-hydroxyvitamin D concentrations in otherwise healthy children and adolescents. *Am J Clin Nutr*. 2007;86:150-158.

6. Administration on Aging. A Profile of Older Americans: 2011. Available at http://www.aoa.gov/aoaroot/aging_statistics/Profile/2011/docs/2011profile.pdf. Accessed August 2, 2012.

7. Position of the American Dietetic Association, Dietitians of Canada and the American College of Sports Medicine: Nutrition and Athletic Performance. Available at www.eatright.org/About/Content.aspx?id=8365. Accessed August 2, 2012.

8. Rodriguez NR, Vislocky LM, Gaine PC. Dietary protein, endurance exercise, and human skeletal-muscle protein turnover. *Curr Opin Clin Nutr Metab Care*. 2007;10:40-45.

9. National Center for Health Statistics. Health, United States, 2011. Available at http://www.cdc.gov/nchs/hus.htm. Accessed August 2, 2012

10. International Food Information Council Foundation. 2011 Food & Health Survey: Consumer Attitudes Toward Food Safety, Nutrition, & Health. Available at www.foodinsight.org/Resources/Detail.aspx?topic=2011_Food_Health_Survey_Consumer_Attitudes_Toward_Food_Safety_Nutrition_Health. Accessed May 30, 2012.

11. Hill JO. Can a small-changes approach help address the obesity epidemic? A report of the Joint Task Force of the American Society for Nutrition, Institute of Food Technologists, and International Food Information Council. *Am J Clin Nutr*. 2009; 89:477-84.

12. Nishida C, Uauy R, Kumanyika S, Shetty P. The Joint WHO/FAO Expert Consultation on diet, nutrition and the prevention of chronic diseases: process, product and policy implications. *Public Health Nutrition*. 2004;7:245-50.

13. Vegetarian Resource Group. How Many Vegetarians Are There? Available at www.vrg.org/press/2009poll.htm. Accessed August 2, 2012.

14. Vegetarian Resource Group. How Many People Order Vegetarian Meals When Eating Out? Available at http://www.vrg.org/journal/vj2008issue3/survey.htm. Accessed August 2, 2012

15. The Jewish Federations of North America. National Jewish Population Survey 2000-01: Strength, Challenge and Diversity in the American Jewish Population, United Jewish Communities. Available at www.jewishfederations.org/page.aspx?id=33650. Accessed August 2, 2012

16. Mintel. Kosher Foods - US - January 2009. Available at http://oxygen.mintel.com/display/393508/. Accessed August 2, 2012.

17. Regenstein JM. Cornell University. The Cornell Kosher and Halal Food Initiative, 2007 Impact statement. Available at http://vivo.cornell.edu/display/TheCornellKosherandHalalFoodInitiative#overview. Accessed August 2, 2012.

Chapter 13

1. Roger VL, Go AS, Lloyd-Jones D, Adams RJ, Berry JD, Brown TM, Carnethon M, Dai S, de Simone G, Ford ES, Fox CS, Fullerton H, Gillespie C, Greenlund K, Hailpern S, Heit J, Ho PM, Howard V, Kissela B, Kittner S, Lackland D, Lichtman J, Lisabeth L, Makuc D, Marcus G, Marelli A, Matchar D, McDermott M, Meigs J, Moy C, Mozaffarian D, Mussolino M, Nichol G, Paynter N, Rosamond W, Sorlie P, Stafford R, Turan T, Turner M, Wong N, Wylie-Rosett J, on behalf of the American Heart Association Statistics Committee and Stroke Statistics Subcommittee. Heart Disease and Stroke Statistics 2011 Update. A Report from the American Heart Association. *Circulation.* Available from http://circ.ahajournals.org/content/123/4/e18.full.pdf+html?sid=f2bb914b-504f-4bba-a5d7-e5bc9971de28. Accessed August 4, 2012.

2. National Health and Nutrition Examination Survey. Available at www.cdc.gov/nchs/nhanes.htm. Accessed August 4, 2012.

3. *Cancer Trends Progress Report – 2009/2010 Update.* National Cancer Institute. National Institutes of Health, Bethesda, MD, April 2010. Available at http://progressreport.cancer.gov. Accessed August 4, 2012.

4. National Diabetes Information Clearinghouse (NDIC). Available at http://diabetes.niddk.nih.gov. Accessed August 4, 2012.

5. The Culinary Institute of America. Worlds of Healthy Flavors, 2010. Available at www.ciaprochef.com/wohf/index.html. Accessed August 4, 2012.

6. Lloyd-Jones DM, Hong Y, Labarthe D, Mozaffarian D, Appel LJ, Van Horn L, Greenlund K, Daniels S, Nichol G, Tomaselli GF, Arnett DK, Fonarow GC, Ho PM, Lauer MS, Masoudi, FA, Robertson RM, Roger V, Schwamm LH, Sorlie P, Yancy CW, Rosamond WD, on behalf of the American Heart Association Strategic Planning Task Force and Statistics Committee. Defining and Setting National Goals for Cardiovascular Health Promotion and Disease Reduction: The American Heart Association's Strategic Impact Goal Through 2020 and Beyond. *Circulation.* 2010;121:586-613. Available at http://circ.ahajournals.org/cgi/content/abstract/CIRCULATIONAHA.109.192703v1. Accessed August 4, 2012.

7. Dickinson BD, Havas S. for the Council on Science and Public Health. Reducing the population burden of cardiovascular disease by reducing sodium intake. *Arch Intern Med.* 2007;167(14):1460-68.

8. Mattes RD, Donnelly D. Relative contributions of dietary sodium sources. *J Am Coll Nutr.* 1991;10(4):383-93.

9. Institute of Medicine of the National Academies. *A Population-Based Policy and Systems Change Approach to Prevent and Control Hypertension.* Washington, DC: The National Academies Press. Board on Population Health and Public Health Practice Committee on Public Health Priorities to Reduce and Control Hypertension in the US Population; 2010.

10. The Culinary Institute of America. Worlds of Healthy Flavors, 2010. Available at www.ciaprochef.com/wohf/ index.html. Accessed August 4, 2012.

11. Kushi LA, Byers T, Doyle C, Bandera EV, McCullough M, Gansler T, Andrews KS, Thun MJ, and The American Cancer Society 2006 Nutrition and Physical Activity Guidelines Advisory Committee. American Cancer Society guidelines on nutrition and physical activity for cancer prevention: reducing the risk of cancer with healthy food choices and physical activity. *CA Cancer J Clin.* 2006;56:254-281. Available at http://onlinelibrary.wiley.com/doi/10.3322/canjclin.56.5.254/pdf. Accessed August 4, 2012.

12. Center for Disease Control and Prevention. NCHS Data Brief. No. 10. Food Allergy Among U.S. Children: Trends in Prevalence and Hospitalizations. October 2008. Available at www.cdc.gov/nchs/data/databriefs/db10.htm. Accessed August 4, 2012.

13. Fasano A, Berti I, Gerarduzzi T, Not T, Colletti RB, Drago S, Elitsur Y, Green PHR, Guandalini S, Hill ID, Pietzak M, Ventura A, Thorpe M, Kryszak D, Fornaroli F, Wasserman SS, Murray JA, Horvath K. Prevalence of celiac disease in at-risk and not-at-risk groups in the United States. *Arch Int Med.* 2003;163(3):268-92. Available at http://archinte.jamanetwork.com/article.aspx?articleid=215079. Accessed August 4, 2012.

14. National Foundation for Celiac Awareness. Gluten-Free Resource Education Awareness Training Program. Available at www.celiaccentral.org/Education/GREAT-Food-Service/Great-Kitchens/234. Accessed August 4, 2012.

Glossary

Absorption The process by which nutrients pass from the digestive tract, through the intestinal walls, and into the bloodstream.

Acceptable Macronutrient Distribution Range (AMDR) A range of intake for carbohydrates, fats and proteins that reduces risk of chronic disease while providing intakes of essential nutrients. If an individual's intake is outside the AMDR, the risk for chronic diseases and/or insufficient intakes of essential nutrients is increased.

Added sugars Sugars, syrups and other caloric sweeteners that are added to foods during processing or preparation or consumed separately. Added sugars do not include naturally occurring sugars such as those in milk or fruits. Names for added sugars include: brown sugar, corn sweetener, corn syrup, dextrose, fructose, fruit juice concentrates, glucose, high-fructose corn syrup, honey, invert sugar, lactose, maltose, malt syrup, molasses, raw sugar, turbinado sugar and sucrose.

Adequate Intake (AI) A recommended average daily nutrient intake level based on estimates of average nutrient intake by healthy people. AI is used when the Recommended Dietary Allowance cannot be determined.

Adipose tissue Fat tissue in the body.

Adobo seasoning A seasoning mix used in Latin American and Southwest American cooking.

Allergy An immune reaction to an ordinarily harmless substance.

Amino acids The building blocks of protein. Chains of amino acids link together to form proteins.

Anaphylaxis An allergic reaction that, in severe cases, can be fatal within minutes either from swelling that shuts off airways or from a dramatic drop in blood pressure.

Animal protein Protein from animal products such as meat, poultry, seafood, eggs, milk and milk products. Animal proteins tend to be higher quality because they contain all the essential amino acids humans need. They are more digestible than most vegetable sources of protein.

Antibodies Proteins generally found in the blood that detect and destroy invaders such as bacteria and viruses.

Aromatics Plant ingredients such as garlic, citrus zest, herbs and spices used to enhance the taste and fragrance of food.

Artificial sweetener A man-made chemical substance that provides sweetness without providing calories or carbohydrates.

Atherosclerosis A disease in which plaque builds up in the arteries, limiting the flow of oxygen-rich blood through the body; can lead to a heart attack or stroke.

Baker's asthma Common occupational respiratory diseases caused by exposure to antigens from flour and/or grain dust in bakeries.

Baking Surrounding food with hot, dry air in a closed environment, usually an oven; a dry-heat cooking method.

Barbecue Grilling food over a wood or charcoal fire. A marinade or sauce is often brushed on the item during cooking.

Batch cooking Preparing small containers of food several times throughout a service period so a fresh supply of cooked items is always available.

Bile A digestive fluid made in the liver and stored in the gall bladder that aids in fat digestion in the intestines; made of cholesterol, bile salts and bilirubin.

Bioavailability The ability of a nutrient to be absorbed; influenced by the condition of the small intestine and presence of other substances needed to transport nutrients through the intestine into the bloodstream.

Biotin A water-soluble vitamin essential for the metabolism of proteins and carbohydrates and in the production of hormones and cholesterol.

Blanching Briefly boiling foods in water; a technique generally used as the first part of a combination cooking method, such as to remove peels from fruits or vegetables.

Body mass index (BMI) A measure of body weight relative to height. BMI is a tool that is often used to determine if a person is at a healthy weight, overweight or obese, and whether a person's health is at risk due to his/her weight. The formula used to calculate BMI is:

$$BMI = \frac{\text{Weight in Pounds} \times 703}{\text{Height in Inches} \times \text{Height in inches}}$$

A BMI of 18.5 to 24.9 is considered healthy. A person with a BMI of 25 to 29.9 is considered overweight; a person with a BMI of 30 or more is considered obese. See Appendix E for a table on Body Mass Index.

Boiling Cooking food by transferring heat from very hot water (around 212° F) to food. The water has large, rolling bubbles rising to the surface.

Bouquet garni A small bunch of herbs, flavorful foods and/or spices tied with string; used to flavor stocks, braises and other preparations. The standard ingredients are parsley stems, thyme, celery and bay leaves. The bouquet is discarded after flavor is imparted to the foods.

Braising Browning food in hot fat and then covering it with liquid and cooking slowly over low heat.

Broiling A dry-heat cooking method using heat radiating from an overhead source.

Broth A flavorful liquid made by simmering water with meat, vegetables and/or spices and herbs.

Calcium A mineral needed by the body to maintain bone health and to regulate functions of the heart, muscles and nerves. Dairy products such fat-free or low-fat milk, yogurt and cheeses are the best sources of calcium.

Calorie A unit of heat in food that produces energy to sustain the body's various functions, including metabolic processes and physical activity. Food calories come from carbohydrates, proteins, fats and alcohol. Carbohydrates and proteins have 4 calories per gram; fat has 9 calories per gram; and alcohol has 7 calories per gram.

Cancer Abnormal cells that create a malignant and invasive growth or tumor that may recur after removal and can spread to other sites.

Capsaicin The chemical compound that puts the heat or pungency in chiles.

Carbohydrate A macronutrient that includes sugars, starches and fibers. Carbohydrates are a major source of energy in the diet. Simple carbohydrates are sugars and complex carbohydrates include both starches and fiber. Carbohydrates provide 4 calories per gram.

Cardiovascular disease Diseases of the heart and blood vessel system (arteries, capillaries, veins) within a person's entire body. The most common cardiovascular disease is atherosclerosis.

Caramelization The process of browning sugar using heat. Sugar caramelizes at approximately 320° F to 360° F.

Celiac disease An immune reaction to gluten, a protein found in wheat, rye and barley. The disease causes damage to the lining of the small intestine and prevents absorption of nutrients; also called celiac sprue or non-tropical sprue.

Cholesterol A fat-like substance that is both made by the body and found naturally in animal foods such as meat, fish, poultry, eggs and dairy products. Some cholesterol is needed for hormone and vitamin production and to make bile. Cholesterol is carried through the blood in small units called lipoproteins. There are two types of cholesterol carriers: low-density lipoproteins (LDL) and high-density lipoproteins (HDL). When cholesterol levels are too high, some of the cholesterol is deposited in the walls of the blood vessels. Over time, the deposits can build up and cause the blood vessels to narrow and blood flow to decrease. Both cholesterol in food and saturated fat tend to raise blood cholesterol, which increases the risk for heart disease.

Coenzyme A small molecule that works with an enzyme to promote the enzyme's activity. Many coenzymes have B vitamins as part of their structure.

Complementary protein A combination of foods, each of which supplies amino acids. The amino acids lacking (or an insufficient supply) in one food are supplied by amino acids found in the second food. Together they supply all the amino acids necessary to build body proteins.

Complete protein A food source that provides all of the essential amino acids in amounts that can be used in the body to create other proteins.

Complex carbohydrates Starches and fiber with many linked sugar units. Complex carbohydrates are usually not sweet. Some fibers are not digested and aid in elimination.

Coulis A thick puree of fruit or vegetables.

Cross-contamination The spread of bacteria, viruses or other harmful agents (like gluten for some individuals) from one surface to another surface.

Deep-frying A dry-heat cooking method submerging food, usually coated first in breading or batter, into very hot fat. Deep-frying creates a crispy-coated surface on the food product.

Deglaze Swirling or stirring a liquid, such as stock or wine, in a pan to dissolve cooked food particles on the bottom of the pan. The resulting mixture usually is used as a base for a sauce.

Dehydration A process of reducing the moisture in foods to levels that inhibit the microbial growth that causes them to rot. Dehydration is done either by heat of the sun or at approximately 120° F to 140° F.

Diabetes mellitus A disease that occurs when the body is not able to form or use blood glucose (sugar) properly. Blood sugar levels are controlled by insulin, a hormone in the body that helps move glucose from the blood to muscles and other tissues. Diabetes occurs when the pancreas does not make enough insulin or the body does not respond to the insulin that is made. There are several types of diabetes mellitus.

Diet What a person eats and drinks. The term diet is also used to mean any type of restricted eating plan.

Dietary Approaches to Stop Hypertension (DASH) A dietary pattern that emphasizes potassium-rich vegetables and fruits and low-fat dairy products; includes whole grains, poultry, fish and nuts and is reduced in red meat, sweets and sugar-containing beverages. As a result, the DASH diet is rich in potassium, magnesium, calcium and fiber and reduced in total fat, saturated fat and cholesterol. It also is slightly increased in protein. This nutrient-rich diet has been shown to lower blood pressure and LDL cholesterol.

Dietary cholesterol A substance found in foods of animal origin, including meat, fish, poultry, eggs and dairy products. Used by the body to produce hormones, vitamin D and bile. Excesses of dietary cholesterol may lead to atherosclerosis over time.

Dietary fiber Complex carbohydrates with chemical bonds that cannot be broken down during digestion by humans. This nondigestible carbohydrate is found in foods such as whole-grain products, fruits, vegetables and legumes (such as dry beans and peas).

Dietary Guidelines for Americans The federal government's science-based advice to promote health and reduce risk of chronic diseases through nutrition and physical activity. The guidelines are developed jointly by the U.S. Department of Agriculture and Health and Human Services and are updated every five years.

Dietary pattern A description of the types of foods and beverages generally consumed on average, over time. For example:
Plant-based – A pattern in which the majority of protein comes from plant products, though some animal products can be included.
Vegetarian – A pattern that is exclusively or almost exclusively composed of plant foods. Some vegetarians may consume specified animal products, such as eggs, milk and milk products (lacto-ovo vegetarians) and processed foods containing small amounts of animal products.
Vegan – A pattern that is exclusively composed of plant foods.

Dietary Reference Intakes (DRIs) Amounts of nutrients based on scientific data. DRIs expand upon and replace the former Recommended Dietary Allowances (RDAs). Sets of DRI data include:
- Acceptable Macronutrient Distribution Ranges (AMDR)
- Adequate Intakes (AI)
- Estimated Average Requirements (EAR)
- Recommended Dietary Allowance (RDA)
- Tolerable Upper Intake Level (UL)

Digestion The process the body uses to break food down in the digestive tract into simple substances for energy, growth and cell repair.

DVs (Daily Values) Healthful levels for daily consumption of nutrients determined by public health experts and based on a 2,000-calorie diet. These values are found in the footnote of the Nutrition Facts label and do not change from product to product.

Electrolyte balance The equilibrium among elements that regulate cell activity by providing positive and negative ions.

Electrolytes Positive and negative ions including sodium, chloride, potassium and sulfate.

Emulsifiers Ingredients that bind together foods or liquids that normally do not mix, such as oil and water. Emulsifiers are used to stabilize solutions so fat and water ingredients do not separate.

Endorphins Peptide compounds in the brain that raise the threshold for pain and produce a feeling of well being.

Energy balance The balance between calories consumed through eating and drinking and those expended through physical activity and metabolic processes. Energy consumed must equal energy expended for a person to remain at the same body weight. Weight gain will result from excess calorie intake and/or inadequate physical activity. Weight loss will occur when a calorie deficit exists, which can be achieved by eating less, being more physically active or a combination of the two.

Energy density The amount of energy per unit of weight of a food, usually expressed as calories per 100 grams.

Energy expenditure The amount of energy, measured in calories, that a person uses. Calories are used to breathe, circulate blood, digest food, maintain posture and be physically active.

Energy nutrients Substances found in foods that can be broken down in the body and used for energy as well as for the growth, repair and replacement of tissues. These substances include carbohydrates, protein and fat. Alcohol provides energy but is not a nutrient.

Enrichment The addition of specific nutrients (iron, thiamin, riboflavin and niacin) to refined grain products to replace nutrient losses that occur during processing/refining.

Enzymes Specialized protein substances that act as catalysts to regulate the speed of the many chemical reactions within cells.

Essential fatty acids (EFA) Fatty acids that cannot be manufactured by the body and must come from food.

Estimated Average Requirement (EAR) The average daily nutrient intake estimated to meet the requirement of half the healthy individuals in a particular life stage and gender group.

Estimated Energy Requirement (EER) The average calorie intake to maintain weight of a healthy adult of a particular age, gender, weight, height and level of physical activity.

Extraction The process of removing juice from fruits and vegetables.

Fat A nutrient that supplies the body with essential fatty acids and calories. Fat is the most concentrated source of calories. Fats in foods are generally triglycerides – linked fatty acids that may be monounsaturated, polyunsaturated, saturated or a combination of these. Fat is stored in the body as adipose tissue. Oil is fat in liquid form.

Fiber Nondigestible carbohydrates and lignin that are part of the structure of plants. Dietary fiber is the fiber naturally occurring in foods, and functional fiber is specific types of nondigestible carbohydrate that have beneficial physiological effects in humans.

Flavor The sensation produced when food comes into the mouth; a result of the complex interplay of experiences from all the senses – smell, taste, touch, sight and sound.

Flavor enhancers Spices, herbs, seasonings and food preparation techniques that improve the taste and aroma of foods.

Fluids All the liquids and water in beverages and foods.

Folate A water-soluble vitamin that works with vitamin B_{12} to help form red blood cells. Folate is necessary for the production of DNA, which controls tissue growth and cell function. Low levels of folate are linked to birth defects such as spina bifida. Folic acid, folacin and folate are slightly different forms of the same vitamin.

Food allergy An abnormal response to a food triggered by the body's immune system.

Food environment The overall food supply and the settings from which a person can obtain food, such as the home, food retail establishments, restaurants, schools and worksites.

Food insecurity The limited availability of nutritionally adequate and safe foods or uncertain ability to acquire acceptable foods in socially acceptable ways. Lack of funds to buy enough food is the most common cause of food insecurity.

Food security Access by all people at all times to enough food for an active, healthy life. Food security includes the ready availability of nutritionally adequate and safe foods, and an ability to acquire acceptable foods in socially acceptable ways (e.g., without resorting to emergency food supplies, scavenging, stealing or other coping strategies).

Foodborne disease Disease caused by consuming foods or beverages contaminated with disease-causing bacteria or viruses. Many different disease-causing microbes, or pathogens, can contaminate foods. Poisonous chemicals or other harmful substances can cause foodborne diseases if they are present in food. The most common foodborne infections are those caused by the bacteria *Campylobacter*, *Salmonella* and *E. coli* O157:H7, and by a group of viruses called calicivirus, also known as Norwalk and Norwalk-like viruses.

Fortification The addition of nutrients to food that did not have these nutrients in their natural state. Milk is fortified with vitamins A and D; some juices are fortified with calcium.

Glucose A simple sugar that is the building block of most carbohydrates. Digestion causes some carbohydrates to break down into glucose. After digestion, all carbohydrates are converted to glucose, which is carried in the blood and goes to cells where it is used for energy or stored as glycogen or body fat.

Gluten A protein found in wheat, rye and barley. In people with celiac disease, gluten damages the lining of the small intestine or causes sores on the skin.

Glycerol A chemical compound that links combinations of fatty acids to form fats.

Glycogen A chain of glucose molecules used for glucose storage in the body, primarily in the liver. The body has limited stores of glycogen, which is released to maintain blood levels of glucose necessary for brain and nervous system cells.

Grill A dry-heat cooking method of heating food from a source (electricity, burning gas or charcoal) below the cooking surface.

Healthy diet A diet that emphasizes a variety of fruits, vegetables, whole grains and fat-free and low-fat milk products; includes lean meats, poultry, fish, beans, eggs and nuts. A healthy diet is low in saturated and trans fats, cholesterol, salt (sodium) and added sugars; and stays within daily calorie needs for a person's recommended weight.

Healthy weight A range of body weight based on gender, age and frame size that is least likely to be linked with weight-related health problems. People above and below healthy weight have increased health risks.

Heirloom plant An open-pollinated (by birds, insects, wind or other mechanisms) plant that was grown in an earlier era.

Herbs The edible leaves of aromatic plants; available fresh, dried and, in some cases, frozen.

Heritage animals Animals that have unique genetic traits, were raised many years ago and are typically grown in a sustainable manner.

Heterocyclic amines Substances in the muscle protein of red meat, poultry or seafood that react under high heat to form carcinogenic compounds.

High blood pressure Another term for hypertension. Blood pressure rises and falls throughout the day. An optimal blood pressure is less than 120/80 mm Hg. When blood pressure stays high – greater than or equal to 140/90 mm Hg – hypertension is diagnosed. With high blood pressure, the heart works harder, arteries are stressed and chances of a stroke, heart attack and kidney problems are greater. Prehypertension is blood pressure between 120 and 139 for the top number or between 80 and 89 for the bottom number. If blood pressure is in the prehypertension range, it is likely that a person will develop high blood pressure unless action is taken to prevent it.

High-density lipoprotein (HDL) A specific fat-protein substance in the bloodstream that transports cholesterol to the liver. HDL is commonly called "good" cholesterol. High levels of HDL cholesterol lower the risk of cardiovascular disease. An HDL level of 60 mg/dl or greater is considered high and is protective against heart disease. An HDL level less than 40 mg/dl is considered low and increases the risk for developing heart disease.

High-fructose corn syrup A sugar syrup made from corn that contains high amounts of the monosaccharide fructose, a sugar sweeter than glucose.

Hormones Chemical messenger proteins that help regulate body functions. Examples of hormones are thyroxin, insulin, estrogen and growth hormone.

Hunger The uneasy or painful sensation caused by a lack of food; the recurrent and involuntary lack of access to food.

Hydrogenation A chemical process in which hydrogen is added to fat to alter and stabilize the fat, which generally turns an oil to a semisolid or solid fat. In hydrogenation, some fat is turned into trans fats.

Hypertension See "high blood pressure."

Inactive lifestyle Lifestyle including only light physical activity during standard day-to-day life, such as getting dressed, preparing food, talking with others and attending class, with much of the time spent sitting.

Infuse To steep an aromatic or flavorful item such as an herb in liquid to extract its flavor.

Inherently healthy foods Foods that are high in nutrients and phytochemicals and low or moderate in calories in their unprocessed or minimally processed forms.

Insoluble fiber Carbohydrates with chemical bonds that are not soluble in water. They usually remain in the digestive tract and are not broken down by digestion for energy. Insoluble fibers provide bulk and aid elimination. Wheat bran and whole grains provide insoluble fiber.

Iron A mineral nutrient that helps build and renew the part of red blood cells (hemoglobin) that carries oxygen to cells.

Jus líe Meat juice thickened lightly with cornstarch or arrowroot.

Kilocalorie (Kcal) 1,000 calories. A food calorie is actually a Kcal.

Lactose intolerance The body's inability to make lactase, the enzyme necessary to digest lactose, which is the natural sugar found in milk. Symptoms are distention, pain and diarrhea.

Lecithin A fatty substance occurring in animal and plant tissues. In cooking, it can be used as an emulsifier and to prevent sticking. Brain and nervous system cells contain lecithin.

Lipids Organic compounds, including fats, oils, sterols and triglycerides, that are insoluble in water. Together with carbohydrates and proteins, lipids constitute the principal macronutrients and energy sources.

Lipoprotein Compounds made up of fat bound to protein that carry fats and fat-like substances, such as cholesterol, in the blood.

Locavore Someone who exclusively or primarily eats foods from his/her local or regional area from a determined radius from home (usually 100 or 250 miles, depending on location).

Low-calorie A specific nutrient content claim about a food indicating 40 calories or less per standard serving.

Low-density lipoprotein (LDL) A unit made up of proteins and fats that carry cholesterol in the body. High levels of LDL cholesterol cause a buildup of cholesterol-containing plaque in the arteries. LDL is commonly called "bad" cholesterol. High levels of LDL increase the risk of heart disease. An LDL level less than 100 mg/dl is considered optimal; 100 to 129 mg/dl is considered near or above optimal; 130 to 159 mg/dl is considered borderline high; 160 to 189 mg/dl is considered high; and 190 mg/dl or greater is considered very high.

Macrominerals Minerals required by humans in amounts of 100 mg/day or more.

Macronutrients Nutrients present in foods in substantial quantities that provide energy; includes carbohydrate, fat and protein.

Maillard reaction A reaction that occurs when heat is applied to a food that contains carbohydrate and protein; causes browning and development of flavor as in toasting or roasting.

Marinate Soaking or coating a food in a seasoned liquid to infuse flavors and tenderize the food prior to cooking.

Metabolism All of the chemical processes that occur in cells of the body that turn food into energy the body can use.

Microminerals Minerals required by humans in amounts of less than 100 mg/day.

Micronutrients A term that includes both vitamins and minerals needed in small quantities necessary for life and health.

Minerals Inorganic substances that include calcium, iron, zinc, chromium, copper, fluoride, iodine, magnesium, manganese, molybdenum, phosphorus, potassium, selenium and sodium. Some minerals regulate body processes while others become part of body tissues.

Minimally processed food Food processed for food safety or storage that retains most of its inherent physical, chemical, sensory and nutritional properties. Many minimally processed foods are as nutritious as the food in its unprocessed form. Plain frozen vegetables or frozen fish are examples of minimally processed foods.

Mirepoix A combination of chopped vegetables used to give flavor to stocks, sauces and gravies as well as to simmered, braised and stewed dishes. The standard ratio is 2 parts onion, 1 part carrot and 1 part celery.

Moderate alcohol consumption Daily consumption of up to 1 drink per day for women and up to 2 drinks per day for men, with no more than 3 drinks in any single day for women and no more than 4 drinks in any single day for men. One drink is defined as 12 fluid ounces of regular beer, 5 fluid ounces of wine or 1.5 fluid ounces of distilled spirits.

Monounsaturated fat A fat that has one double bond in its carbon chain. Monounsaturated fat is found in canola oil, olives and olive oil, nuts, seeds, and avocados. Monounsaturated fats may help lower cholesterol and reduce heart disease risk. Monounsaturated fat has the same number of calories as other types of fat and can still contribute to weight gain if eaten in excess.

MyPlate *MyPlate* is the visual image developed by the U.S. Department of Agriculture as a guide to healthful eating.

MyPyramid *MyPyramid: Steps to a Healthier You* was the infographic developed by the U.S. Department of Agriculture to guide healthful eating and active living. It has been replaced by *MyPlate*.

Niacin A water-soluble B vitamin that helps maintain healthy skin and nerves. As a supplement in high doses, niacin has cholesterol-lowering effects but some side effects.

Nitrates Compounds containing nitrogen and oxygen. Some nitrates are used as food preservatives. At high concentrations, nitrates can have harmful effects on humans and animals.

Nonessential amino acids Amino acids that the body is able to produce from other amino acids to meet its requirements.

Non-heme iron The form of iron found in plants that is less well absorbed than iron from animal sources.

Nutrient-dense foods Foods that are naturally rich in vitamins, minerals and phytochemicals; lean or low in solid fats; without added solid fats, sugars, starches or sodium; and retain naturally occurring components such as fiber. All vegetables, fruits, whole grains, fish, eggs and nuts prepared without added solid fats or sugars are considered nutrient-dense, as are lean or low-fat forms of fluid milk, meat and poultry prepared without added solid fats or sugars. Nutrient-dense foods provide substantial amounts of vitamins and minerals (micronutrients) and relatively few calories per standard serving; also called "healthful foods."

Nutrients Compounds supplied by food that are required by the body to maintain life. Carbohydrates, fat, protein, vitamins, minerals and water are nutrients.

Nutrition The study of food and diet.

Nutrition Facts label The part of the food label that lists the serving size, servings per container, calories per serving and information on some nutrients in a standard format.

Obesity Excess body fat. Because total body fat is difficult to measure, a ratio of body weight to height (body mass index or BMI) is often used instead. An adult who has a BMI of 30 or higher is considered obese. See "body mass index."

Oils Fats that are liquid at room temperature. Oils come from many different plants and from fish. Common oils include canola, corn, olive, peanut, safflower, soybean and sunflower. Foods that are naturally high in oils include nuts, olives, fish and avocados.

Omega-3 fatty acids Polyunsaturated essential fatty acids found in fish, flax, canola oil, pumpkin seeds and walnuts. A diet rich in omega-3 fatty acids raises HDL cholesterol levels and may help to prevent cardiovascular disease.

Omega-6 fatty acids Polyunsaturated essential fatty acids found largely in plant and vegetable oils including soy, corn and safflower oils.

Omega-9 fatty acids Nonessential polyunsaturated fatty acid that can be created chemically or by the human body from unsaturated fat.

Osteoporosis The thinning of bone tissue and loss of bone density over time. A diet inadequate in calcium and other minerals, vitamin D and protein plus hormonal deficits contribute to the development of osteoporosis, which leads to weakened bones that break easily.

Overweight A body mass index (BMI) of 25 to 29.9. Body weight comes from fat, muscle, bone and body water. Although BMI correlates with amount of body fat, BMI does not directly measure body fat. As a result, some people, such as muscular athletes, may have a BMI that categorizes them as overweight even though they do not have excess body fat.

Oxalic acid An organic acid, found in some leafy vegetables, that binds calcium and inhibits its absorption.

Pan-fry A dry-heat cooking method in which food is cooked quickly in a shallow pan with some hot fat.

Pantothenic acid A water-soluble vitamin essential for the metabolism of food. Pantothenic acid plays a role in the production of hormones and cholesterol.

Papillae The bumps on top of the tongue that help grip food and move it around while chewing; contain the taste buds.

Peptide bonds Chemical bonds that link two amino acids.

Percent Daily Values (%DVs) The percentage of the Daily Values found in a specific serving of a food. %DVs are based on Daily Value recommendations for key nutrients in a 2,000-calorie diet. %DVs help determine if a serving of food is high or low in a nutrient. Created for food labels, %DVs make it easier to compare the amount of nutrients in a food and to know which foods contribute a lot or little to meeting the daily need for key nutrients.

Phospholipids Chemical structures combining a fat with a phosphorus compound. Phospholipids circulate in the bloodstream and can be used for energy by most types of cells.

Physical activity Any form of exercise or movement. Physical activity may include planned activities such as walking, running, strength training, basketball or other sports. Physical activity may also include daily activities such as household chores, yard work, walking the dog, etc. It is recommended that adults get at least 30 minutes of moderate-intensity physical activity daily for general health benefits. Children should get at least 60 minutes of moderate-intensity physical activity most days of the week. Moderate-intensity physical activity is any activity that uses as many calories as walking 2 miles in 30 minutes.

Phytic acid A phosphorus-containing compound, found in the outer husks of grains, that binds with iron, calcium and other minerals and inhibits absorption of these nutrients.

Phytochemicals Certain organic components of plants that are thought to promote human health. Fruits, vegetables, grains, legumes, nuts and teas are rich sources of phytochemicals. Also called phytonutrients.

Plant sterols and stanols Naturally occurring substances found in plants that may reduce risk for heart disease by blocking the absorption of cholesterol in the small intestine. They are present in small quantities in many fruits, vegetables, vegetable oils, nuts, seeds, cereals and legumes.

Plaque Deposits composed primarily of cholesterol that collect on the inner walls of blood vessels and narrow the vessels, increasing risk of heart attacks and strokes.

Poach A moist-heat cooking method in which food is submerged into a hot liquid (approximately 160° F to 180° F).

Polycyclic aromatic hydrocarbons Compounds produced when meats are grilled or broiled over a direct flame; thought to be cancer causing.

Polyunsaturated fat A triglyceride in which most of the fatty acids have two or more points of unsaturation. Polyunsaturated fats are found in greatest amounts in corn, soybean and safflower oils and in many types of nuts.

Portion The amount of food eaten in one eating occasion.

Portion size The amount of a food served or to be eaten in one eating occasion. A portion is not a standardized amount. The amount served as a portion is subjective and varies.

Prebiotics Nondigestible food ingredients that are helpful in stimulating the growth or activity of beneficial bacteria in the colon.

Probiotics Live microorganisms added to food to promote intestinal health; also called "friendly bacteria."

Processed food Any food other than a raw agricultural commodity. Any food that has been washed, cleaned, milled, cut, chopped, heated, pasteurized, blanched, cooked, canned, frozen, dried, dehydrated, mixed, packaged or undergone any procedure that alters it from its natural state is a processed food. Processing also may include the addition of other ingredients to the food, such as preservatives, flavors, nutrients and other food additives or food ingredients. Processing may reduce, increase or have no affect on the nutritional characteristics of raw agricultural products.

Protein Large molecules composed of many amino acids. This essential macronutrient helps build all parts of the body, including muscle, bone, skin and blood. Protein provides 4 calories per gram and is abundant in foods such as meat, fish, poultry, eggs, dairy products, beans, nuts and tofu.

Recommended Daily Allowance (RDA) The average daily dietary nutrient intake needed to meet the nutrient requirement of nearly all (97% to 98%) healthy individuals of a particular life stage and gender group.

Reduce or reduction To cook a liquid long enough to reduce its original volume, concentrating the flavor, color and amount of the original liquid.

Refined grains Grains and grain products processed to remove the bran, germ and/or endosperm; any grain product that is not a whole grain. Many refined grains are low in fiber but enriched with thiamin, riboflavin, niacin and iron and fortified with folic acid.

Registered Dietitian (RD) A person who has studied diet and nutrition at a college program approved by the Academy of Nutrition and Dietetics (formerly The American Dietetic Association), completed 900 hours of supervised practical experience accredited by the Accreditation Council for Education in Nutrition and Dietetics and passed an exam to earn the RD credential.

Riboflavin A water-soluble vitamin that is part of the B-complex. Riboflavin is important for the production of red blood cells and many chemical reactions within cells.

Roast A dry-heat cooking method in which food is surrounded with hot air, either in an oven or over a fire; usually applies to meat, poultry, game, vegetables or potatoes.

Satiety The pleasant feeling of fullness after eating.

Saturated fat A fat composed primarily of saturated fatty acids; found in high-fat dairy products (like cheese, whole milk, cream, butter and regular ice cream), meats, lard, palm oil and coconut oil. Eating a diet high in saturated fat raises blood cholesterol and risk of heart disease. The *Dietary Guidelines for Americans* recommend limiting saturated fat to 7% of calories.

Saute A dry-heat cooking method in which heat is transferred from a hot pan to the food with a small amount of fat; usually done at very high temperatures.

Sear Browning food surfaces quickly over very high heat; usually the first step in a combination cooking method.

Serum cholesterol A lipid that travels in the blood as part of particles containing both lipids and proteins (lipoproteins). High serum cholesterol levels can be caused by genetics and internal production of cholesterol and/or from the cholesterol in foods eaten. High serum cholesterol levels increase the risk of atherosclerosis.

Serving size A standardized amount of a food in volume or weight, such as a cup or an ounce, used to provide information about food, such as on the Nutrition Facts label, in diabetic exchanges or in dietary guidance. Standard serving sizes aid comparisons among similar foods. Portion size consumed may differ from the standard serving size.

Servings per container Total number of servings in a food package based on the standard serving size for that type of food as listed in the Federal Register; listed on the Nutrition Facts label directly below the serving size.

Shortfall nutrients Nutrients that are consumed in amounts low enough to be of concern for adults and children. Shortfall nutrients identified in the *Dietary Guidelines for Americans, 2010* for children include vitamins A, C, D and E, and calcium, phosphorus and magnesium. Shortfall nutrients in adults are vitamins A, C, D, E and K, and choline, calcium, magnesium, potassium and dietary fiber.

Simmer Cooking food in a hot liquid that is heated to just below the boiling point. Small bubbles may rise to the surface of the liquid, but the liquid is much calmer than boiling.

Simple carbohydrates Sugars, monosaccharides or disaccharides that are usually sweet. Glucose, fructose and sucrose are examples.

Slurry Starch dispersed in a cold liquid to prevent it from forming lumps when added to hot liquid as a thickener.

Smoke roasting Method for cooking and flavoring food by exposing it to smoke in a closed container.

Sodium A mineral nutrient that helps balance the movement of fluid in and out of body cells, regulate blood pressure and transmit nerve impulses. Table salt is 40% sodium and 60% chloride. Most Americans eat too much sodium.

SoFAS An abbreviation for solid fats and added sugars. This term is used when calculating the number of calories that come from these two food components together. Limits for the amount of calories from SoFAS are included in U.S. Department of Agriculture food patterns and guidance beginning in 2010.

Solid fats Fats that are usually not liquid at room temperature. Solid fats are found in most animal foods but also can be made from vegetable oils through hydrogenation. Some common solid fats are butter, beef fat (tallow, suet), pork fat (lard), stick margarine and shortening. Foods high in solid fats include many cheeses, creams, whole milk, ice creams, well-marbled cuts of meats, regular ground beef, bacon, sausages and many baked goods (such as cookies, crackers, doughnuts, pastries and croissants). Most solid fats contain saturated fat, cholesterol and/or trans fats.

Soluble fiber Food components that readily dissolve in water and often impart gummy or gel-like characteristics to foods, such as pectin. Soluble fibers are indigestible by human enzymes but may be broken down to absorbable products by bacteria in the digestive tract.

Sous vide Method of cooking that is intended to maintain the integrity of ingredients by heating them for a long period at relatively low temperatures sealed in an airtight plastic bag placed in hot water.

Sphincter (esophageal) The muscular ring at the opening between the esophagus and stomach.

Starches Many glucose units linked together. Examples of foods containing starch include breads, pastas, potatoes, dry beans and peas, and grains (e.g., rice, oats, wheat, barley and corn).

Steam or steaming A moist-cooking method in which food is exposed directly to vaporized liquid, usually by placing it in a basket or rack above a boiling liquid in a covered pan or in a commercial steamer.

Sterols A type of fat with a specific ring-like chemical structure, the most abundant being cholesterol.

Stock A liquid made by simmering bones and flavorful ingredients in water to extract flavor and color. Stock is often a base for soups and sauces and can be used for cooking grains.

Sugar A simple carbohydrate composed of 1 unit (a monosaccharide, such as glucose and fructose) or 2 joined units (a disaccharide, such as lactose and sucrose). There are many forms of sugar; their names often end in -ose.

Sugar substitute A calorie-free sweetener that does not contain carbohydrates.

Supplement A product that provides concentrated nutrients such as vitamins, minerals, amino acids and fiber. Herbal products and many other chemicals that have (or are purported to have) health benefits are also sold as supplements. A dietary supplement can be taken by mouth as a pill, capsule, tablet or liquid.

Sustainable agriculture An integrated system of plant and animal production practices having a site-specific application that will, over the long term, satisfy human food and fiber needs, enhance environmental quality and natural resources, make the most efficient use of nonrenewable resources, sustain the economic viability of farm operations and enhance the quality of life for farmers and society as a whole.

Sweat To cook a food such as onions over low heat in a small amount of fat or stock, covered, until the food releases its own juices and becomes limp and tender.

Thiamin A water-soluble B vitamin that helps cells change carbohydrates into energy; essential for heart function and healthy nerve cells.

Tolerable Upper Intake Level (UL) The highest daily intake of a nutrient likely to pose no risk of adverse health effects for nearly all individuals in a particular life stage and gender group. As intake increases above the UL, the potential risk of adverse health effects increases.

Trans fatty acids A fat that is produced when oil is turned into solid fat through a chemical process called hydrogenation that rearranges molecules in the structure of fatty acids. Eating trans fatty acids raises blood cholesterol and risk of heart disease. Most trans fats are created by food processing, and trans fat levels must be listed on food labels. Trans fatty acids are found in some margarines and shortenings and in some commercial baked foods like cookies, crackers, muffins and cereals.

Triglycerides Three fatty acids joined to a glycerol molecule; the most common form of fat in foods.

Type 1 diabetes Previously known as "insulin-dependent diabetes mellitus," or "juvenile diabetes." Type 1 diabetes is a life-long condition in which the pancreas does not make insulin. To treat the disease, a person must get insulin from an external source, follow a specific eating plan, exercise daily and test blood sugar several times a day. Type 1 diabetes usually, but not always, begins before the age of 30.

Type 2 diabetes Previously known as "noninsulin-dependent diabetes mellitus" or "adult-onset diabetes." Type 2 diabetes is the most common form of diabetes mellitus. People with type 2 diabetes produce insulin, but either do not make enough insulin or their bodies do not efficiently use the insulin they make. Although Type 2 diabetes commonly occurs in adults, an increasing number of children and adolescents who are overweight also develop type 2 diabetes.

Umami A savory, meaty taste often associated with glutamate in foods and monosodium glutamate.

Unsaturated fat A fat that is composed primarily of unsaturated fatty acids. Unsaturated fats include polyunsaturated and monounsaturated fats. Most vegetable oils, nuts, olives, avocados and fatty fish such as salmon contain unsaturated fat.

Vegetable protein Protein from plants such as legumes, dry beans, grains, nuts, seeds and vegetables. Vegetable proteins tend to have lower protein quality than animal proteins because they are usually lacking one or more of the essential amino acids. Soybean products provide relatively complete protein from vegetable sources.

Villi Tiny, fingerlike projections on the inside surface of the small intestine that increase surfaces for nutrient absorption.

Vitamin A A fat-soluble vitamin that helps form and maintain healthy teeth, bones, soft tissue, mucous membranes and skin.

Vitamin B$_{12}$ A water-soluble vitamin, like the other B vitamins, that is important for metabolism. Vitamin B$_{12}$ also helps form red blood cells and maintain the central nervous system.

Vitamin B$_6$ A water-soluble vitamin also called pyridoxine, pyridoxal or pyridoxamine. The more protein consumed, the more vitamin B$_6$ needed to help the body use it. Vitamin B$_6$ helps form red blood cells and maintain brain function.

Vitamin C A water-soluble vitamin; also called ascorbic acid. Vitamin C is an antioxidant that promotes healthy teeth and gums, connective tissues between cells and wound healing. Vitamin C helps the body absorb iron from plant sources.

Vitamin D A fat-soluble vitamin known as the "sunshine vitamin," because the body can make it after being in the sun. Many people do not make enough vitamin D and need more from their diet or from supplements. Vitamin D helps the body absorb calcium and is needed for the normal development and maintenance of healthy teeth and bones and other body functions. Vitamin D has several forms – calciferol, cholecalciferol (D$_3$) and ergocalciferol (D$_2$). Most milk is fortified with vitamin D.

Vitamin E A fat-soluble vitamin that is an antioxidant; also known as tocopherol. Vitamin E plays a role in the formation of red blood cells and helps the body use vitamin K.

Vitamin K A fat-soluble vitamin that that helps blood coagulate; also known as phylloquinone.

Vitamins Nutrients that do not provide energy or build body tissue but are needed in small quantities to help regulate body processes. Vitamins include biotin, choline, folate, niacin, pantothenic acid, riboflavin, thiamin, vitamin A, vitamin B$_6$, vitamin B$_{12}$, vitamin C, vitamin D, vitamin E and vitamin K.

Waist circumference A measurement of the waist in inches or centimeters. Women with a waist measurement of more than 35 inches and men with a waist measurement of more than 40 inches have a higher risk of developing obesity-related health problems, such as diabetes, high blood pressure and heart disease.

Weight control Achieving and maintaining a healthy weight by eating healthful foods and being physically active.

Weight-cycling A pattern of losing and gaining weight over and over again; commonly called "yo-yo dieting."

Whole grains Grains and grain products made from the entire grain seed, usually called the kernel, which consists of the bran, germ and endosperm. If the kernel has been cracked, crushed or flaked, it must retain nearly the same relative proportions of bran, germ and endosperm as the original grain in order to be called whole grain. Whole grains are a good source of dietary fiber, vitamins, minerals and complex carbohydrates.

Index

See also Glossary on pages 383-391